Color Doppler in
Obstetrics and Gynecology
Text and Atlas

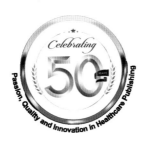

Color Doppler in Obstetrics and Gynecology Text and Atlas

Sonal Panchal MD
Ultrasound Consultant
Dr Nagori's Institute for Infertility and IVF
Ahmedabad, Gujarat, India

Chaitanya Nagori MD DGO
Director
Dr Nagori's Institute for Infertility and IVF
Ahmedabad, Gujarat, India

Foreword
Asim Kurjak

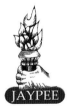

JAYPEE BROTHERS MEDICAL PUBLISHERS
The Health Sciences Publisher
New Delhi | London | Panama

Jaypee Brothers Medical Publishers (P) Ltd

Headquarters

Jaypee Brothers Medical Publishers (P) Ltd
4838/24, Ansari Road, Daryaganj
New Delhi 110 002, India
Phone: +91-11-43574357
Fax: +91-11-43574314
Email: jaypee@jaypeebrothers.com

Overseas Offices

J.P. Medical Ltd
83 Victoria Street, London
SW1H 0HW (UK)
Phone: +44 20 3170 8910
Fax: +44 (0)20 3008 6180
Email: info@jpmedpub.com

Jaypee-Highlights Medical Publishers Inc
City of Knowledge, Bld. 235, 2nd Floor
Clayton, Panama City, Panama
Phone: +1 507-301-0496
Fax: +1 507-301-0499
Email: cservice@jphmedical.com

Jaypee Brothers Medical Publishers (P) Ltd
Bhotahity, Kathmandu, Nepal
Phone: +977-9741283608
Email: kathmandu@jaypeebrothers.com

Website: www.jaypeebrothers.com
Website: www.jaypeedigital.com

Color Doppler in Obstetrics and Gynecology: Text and Atlas

First Edition: **2019**

ISBN 978-93-5270-895-6

Printed at: Samrat Offset Pvt. Ltd.

Foreword

Medicine today is still a strange mixture of empiricism, unexpurgated tradition and advanced technology, of clinical guesswork and scientific measurement.

In the midst of all this change from the human to the more precise, ultrasound is remarkable for its unique ability to glean diagnostic information without discomfort, indignity or known hazard to the patient. It is not surprising, therefore, that from an exciting novelty, ultrasound has now become an irreplaceable diagnostic tool. Color Doppler sonography represents further "breakthrough" in ultrasound imaging. This technique has radically changed the approach to noninvasive vascular diagnostic. For the first time, it is possible to obtain truly useful information about functional hemodynamic events. Impressive results are particularly encouraging in differentiating tissue characteristics in pelvic tumors and in visualizing blood vessels in tumors. This book clearly shows the dramatic development in the clinical application and I strongly believe will find many grateful readers.

In 1987, my team from University of Zagreb (Croatia) pioneered the use of color Doppler ultrasound in obstetrics and gynecology. A few years ago at the national congress of Indian gynaecologists, I met a young lady asking me to write a dedication for her book Transvaginal color Doppler. Her name was Sonal Panchal and after this very important meeting we made many contacts becoming close co-workers and even friends. One of the most admirable co-worker, she made impressive scientific career, becoming world leader in ultrasound. She is also an excellent teacher and together with Dr Chaitanya Nagori she is running one of the best world institutes for infertility. It is, therefore, my great pleasure and honor to write this foreword for the book of Sonal Panchal wishing to the authors' best success among the readers. I have no doubt that the readers will like written text from experienced authors and first-class practitioners.

Asim Kurjak MD PhD
Professor
Department of Obstetrics and Gynecology
Medical School University of Zagreb
Zagreb, Croatia
Founder Director
Ian Donald Inter University School of Medical Ultrasound

Preface

This book is a practical guide and a quick reference for the obstetricians and gynecologists, to ease out the use of Doppler technology for better diagnosis with ultrasound. It indicates the use of Doppler for the differential diagnosis of different endometrial and myometrial lesions, as well as ovarian and tubal lesions. It gives an idea about Doppler findings that would differentiate between malignant and benign lesions. The important role of Doppler in deciding stimulation protocols for patients on assisted reproductive technology treatment, for assessment of functional maturity of the follicle and endometrium, and also the correlation of these Doppler changes with hormonal level fluctuations have also been described. Doppler has a major role to play for suspected chromosomal and cardiac abnormalities in the first trimester, detection, and differential diagnosis of abnormalities of structural abnormalities in the second trimester. Role of Doppler cannot be underestimated in fetal growth restriction and pregnancy-induced hypertension (PIH) cases, and all these have been discussed in depth in a very simple way.

Sonal Panchal
Chaitanya Nagori

Acknowledgments

I sincerely thank my friends and colleagues who have helped me in the process of conceptualizing this book and also helping me by contributing for ultrasound images of a few not very common conditions. Dr Sridevi Kolli (Visakhapatnam, Andhra Pradesh), Dr Kuldip Jasoliya and Dr Sanjay Vasoya (Surat, Gujarat) have always been of a great support to me for the same. Friends, I sincerely thank you for the images that you have contributed for this book to make it complete.

I am grateful to my patients for their support in my Doppler studies. I sincerely acknowledge the encouragement, support, and guidance of my "Guru" Dr Chaitanya Nagori, without which it would have not been possible to complete this project.

Lastly, I would like to thank Shri Jitendar P Vij (Group Chairman), Mr Ankit Vij (Managing Director), Ms Chetna Malhotra Vohra (Associate Director-Content Strategy), Prerna Bajaj (Development Editor) of M/s Jaypee Brothers Medical Publishers (P) Ltd, New Delhi, India, for their untiring support.

Sonal Panchal

Contents

Doppler Basics for a Gynecologist

WHAT IS DOPPLER?

Doppler is an effect produced on the frequency of a sound wave when it hits a moving object. This can be most simply explained by the difference in the sound quality perceived by an individual who is standing on the road and hears the voice of the siren of the moving ambulance. The intensity of the sound increases as the sound source moves toward the individual and decreases as it moves away from the individual. When the receiver and the sound source move toward each other, the frequency of the heard sound wave is higher than sent by the sound source and if the two move away from each other, the frequency of the heard sound is lower than that produced by the sound source. The difference in the emitted and the received frequency is known as Doppler shift. This effect was first described by Christian Johann Doppler in 1842. But it was only in 1959 that Satomura demonstrated the use of this technology for demonstration of blood flows.

Translating the Doppler effect in the body for blood flow assessment: The sender and receiver are both static and the target [red blood cells (RBCs)] moves. The first frequency shift occurs when the sound beam hits the moving RBC and the frequency shift again occurs when it returns.

The shift depends on the angle at which the sound beam hits the moving object.

$$\text{Doppler frequency } (f_d) = \frac{2 \times f_t \times V \times cos\,\theta}{c}$$

Where,
f_d = Doppler shift
f_t = Transmitted beam
c = Speed of sound in tissue
V = Velocity of blood flow

θ = Angle of incidence between the ultrasound beam and the direction of flow.

Considering this equation, it is important to notice that the frequency of the received beam is dependent on the frequency of incident beam, velocity of the moving object, and the angle of incidence. But more importantly, it is not dependent on the absolute value of the angle of incidence, it is on the "cos" value of this angle. Therefore, for correct calculation of the frequency, or any one of the unknown variable out of these above-mentioned four, the "cos" value of the angle (cos θ) should be within acceptable limits (Table 1.1).[1]

The precise Doppler frequency is calculated, taking into account an angle correction factor of 1/cos θ (Table 1.2).

The Doppler effect can be displayed as color Doppler, power Doppler, and spectral Doppler.

Color Doppler

Doppler is most commonly used term for color Doppler. It displays the blood flow in two colors, and these are conventionally red and blue. The color indicates the direction of the flow. Flow towards the probe is red and

TABLE 1.1: The angle of incidence of the sound beam, their "cos" values, and the percentage deviation these lead to in the velocity value.[1]

Angle	"cos" value	% deviation
0°	1	0
30°	0.866	13
45°	0.707	29
60°	0.5	50
90°	0	100

away from the probe is blue (Fig. 1.1). But these can be interchanged by using the invert switch (Fig. 1.2). When the flow is perpendicular to the sound beam, not towards or away from the probe, no color will be displayed in spite of presence of the flow. The cause for this has already been explained earlier. When the flow is perpendicular to the sound beam, the Doppler angle is 90° and the cos θ value is 0, so the flow cannot be displayed. The arterial flow is pulsatile and the venous flow is nonpulsatile. The brightness of the color depends on the velocity of the flow. The higher flow velocities display bright colors and the lower flow velocities display dull colors (Fig. 1.3). Though color Doppler does not give exact velocity values. So, it is a directional semiquantitative Doppler.

Power Doppler

Though a Doppler, power Doppler is not an angle-dependent technology. It is known that movement of any object produces energy and this is used to depict the blood flow signals in power Doppler. This means that wherever there is a movement of blood or of body tissues, color signals will be generated. It is not an angle-dependent technology and so the advantage is that it displays color signals even in vessels perpendicular to the sound beam. But the disadvantage is that it is a single color display and does not show the flow direction. It indigenously potentiates the signals and therefore is a useful technology for documentation of low velocity blood flows. The main application of the power Doppler therefore is to pick up low velocity blood flow and the blood flows in the vessels perpendicular to the sound beam (Fig. 1.4).

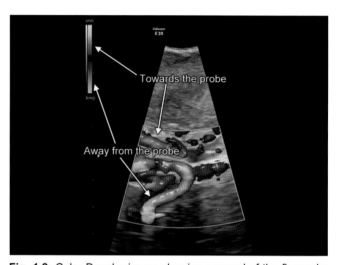

Fig. 1.2: Color Doppler image showing reversal of the flow color against direction. The inversion can be seen on the color bar also as shown by the arrows.

TABLE 1.2: The angle of incidence of the sound beam, correction factors used for calculation of velocity and the correction error.[1]

Angle	Correction factor 1/cos θ	Correction error
30°	1.15	±3%
45°	1.41	±6%
60°	2.00	±9%
70°	2.92	±14%
75°	3.86	±21%
80°	5.76	±30%

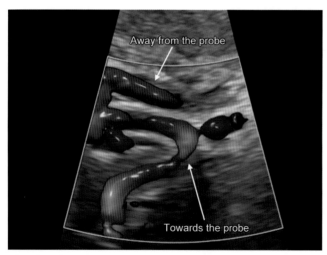

Fig. 1.1: Color Doppler image showing flow toward the probe is red and away from the probe is blue.

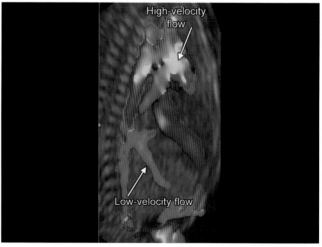

Fig. 1.3: Color Doppler image showing brighter color for high-velocity flows and dull color for low-velocity flow.

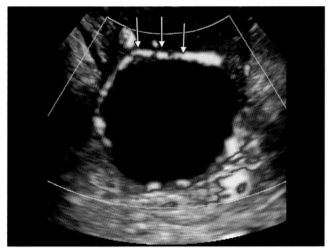

Fig. 1.4: Power Doppler image showing color in the vessels perpendicular to the sound beam—sound beam is shown by white arrows.

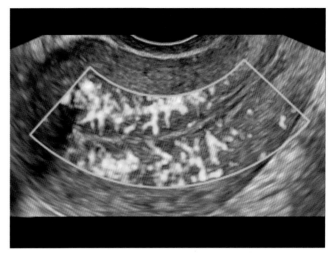

Fig. 1.6: High-definition (HD) flow image showing color of the flow according to its direction.

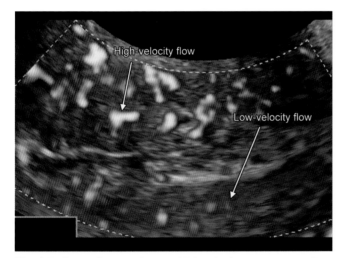

Fig. 1.5: Power Doppler image: high-velocity movements show a bright color and the low-velocity movements display dull color.

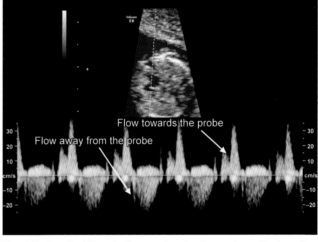

Fig. 1.7: Spectral Doppler image showing trace above the baseline in the spectrum is the flow toward the probe and the trace below the baseline is the flow away from the probe.

Like color Doppler, the color display of the power Doppler signals also varies depending on the velocity of the moving object. High-velocity movements show a bright color and the low-velocity movements display dull color (Fig. 1.5).

High-definition Flow

High-definition (HD) flow is a new addition to the basic power Doppler technology. It is a directional power Doppler. Apart from high-flow sensitivity, HD flow also has a color coding for the flow toward or away from the probe as in color Doppler (Fig. 1.6). Like color and power Doppler, the brightness of the color correlates with the velocity of the moving object.

Spectral Doppler

Spectral Doppler is the spectral display of the flow/ movement of a moving object. Trace above the baseline in the spectrum is the flow towards the probe and the trace below the baseline is the flow away from the probe (Fig. 1.7) on the spectrum. Like in color Doppler, the invert switch can reverse the flow display. On the spectral Doppler, the arterial

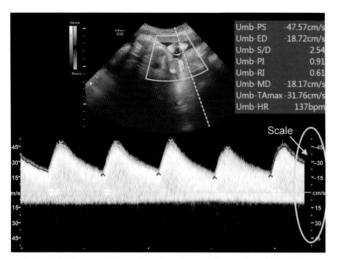

Fig. 1.8: Spectral Doppler showing scale on the side of the spectrum, for calculation of the flow velocities.

flow appears spiky and the venous flow appears flat. There is a scale on the side of the spectrum and it is by this scale that the exact velocities of the flows can be calculated (Fig. 1.8).

The spectrum can be displayed for pulsed wave Doppler and the continuous wave Doppler. In pulsed wave Doppler, the transducer is dedicatedly used for emitting the sound wave and then dedicatedly to receive the sound wave alternatively. As the sound waves are emitted in pulses, it is called a pulsed wave Doppler. The limitation of the pulsed wave Doppler is that the maximum frequencies recorded correctly are smaller than half that of the pulse repetition frequency (PRF). This limit of any PRF is called Nyquist limit/frequency. The PRF therefore should at least be double the frequency to be measured. Therefore, to record different velocities, the pulse repetition frequencies have to be accordingly selected. Pulsed Doppler therefore has a limitation to maximum velocities that it can record. This can be overcome by continuous wave Doppler. This uses dedicated elements for emitting and receiving sound waves and therefore has no higher limit for velocities recorded. This is used chiefly for adult echocardiography. Since continuous wave Doppler is not used for the Doppler studies in gynecology and obstetrics, we shall not include it in further discussion here.

To obtain the correct information about flow velocities with Doppler, certain settings and adjustments on the scanner are required. Though most of these are set on the dedicated presets, it is important to understand that how can we manipulate certain switches/knobs to achieve best flow information.

These are the Doppler box size, color gains, PRF, wall motion filter (WMF), and balance on color and power

Doppler and sample volume, gains, PRF, WMF, and angle correction for the pulsed wave Doppler.

Color/Power Doppler Settings

Box Size

When one switches on the color Doppler, a box appears on the screen, on the B-mode image. This box defines in which area of the B-mode image, the blood flow information will be displayed. It is important to consider here that when the Doppler is switched on, the machine has to process the B-mode information as well as the flow information and therefore the frame rate significantly decreases.

What is this frame rate?

The ultrasound scan that we are doing gives us continuous live, real time information of the area scanned. This we call real time because it matches with the live movements of the human body. This is done by compilation of multiple B-mode images. Only if the B-mode images are processed fast enough to match the real time changes, this scan can be seen like a continuous scan as in a video. The number of B-mode images produced in a unit time is called a frame rate. This clearly means that the higher the frame rate, better would the scan quality be considered. This frame rate can be increased, if the machine has to process less. Though it is known that starting the color Doppler decreases the frame rate, the frame rate with color Doppler can be optimized, if the color box size is planned just large enough to cover the area of interest. I would add here that before switching on the color Doppler, the B-mode image also should be optimized for its angle and depth to concentrate only on the area of interest. The color box can be moved all across the B-mode image and the size can be altered based on the requirement (Fig. 1.9).

Gains

When the Doppler is switched on, it should show the blood vessels filled up with color and no color spilling out of the vessels. This is done by gain adjustment. When the gains are too high, the color will be seen spilling out of the vessels (Fig. 1.10). Whereas when the gains are low, the color will not completely fill up the vessels (Fig. 1.11). This is because when the gains are low, the low-velocity signals will not be picked up by Doppler. It is important to mention at this stage that in a vessel the central stream has the highest velocity flow whereas close to the walls the velocity is lower due to friction with the walls. The correct gain setting therefore is when the entire lumen of the vessel is filled with color and there is no spill outside.

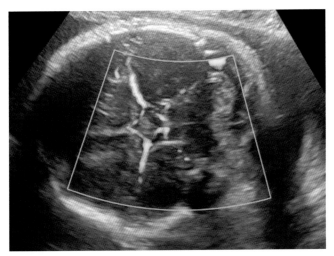

Fig. 1.9: Color Doppler image showing the box in green outline in which the flow is assessed.

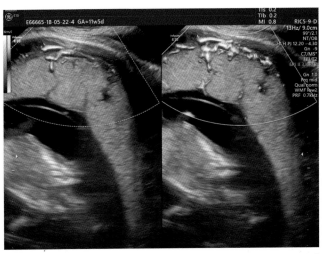

Fig. 1.11: High-definition (HD) flow image: the image in the left shows hardly any vessels as the gains are low, whereas that on the right shows adequate filling of the vessels.

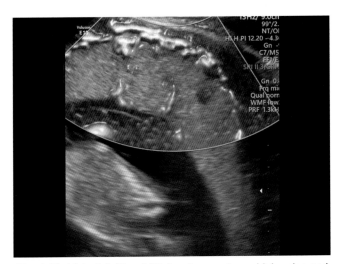

Fig. 1.10: High-definition (HD) flow image shows high gains and the color is seen spilling out of the vessels.

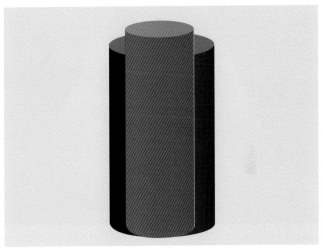

Fig. 1.12: Diagrammatic demonstration of the color flow in presence of low gains—black area between the vessel wall and the color column due to nonvisibility of the low-velocity flow information close to the walls due to low gains or high-wall filter.

How to set?

Increase the gains to maximum, there will be a lot of spill of color. Start decreasing the gains till the color is contained in the vessel, further decrease the gains and there will be black (anechoic) areas between the color column and the vessel wall (Fig. 1.12). This means that the gains are over-reduced. Now increase gains till the vessel again fills up fully and this is your correct setting. Gain settings for color and power Doppler once set and placed in the presets are not to be changed.

Pulse Repetition Frequency

It has already been discussed that the PRF decides what is maximum receiving frequency of the sound wave (indirectly velocity) that is recordable at a particular setting[2] (Nyquist frequency). Therefore, it is important to select an optimum PRF for the velocity of the blood vessels flow studied. High PRF, if used for low-velocity flow, it will not be possible to pick up the color where there are flows (Fig. 1.13). Instead if low PRF is used for high-velocity flows, there will be

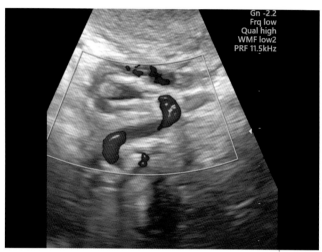

Fig. 1.13: High pulse repetition frequency (PRF) for low-velocity flow—showing empty vessel lumen without the flow.

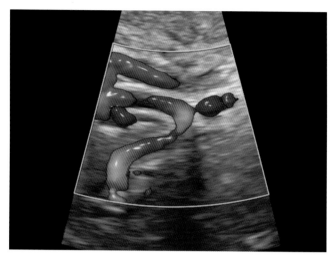

Fig. 1.15: Optimum pulse repetition frequency (PRF) setting gives unicolor filling of the vessel.

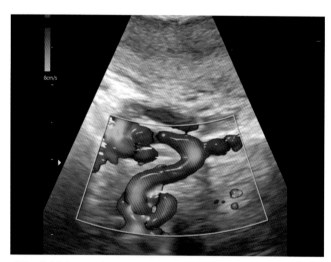

Fig. 1.14: Low pulse repetition frequency (PRF) when used for high-velocity flow shows mixing of colors.

aliasing—mixing of red and blue colors—appears like turbulence (Fig. 1.14). The PRF setting would be optimum when the color homogenously fills the entire vessel with single color—red or blue (Fig. 1.15).

Wall Motion Filter

It is known that Doppler produces color signals wherever there is a movement. And, the brightness of the color depends on the velocity of the moving object. This means that the color signals are produced by the red blood corpuscles in the blood, but are also produced by the wall movement of the artery and also by the pulsations transmitted to the surrounding tissues. The color signals

of the blood flow are the brightest, those of wall motion are dull and those due to transmitted pulsations from the surrounding tissues are the dullest, for the reasons explained earlier.

But these dull signals produced by low-velocity movements corrupt the flow information and can be eliminated only if a low-velocity filter is used. This filter is named as WMF. WMF can be adjusted at various levels depending on the level of sound signals that need to be eliminated to produce clear flow velocity signals. For larger vessels with high-velocity flows, the arterial flow movement is more and higher WMF is required, whereas for small vessels with low-velocity signals, the arterial wall movements are less and so low-wall filters are required. Using higher wall filter for a low-velocity blood flow vessel will eliminate the slow flow information. This will lead to a typical color flow signal with a color column seen in the center of the vessel, with a black line seen on both the sides between the vessel wall and the color column, similar to that produced by low gains (*see* Fig. 1.12).

Balance

As the name suggests, this is a balancing tool between the two modalities—the B-mode and the color Doppler. As discussed earlier, when Doppler is switched on, the scanner computer processing is doubled and so scanner is to be advised as to which of the two modalities should be given predominance. This can be decided by the balance. When color/power Doppler is switched on, a gray bar and a color bar appear on the left side of the screen. On the gray bar

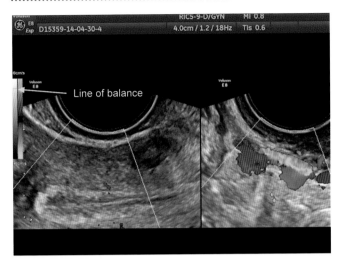

Fig. 1.16: Color Doppler image showing gray bar and the color bar on the left upper corner of the image, with gray bar showing green "line of balance".

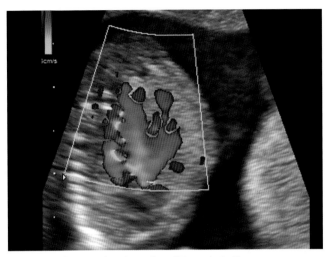

Fig. 1.18: Decreasing the gains of B-mode in the same case as in Figure 1.17, the color pick up becomes bold and smooth.

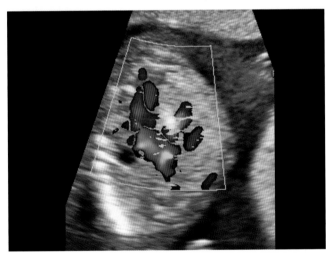

Fig. 1.17: Color Doppler image showing white patches in the color, due to low balance.

is a green line (Fig. 1.16). This line indicates the balance adjustment. When the brightness of the gray scale on the image matches the brightness below the green line on the gray bar, the color predominates and the color filling is normal, but when the brightness on the gray scale image matches the brightness above the green line on the gray bar, the B-mode predominates and therefore in these areas if the color is present to show the flows, the color will be patched up with white (Fig. 1.17). Increasing color gain is surely not an answer to this problem.

Very importantly, when this happens, the correct thing to do is to change the balance to higher that allows the color pick up even with bright gray scale. But the balance setting on many scanners are on the submenu of color Doppler. This makes it clumsy because when the operator is assessing flow in a relatively small vessel on the scan, to open the submenu and change the balance is difficult. Therefore, a practical solution to this is to reduce the B-mode gains that will match the brightness of the image to a gray shade below the green line on the gray bar and allows good color pick up (Fig. 1.18).

SETTINGS FOR PULSED WAVE DOPPLER

Sample Volume

Sample volume is the selected length of the vessel to assess the flow. When pulsed wave Doppler is switched on, a dotted line appears on the screen. This line can be swapped across the entire image. Two parallel short horizontal lines (= sign) appear on this line (Fig. 1.19). This indicates the sample volume. This "= sign" can be moved up and down on the dotted line anywhere. This sign is to be placed on the vessel in which the flow is to be measured. The distance between the two lines decides—what length of the vessel will be evaluated for the flow assessment. If the vessel is not absolutely parallel to the sound beam (overlapping on the dotted line), the distance between the two line (sample volume) should be equal to the diameter of the vessel. A sample volume smaller than the diameter will lead to error in the velocity assessment, because then it will not evaluate the flow in the entire stream (Fig. 1.20). When that happens, correct velocity readings are not possible because flow

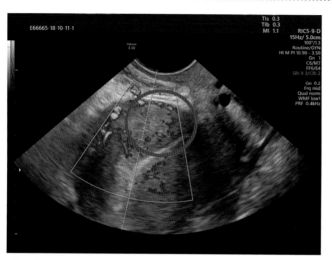

Fig. 1.19: Two parallel short horizontal lines (= sign) is seen on the dotted line on activation of the spectral Doppler.

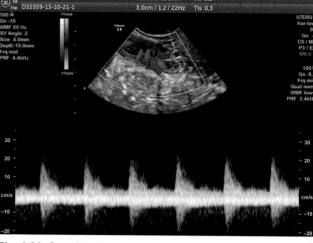

Fig. 1.21: Sample volume, larger than the diameter of the vessel, shows flow information from neighboring vessels.

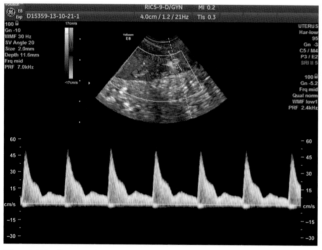

Fig. 1.20: A sample volume smaller than the diameter will not evaluate the flow in the entire stream, and will give erroneously higher velocity.

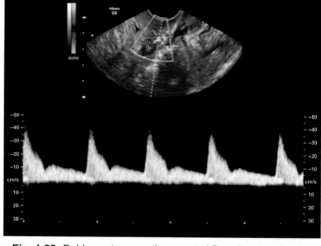

Fig. 1.22: Bold spectrum on the spectral Doppler showing the flow information.

velocities in the central stream and at the sides are not the same. If the sample volume is larger than the diameter of the vessel, the vessel wall movement or flow information from neighboring vessels may corrupt the flow information details (Fig. 1.21).

Gains

Gain settings on the pulsed wave Doppler should be such that it produces a clear well-defined bold spectrum of blood flows (Fig. 1.22). If the gains are too high, the flow information will be corrupted by lot of noise (Fig. 1.23). If the gains are too low, the entire spectrum will appear scarce and scattered (Fig. 1.24).

Pulse Repetition Frequency

As it has been discussed earlier that the Nyquist frequency of a sound wave decides what maximum flow velocities can be recorded by a sound wave of certain frequency. Therefore, the PRF is adjusted according to flow velocity to be assessed. If high PRF is used for low-velocity flow, it will not be possible to differentiate between the systolic and diastolic flows, as the systolic flow recordings will be subdued (Fig. 1.25). If low PRF is selected for high-velocity blood flows, there will be an overlapping of systolic and diastolic signals, which is known as aliasing (Fig. 1.26). The correct PRF setting would therefore be when the spectrum will fill up two-thirds of the spectral area (above the baseline) (Fig. 1.27). Though when

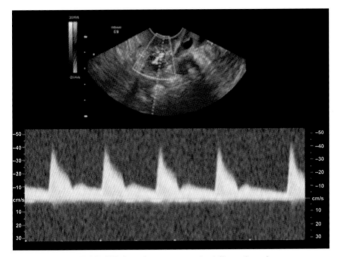

Fig. 1.23: High gains on spectral Doppler show noise on the spectrum.

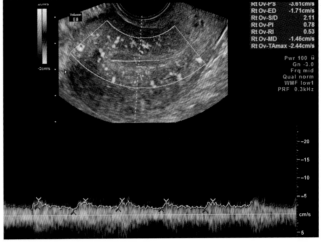

Fig. 1.25: Spectral Doppler image of a low-velocity flow documented by high pulse repetition frequency (PRF) showing minimal difference in the systolic peak and diastolic flow.

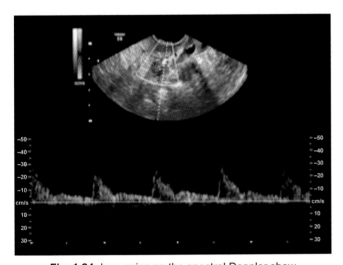

Fig. 1.24: Low gains on the spectral Doppler show scattered spectrum.

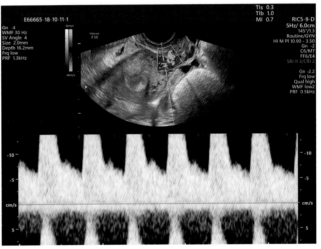

Fig. 1.26: If low pulse repetition frequency (PRF) is selected for high-velocity blood flows, there will be overlapping of systolic and diastolic signals.

there is minimal adjustment required to achieve this, moving the baseline up or down would also solve the purpose.

Wall Motion Filter

Like in color and power Doppler, the function of wall motion filter in pulsed Doppler also is to eliminate signals from low-velocity movements, chiefly not to corrupt the image with wall motions and also with venous flows, adjoining the artery. Again like color and power Doppler, the settings are low for low-velocity vessels and high for high-velocity vessels. But the wall filter setting in a pulsed Doppler

spectrum is known to be correct, only if the spectrum touches the baseline (Fig. 1.28). When there is a black line or a gap between the baseline and the spectrum (Fig. 1.29), this trace is not to be accepted as this clearly indicates high-wall filter for the case. In that case, if we say it eliminates low-velocity information—means it interferes with the diastolic flow information and may lead to false diagnosis of absent end-diastolic flow and naturally then wrong interpretations. Spectral Doppler being a quantitative Doppler, the wall filter settings on this modality are in numbers 30 Hz, 60 Hz, 90 Hz, etc. Wall filters as a rule for gynecological and infertility assessment are set at the lowest 30 Hz; and for

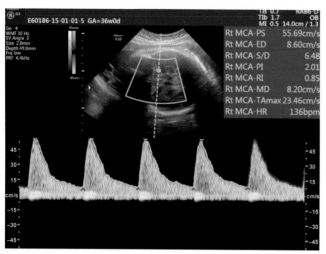

Fig. 1.27: Spectral Doppler showing the spectrum above the baseline, using two-thirds of the area dedicated to spectrum.

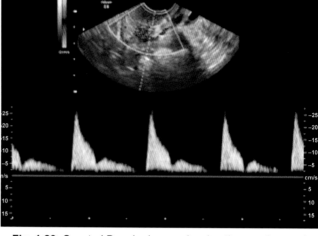

Fig. 1.29: Spectral Doppler image showing the spectrum not touching the baseline and that is high setting of wall filter.

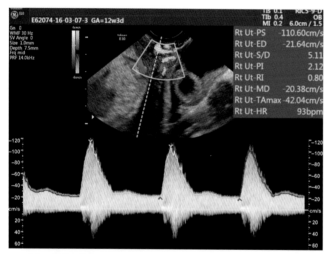

Fig. 1.28: Spectral Doppler image showing the spectrum touching the baseline and that is optimum setting of wall filter.

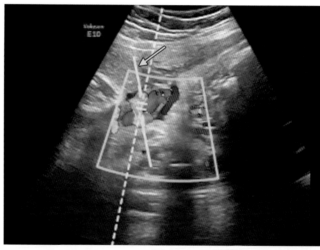

Fig. 1.30: Activation of the spectral Doppler shows a dotted line, the sample volume seen as an "= sign" and the short yellow line is the line that can be aligned to the long axis of the vessel.

fetal echocardiography, this is set high, may be 90–120 Hz, depending on the fetal gestational age.

As is discussed earlier considering the equation for derivation of the blood flow velocity from frequency of incident sound beam, frequency of received sound beam and cos θ of the angle of incidence, if the angle of incidence is 90° then the cos θ is 0, the velocity value will be calculated as 0 and also that with increasing angle from more than 60°, the percentage of error in calculation is highly significant and so the Doppler angle is always set between 0° and 60°, preferably less than 30°. When the pulsed wave Doppler is switched on, the dotted line and the "= sign" appears. The Doppler angle can be considered or set at 0 when the vessel

is parallel to the dotted line. This is often times possible because the dotted line can be swapped across the entire B-mode image and the probe manipulation may also help in the alignment of the two. But if it is still not possible, after achieving the smallest angle between the vessel and the dotted line, angle correction is used. This deviates out a short line from the dotted line, and is tried to align this short line to the vessel (Fig. 1.30). In trying to do this, the angle between the dotted line and the short line is the Doppler angle. It is displayed on the screen or the touch pad of the scanner (Fig. 1.31). This angle is to set as less than 30° preferably and maximum of 60° may be allowed.

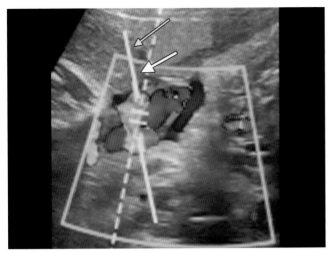

Fig. 1.31: The angle between short line and the dotted line is shown by the white blocked arrow.

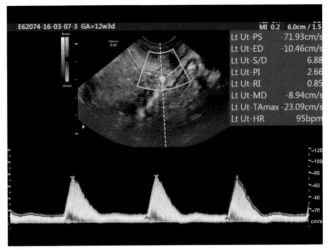

Fig. 1.33: Spectral Doppler traced on higher speed showing trace of multiple cardiac cycles.

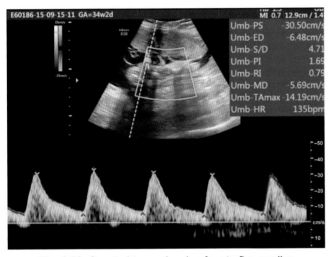

Fig. 1.32: Spectral trace showing four to five cardiac cycles on a single trace.

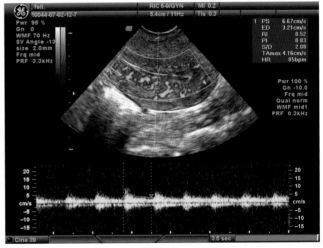

Fig. 1.34: Spectral Doppler traced on lower speed showing trace of less than five cardiac cycles.

SETTING THE SPEED OF THE TRACE

An ideal spectral trace is, when there are 4–5 cardiac cycles (Fig. 1.32), recorded on any one spectrum image. This can be done by scaling the time axis, or in simpler words, setting the speed of the trace. For most scans, this is possible when the speed is set as 4 or 5. Higher speed gives trace of too few cardiac cycles (Fig. 1.33) and lesser speed gives too many cardiac cycles traced (Fig. 1.34).

ARTIFACTS

In spite of all these settings used to optimize the Doppler images, certain artifacts still cannot be completely eliminated. And these are aliasing, mirror image artifacts, and artifacts due to electrical interferences.

Aliasing

When the Doppler frequency exceeds the Nyquist frequency, it results in aliasing. This is overlapping effect of systolic and diastolic velocities across the baseline on both the sides of the spectrum. This effect is similar to what we have often observed especially in movies. The car wheels suddenly appear to start rotating in the opposite direction when the car speeds up.

If the frequency of the oscillations is 5 Hz but the PRF is 2 per second the signal will see this movement only twice in a second and not only miss the intermittent information but also will interpret that the flow is in both directions. Adjusting the optimum PRF sorts out this problem.

Mirror Image Artifacts

Mirror image artifact is when a similar spectrum is seen on both the sides of the baseline. This is especially possible when the sample volume is large and is tracing the flow in two vessels or two loops of the same vessel positioned, side-by-side (Fig. 1.35), second possibility is that a large sample volume is placed on the curve of the loop, when in the proximal half of the loop, the blood flow is observed away from the probe by the transducer and in the distal half of the sample volume, the flow is perceived toward the probe. Decreasing the sample volume and planning to place it on one vessel only will sort out this problem.

Electrical Interferences

These may appear as random signals on color, power, or spectral Doppler (Fig. 1.36), especially when the scanner is sharing the same electrical line as some high-voltage gadget and the only way to get rid of this is to plan the electrical supply to the scanner wisely.

SAFETY OF DOPPLER

There is a big scare against using Doppler in the people who are aware of the ill effects of Doppler and a false sense of safety in those who are not aware of these side effects. The two major effects of sound wave when it passes through the human body are:
- *Thermal effect*: Production of heat that may damage the cells.
- *Mechanical effect*: Due to pressure changes on the molecule.

Thermal Effects

As the sound waves pass through the body tissues, there is absorption of energy and transformation of ultrasound energy into heat. The energy absorption is minimal in fluid and maximum in bones. It is also dependent on the frequency of the ultrasound waves. The absorption is higher with higher frequency waves and lower with low-frequency sound waves. A temperature rise of up to 1°C is considered absolutely safe, whereas if it is more than 2.5°C, it can lead to significant tissue damage. This thermal effect is measured as and displayed as thermal index on the screen. It is generally found that the temperature rise of 2°C is thermal

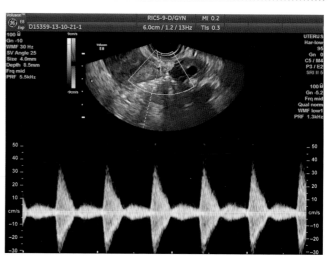

Fig. 1.35: Mirror image artifact showing similar flow trace on both the sides of baseline.

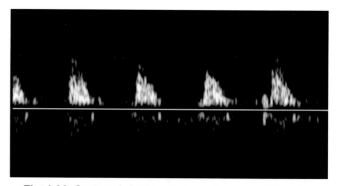

Fig. 1.36: Scattered shadows seen on the spectral Doppler, possibly due to electrical interference.

index 2. We know that the temperature rise of 1°C is safe, so thermal index should be limited at maximum 1. Though it is important here to understand that with higher thermal indices also the damage can occur only after exposure of a certain period of time. Unfortunately, this time is difficult to define confidently. Moreover, since the energy-absorbing capacity of different tissues is different, thermal index for soft tissues (TIs) and bones (TIb) is different.[3]

Mechanical Effect

When the sound wave passes through the body tissues, it leads to oscillations of the body molecules, resulting in cavitating (low pressure) phase and a compressing (high pressure) phase. In the negative pressure phase or the cavitation phase, large microbubbles are formed. Once the oscillations reach a certain level, fluid medium incorporating gas microbubbles is set in motion called microstreaming. This generates very strong pressure and leads to bursting of cell membranes. This effect is pronounced, if the high-frequency, high-intensity ultrasound is aimed on a small focus.[1]

The second possible mechanism explained is as follows—existing microbubbles or cells undergoing cavitation inflate under the influence of negative pressure and implode abruptly. This takes microseconds but causes sudden rise in temperature or pressure and results in tissue destruction. This is transient cavitation and occurs only when energy levels are beyond certain thresholds. This threshold may be quantitatively documented as mechanical index (MI). MI is defined as "maximum estimated in situ rarefaction pressure or maximum negative pressure (in MPa) divided by the square root of the frequency (in MHz). MI of up to 0.3 can be considered safe and more than 0.7 can lead to cavitation.[4]

CONCLUSION

Doppler is a very useful modality for assessment of circulation in the human body. Correct settings on the scanner only can give optimum results and therefore it is very important to understand the basic principles and settings of the ultrasound scanner before starting to use Doppler for interpretation of vascular flows and information of oxygenation in human fetus. Ultrasound and Doppler are generally safe modalities. Their safety can be related to frequency used and the length of exposure. Therefore, Doppler should not used for long times on a single focus and therefore ALARA[5] (as low as reasonably achievable) principle is now applied for all ultrasound scan.

REFERENCES

1. Frey H. Physical and technical fundamentals of ultrasound and Doppler ultrasound. In: Sohn C, Voigt HJ, Vetter K, (Eds). Doppler Ultrasound in Gynecology and Obstetrics, 1st edition. Germany: George Thieme Verlag; 2004.
2. Burns PN. Principles of Doppler and colour flow. Radiol Med. 1993;85(5 Suppl 1):3-16.
3. Duck FA. Biological effects and safety aspect. In: Wladimiroff JW, Eik-Nes S (Eds). Ultrasound in Obstetrics and Gynaecology. China: Elsevier Publishers; 2009. pp. 21-30.
4. The British Medical Ultrasound Society. (2010). Safety of ultrasound. [online] Available from: www.bmus.org/public-info/pi-safety01.asp. [Accessed October, 2018].
5. Auxier JA, Dickson HW. Guest editorial: Concern over recent use of the ALARA philosophy. Health Phys. 1983;44(6):595-600.

Endometrial Lesions and Doppler

INTRODUCTION

Uterus is the central pelvic organ suspended by several ligaments. Endometrium is central in the uterus. It outlines the potential cavity of the uterus. It has cell-rich connective tissue composed of superficial functional layer and inner basal layer (Fig. 2.1). It is the most dynamic anatomical structure in the uterus. In response to the hormonal changes during the menstrual cycle, the functional layer of the endometrium sheds off completely during the menstruation, then grows gradually during the proliferative phase under the effect of estrogen, gets compacted when exposed to progesterone and then again under the effect of progesterone and estrogen in luteal phase grows to maximum till mid-luteal phase and then again starts regressing in a nonconception cycle to breakthrough during menstruation (Fig. 2.2). Endometrium also has different appearances from neonatal life to menopause. Interestingly, the appearance of the endometrium is almost similar in the neonatal life and at menopause. The endometrium is thin and at times ill defined and may also at times contain fluid in the cavity.

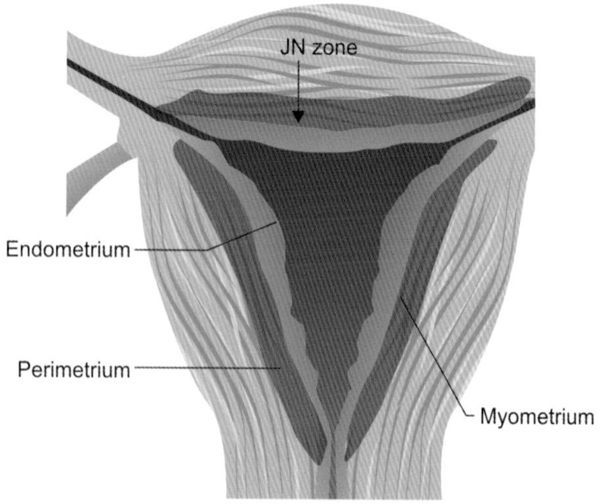

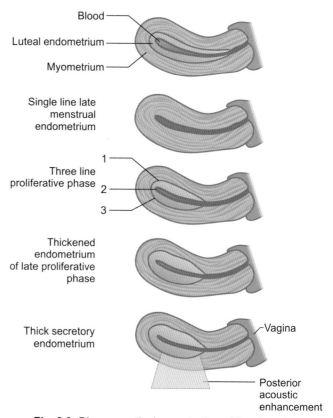

Fig. 2.2: Diagrammatic demonstration of the changing morphology of the endometrium during the menstrual cycle.

Fig. 2.1: Diagrammatic demonstration of the layers of uterine wall. (JN: junctional zone)

Endometrium is best evaluated on transvaginal scan, but a prior abdominal scan is recommended for evaluation of the pelvic anatomy.[1]

In cases when transvaginal scan is not possible or denied by the patient, transrectal scan is preferred to transabdominal route. Doppler must be used for assessment of the vascularity. 3D ultrasound is useful for evaluation of the coronal plane and is a modality with proved ability for assessment of the endometrial–myometrial junction. Endometrial thickness is measured from outer margin of the hyperechoic line to the outer margin of the hyperechoic line, at the broadest part of the endometrium, perpendicular to the central line of the endometrium (Fig. 2.3).

Endometrial pathologies may be inflammatory, may be due to abnormal response to hormones, or may be benign or malignant neoplasms.

But before initiating the discussion on the endometrial lesions and their vascular patterns, it is essential to get acquainted with the standard terminology used worldwide. This is described under the International Endometrial Tumor Analysis (IETA) consensus.[2] It can be used to describe the endometrial appearance on B-mode

ultrasound, on sonohysterography and also on Doppler. There are specific terms used for description of each aspect of the endometrium. Figures 2.4 to 2.8 illustrate the appearances with the text mentioned in the figures narrate the terms to be used.

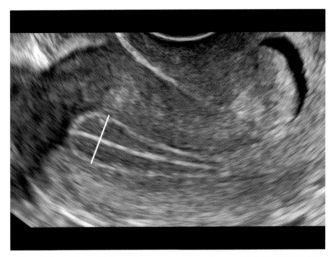

Fig. 2.3: Midsagittal section of the uterus showing endometrial measurement.

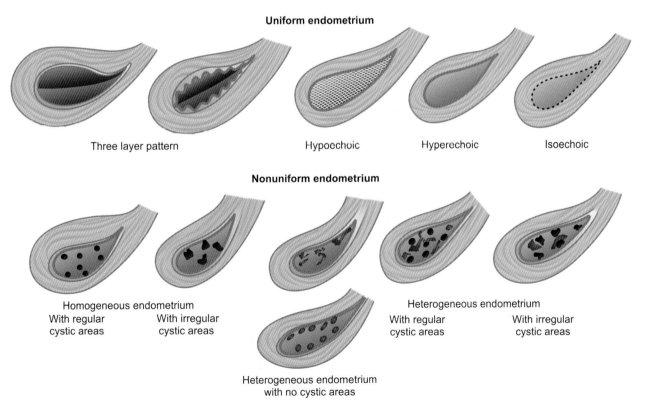

Fig. 2.4: Diagrammatic demonstration of the uniform and nonuniform endometrium on B-mode—International Endometrial Tumor Analysis (IETA) terminology.

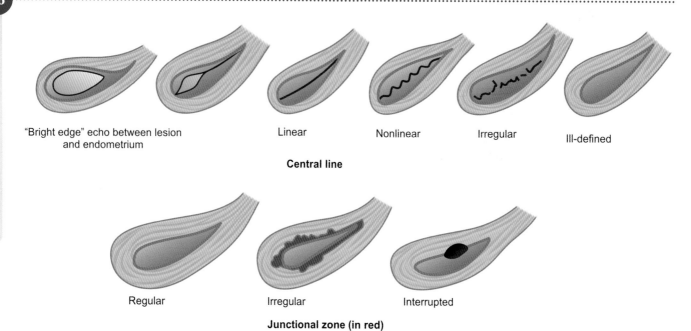

Fig. 2.5: Diagrammatic demonstration of junctional zone, central line, and edges of the endometrial lesion on B-mode—International Endometrial Tumor Analysis (IETA) terminology.

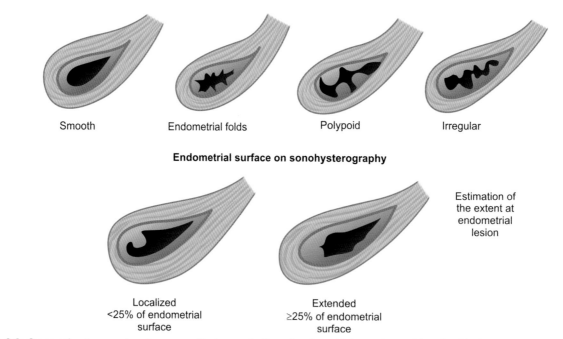

Fig. 2.6: On sonohysterography, diagrammatic demonstration of endometrial margins and localized lesion on B-mode—International Endometrial Tumor Analysis (IETA) terminology.

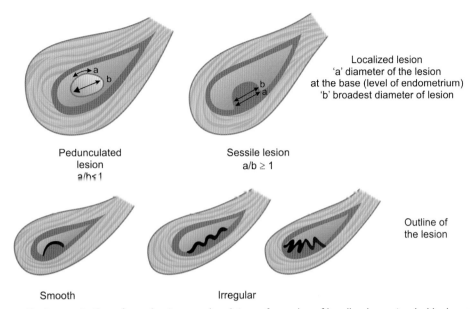

Fig. 2.7: Diagrammatic demonstration of sonohysterography picture of margins of localized or extended lesion and differentiation between sessile or pedunculated localized lesion on B-mode—International Endometrial Tumor Analysis (IETA) terminology.

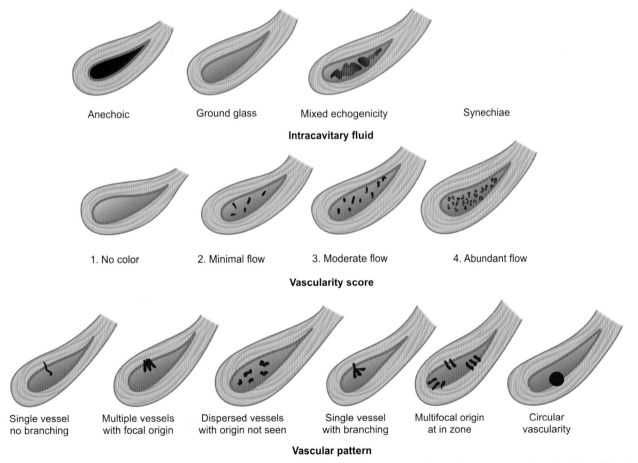

Fig. 2.8: Diagrammatic demonstration of endometrial contents, vascularity score, and vascular arrangement as by International Endometrial Tumor Analysis (IETA).

INFLAMMATORY LESIONS

Endometrium is easily susceptible to infections because of its possibly easy access to infections through vagina and cervix. Inflammation of the endometrium may be related to pregnancy or to pelvic inflammatory disease (PID). Inflammation related to pregnancy—postpartum endometritis is more florid and may present with fever, pain, bleeding (secondary hemorrhage) and foul-smelling lochia.

Chronic endometritis may be due to retained products of conception, but also may be due to tuberculosis, intrauterine contraceptive devices, or neoplastic masses like endometrial carcinoma or a submucous fibroid. This inflammation may be acute or chronic. Patients with acute endometritis may complain of bad odor in the menstrual discharge. At times, inflammation may also present as menorrhagia or metrorrhagia, often associated with acute pelvic pain. Whereas, patients with chronic endometritis more commonly present with scanty bleeding or amenorrhea.

Acute Endometritis

Acute inflammatory process leads to edema and hyperemia due to neoangiogenesis. Edema includes the endometrium and also the subendometrial tissue due to its close anatomical vicinity. But the subendometrial layer is also likely to be affected because it is this layer that hosts the dilated spiral vessels, the parent vessels of the endometrial vessels. Extravasation of the fluid from these dilated vessels may also be the cause of edema in the subendometrial layer.

This leads to irregularly increased thickness of the endometrial–myometrial junctional zone (JZ) (Fig. 2.9). Endometrial edema may appear as increased thickness of the endometrium with a homogeneous texture. It may have a ground-glass-like echogenicity and both because of its echogenicity similar to that of the normal myometrium and also because of irregularity of the JZ, and may be difficult to distinguish from the myometrium. There may be fluid in the endometrial cavity that is turbid (blood/pus) (Fig. 2.10).

If it is due to a foreign body like a gauze or retained products of conception, one may see heterogeneous shadows in the cavity. If it is postpartum, a subinvoluted uterus is seen, that appears bulky and vascular. In presence of anaerobic infections, air may be seen in the endometrial cavity as bright scattered echoes. If associated with PID, adnexa also will present signs of inflammation like free fluid (Fig. 2.11), hydrosalpinx, or oophoritis.

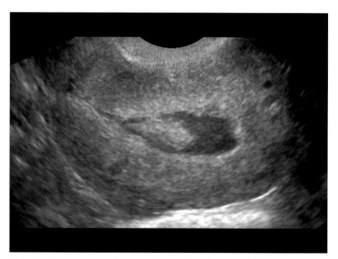

Fig. 2.10: B-mode ultrasound showing irregular junctional zone endometrial fluid with heterogeneous echogenicity of acute endometritis.

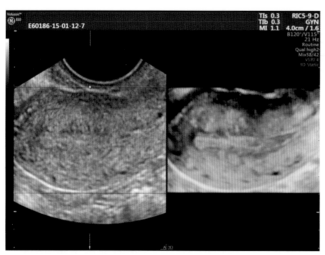

Fig. 2.9: B-mode and volume contrast imaging (VCI) A showing irregularity of the junctional zone.

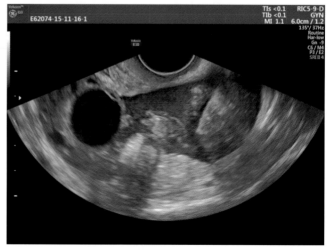

Fig. 2.11: Acute pelvic infection showing free fluid with low level internal echogenicities in it.

The neoangiogenesis of inflammation is documented on ultrasound as increased vascularity in the endometrium. These vessels typically have larger diameter than the normal spiral vessels and also have low resistance (RI < 0.5) blood flow. The vascular distribution may be heterogeneous due to nonuniform involvement of the endometrium in the inflammatory process.

But interestingly, the low-resistance blood flow in the endometrium cannot always be used as diagnostic criteria for diagnosis of acute inflammatory process. This is so because it is known that normally also during the preovulatory and secretory phase—there is physiological neoangiogenesis in the endometrium. Therefore, this sign can be used only in a phase of the cycle when normally the endometrium is avascular or has high-resistance blood flow. This phase is early proliferative phase.

Thickened endometrium also cannot be used as "the" diagnostic criteria for acute inflammation in preovulatory and secretory phases for the reasons described earlier. Though thickened irregular endometrial–myometrial junction can be used a strong supportive sign for inflammatory reaction.

Chronic Endometritis

Chronic inflammatory process instead results into fibrosis and compromise of the normal endometrial tissue. This does not allow the endometrium to grow in thickness under estrogenic or progesterone stimulation. This means endometrium remains thin even during the preovulatory and the secretory phases when it should otherwise grow in thickness. As a result of chronic inflammation, the endometrium also shows scanty high-resistance vascularity. Normally, the endometrium shows vascularity reaching the inner layers of the endometrium in the preovulatory and secretory phases with vascular resistance index (RI) of less than 0.6 and less than 0.5, respectively. The vascular abundance and resistance may vary according to the severity of the inflammation. It is important to clarify here that the endometrium normally also is thin and avascular or has scanty vascularity in the early proliferative phase. Similar to acute inflammation—acute endometritis, even the chronic endometritis shows irregular endometrial–myometrial junction and this may help to suspect chronic endometritis in the early proliferative endometrium (Fig. 2.12).

Tuberculous Endometritis

One of the most commonly found, feared of, and difficult to treat infection in the developing countries is tuberculosis.

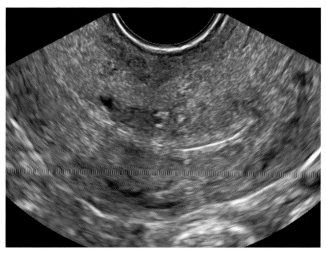

Fig. 2.12: Irregular endometrial–myometrial junction, and thin endometrium of chronic endometritis.

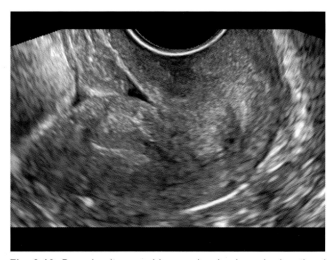

Fig. 2.13: B-mode ultrasound image showing irregular junctional zone and thin endometrium and hyperechoic flecks in junctional zone.

In the acute state of the disease, it is not possible to differentiate other infections from tuberculosis. Ultrasound shows irregular endometrial-myometrial junction and thickening at times. Sometimes, one may find a fairly normal looking endometrium in patients with tuberculosis.

But typically acute tubercular endometritis does not show low-resistance blood flow. This may be so because tuberculosis commonly affects end-arteries. Chronic tuberculous endometritis though like other chronic inflammatory endometritis shows persistently thin endometrium with irregular JZ, it also presents with certain features that are much more commonly seen in tubercular infection as compared to other infections (Fig. 2.13).

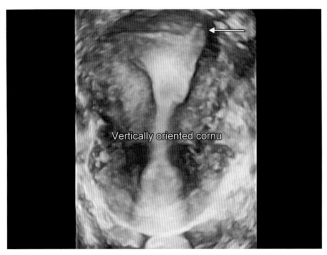

Fig. 2.14: 3D ultrasound of the uterus—coronal plane showing vertical orientation of the cornu (arrow).

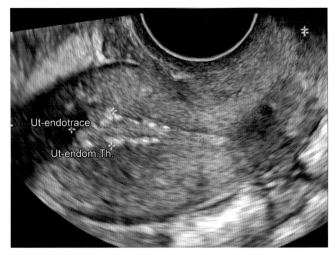

Fig. 2.16: Endometrial–myometrial junctional calcifications seen on B-mode ultrasound.

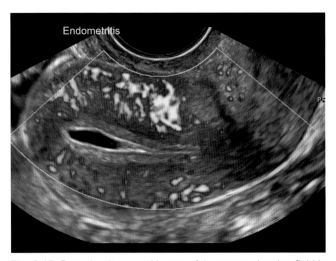

Fig. 2.15: B-mode ultrasound image of the uterus showing fluid in the endometrial cavity, with hyperechoic endometrial margin and absent vascularity in the subendometrial area—chronic endometritis possibly tuberculous.

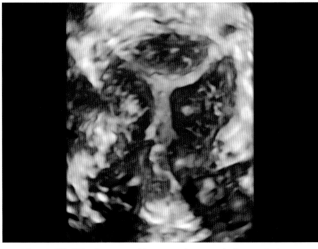

Fig. 2.17: 3D ultrasound image of coronal plane of uterus showing grossly contracted scarred endometrial cavity.

The most consistent is vertical orientation of the interstitial part of the tube (Fig. 2.14). Fluid collection may be seen in the endometrium but typically the inner layer of the endometrium typically appears hyperechoic with irregular endometrial-myometrial junction and no vascularity beyond the JZ (Fig. 2.15). Endometrial, myometrial, and endometrial-myometrial JZ calcifications may be seen (Fig. 2.16). Endometrial scarring and synechiae occur due to healing with fibrosis (Fig. 2.17). Tuberculous endometritis may also at times present as multiple micropolyps in the endometrium (Fig. 2.18). Tuberculosis may also affect the myometrium and cause myometrial cysts. Though

like endometrium, the myometrium also is typically hypovascular in patients with tuberculosis.

Abnormal Response to Hormones

As described earlier in this chapter, it is known that the endometrium has a changing morphology throughout the menstrual cycle. It is the receptor organ for estrogen and progesterone. For the normal menstrual cycle, an alternate predominance of estrogen and progesterone is essential. Moreover, it is withdrawal of both that leads to breakthrough of the endometrium. Break in this hormonal cycle may lead to abnormalities in the endometrium or even abnormal

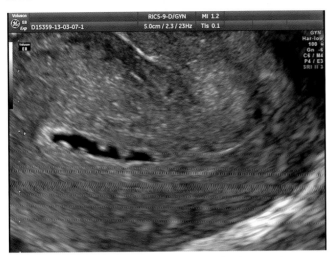

Fig. 2.18: Micropolyposis seen on sonohysterography on B-mode ultrasound.

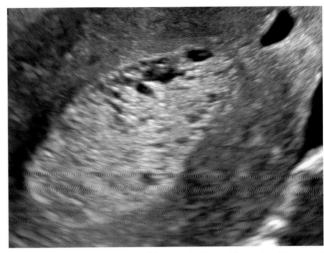

Fig. 2.19: Cystic endometrial hyperplasia on B-mode ultrasound showing thickened endometrium with hyperechogenicity and multiple anechoic cystic areas.

response of the endometrium to normal hormonal changes may lead to pathologies of the endometrium.

It is due to persistent estrogen exposure that the endometrium keeps on growing to a thickness beyond physiological limits. This is mentioned as 15 mm in literature but we have observed the endometrium growing to 18 mm thickness in some patients with normal endometrial morphology. But apart from the thickness, endometrium changes its morphology in presence of persistent estrogen exposure. Under the influence of rising estrogen levels, the endometrium grows from single line to multilayered endometrium. With rising estrogen level, the endometrium changes its morphology from multilayered pattern to homogeneous endometrium. This is due to proliferation of endometrial glands. Persistently, high levels of estrogen load to endometrial hyperplasia resulting into increased endometrial gland to stroma ratio, mildly hyperechoic endometrium, with multiple well-defined round anechoic areas. These anechoic areas are hyperplastic glands. Patients with endometrial hyperplasia present with a period of amenorrhea followed by spotting. As is known, endometrium has glandular and stromal components. The abundance of anechoic areas in the thickened endometrium indicates it is a predominantly *glandular hyperplasia* (Fig. 2.19), and if it has chiefly solid look with only few anechoic areas, it is predominantly *stromal hyperplasia* (Fig. 2.20). Endometrial hyperplasia may show polypoid endometrium at times. This shows irregular central line on B-mode and a polypoid endometrium on sonohysterography. The endometrial–myometrial junction

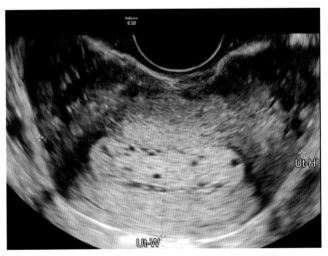

Fig. 2.20: Hyperechoic endometrium with very few cystic areas—endometrial hyperplasia with stromal predominance.

is typically intact in endometrial hyperplasia. Endometrial hyperplasia on Doppler shows regularly distributed blood vessels throughout the endometrium (Fig. 2.21). These blood vessels have a moderate-resistance flow with RI: 0.60–0.70.

Persistent progesterone exposure leads to a compact hyperechoic endometrium, with intact endometrial-myometrial JZ. It is the hyperechogenicity that differentiates a hyperestrogenic endometrium from the hyperprogesteronic endometrium. On Doppler, the endometrium that is hyperprogesteronic shows variable vascularity. Actually, the vascularity of the progesterone-exposed endometrium depends on the estrogen–progesterone ratio.

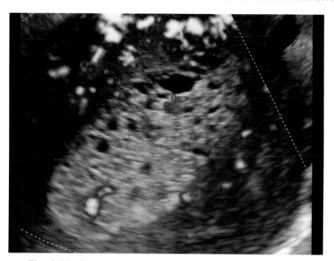

Fig. 2.21: Cystic glandular hyperplasia on power Doppler showing scanty endometrial vascularity.

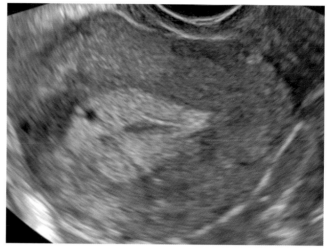

Fig. 2.22: Endometrium showing well-defined round anechoic lesion—endometrial cyst of endometrial metaplasia.

Endometrial Metaplasia

Apart from this, endometrial hyperplasia may also be seen as an effect of tamoxifen. Hyperplastic endometrium seen is in the tamoxifen exposed patients as well as endometrial metaplasia. Tamoxifen is widely used for treating breast cancer and has a proestrogenic effect on endometrium. Endometrial metaplasia due to tamoxifen exposure is about progressive changes in the endometrium when the patient is on tamoxifen therapy. On ultrasound, the endometrium shows different pictures at different stages of this progressive change. The changes seen are as follows:

- Echogenic endometrium with good halo and homogeneous echo pattern.
- Echogenic endometrium, good boundaries with small echo-free cysts (Fig. 2.22).
- Echogenic nonhomogeneous endometrium with small cystic structures, blurred boundaries.
- Echogenic nonhomogeneous endometrium, blurred boundaries, interrupted halo (Fig. 2.23).
- This last is the nonreversible stage to endometrial malignancy.

On Doppler, high-velocity, low-resistance flow is seen where RI may be as low as 0.39. Lower is the resistance, higher is the risk of atypia and malignancy.

NEOPLASTIC LESIONS

Polyps

Endometrial polyps are solid projectile lesions of endometrium. They are often diagnosed as an incidental

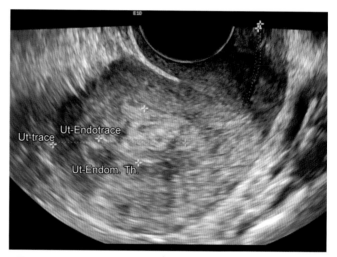

Fig. 2.23: Echogenic nonhomogeneous endometrium, blurred boundaries, interrupted halo—tamoxifen effect.

finding. But some patients may present with spotting and infertility. Sonographically, these are seen as solid echogenic lesions in the endometrial cavity, in-between the endometrial lines. Polyps can be diagnosed on B-mode scan and are best visible in the periovulatory phase of the menstrual cycle. The endometrium in this phase is multilayered with the intervening area being hypoechoic. Against this background, these solid soft tissue lesions stand out as echogenic round or ovalish lesions with smooth margins (Fig. 2.24). In the early proliferative phase, before endometrium becomes multilayered, polyp is only seen deshaping the endometrial cavity. Though at times, if there is fluid in the endometrial cavity, it may help as a negative contrast media and show the polyp as solid soft tissue projectile lesion in the cavity (Fig. 2.25). But I would prefer not to use the menstrual period as a scanning time for endometrial lesions, as there is a strong possibility to misinterpret blood or blood products as endometrial lesions. Pedunculated fibroids also move with peristalsis, like blood clots. Blood clots may appear as solid echogenic structures in the endometrial cavity. In the secretory phase, the endometrium is hyperechoic and obscures the visibility of the polyp. Though Doppler shows a feeding vessel in polyp unlike the clot and that is diagnostic. When the endometrial cavity fills up the endometrial cavity, it is a thin slit of fluid between the solid lesion and the endometrial

hyperechoic line that indicates the correct diagnosis (Fig. 2.26). Polyps may vary in size from very small ones, that may be difficult to visualize on ultrasound, to large ones that may mimic thickening of the entire endometrium, like in hyperplasia or malignancy (Fig. 2.27). Very small polyps may be isoechoic or mildly hyperechoic to the endometrium and sometimes can barely be seen on B-mode ultrasound. Sometimes, polyps may show tiny anechoic cystic areas, due to dilated endometrial glands. This may be seen in the polyps in patients on tamoxifen therapy also. The diagnostic clue to such a polyp is an abnormal curve in the central line of the endometrium (Fig. 2.28). Polyps may be pedunculated or sessile. Polyps may often be multiple

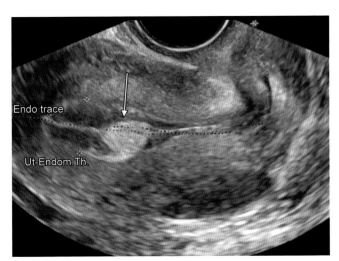

Fig. 2.24: B-mode ultrasound image of endometrial polyp (arrow).

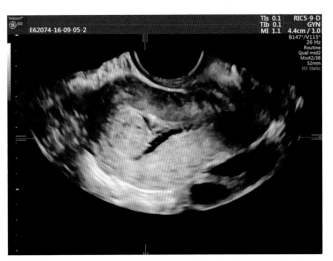

Fig. 2.26: Large endometrium polyp identified on sonohysterography as the fluid fills up surrounding it—on B-mode ultrasound.

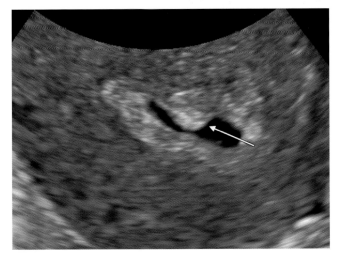

Fig. 2.25: Endometrial polyp (arrow) as seen on B-mode ultrasound with saline infusion sonohysterography.

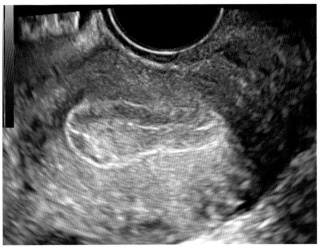

Fig. 2.27: Large polyp with subtle echogenicity—difficult to differentiate from hyperplasia on B-mode ultrasound.

(Fig. 2.29). In spite of this huge variability in types of polyps and their appearances on ultrasound, its typical vascular supply is diagnostic. Polyp has a characteristic blood supply by a single feeding vessel or maximum two vessels very closely placed (pedicular vessels especially in sessile polyps). Even when there are multiple polyps, each one has an individual single feeding vessel. Interestingly, when polyps are seen in the cervix, even these show a similar vascular pattern (Fig. 2.30). Polyps being benign lesions, these vessels have a high-resistance flow (RI is about 0.6). But with RI less than 0.45, atypia may be suspected in these polyps.[3] Infection, necrosis, or atypia in the polyp leads to heterogeneous echogenicity on the B-mode and Doppler shows abundant branching of the vessels inside the polyp mass (Figs. 2.31A and B).

Adenomyomatous polyp also shows abundant branching of blood vessels (Figs. 2.31A and B) inside the polyp mass, but the RI of these vessels is almost always more than 0.5. Vascular pattern has a high accuracy for differential diagnosis of endometrial lesions.

Single vessel pattern for polyp[4]: It has a sensitivity of 81.2%, specificity of 88.2%, positive predictive value (PPV) of 92.9%, and negative predictive value (NPV) of 71.4% for

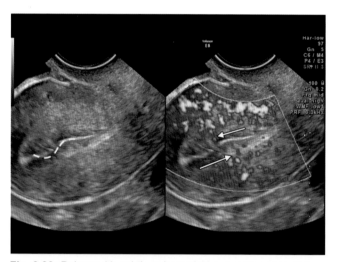

Fig. 2.28: Polyps with subtle echogenicities can be suspected on B-mode by abnormal curvature of the central line and differentiated from hyperplasia by single feeding vessels (arrows).

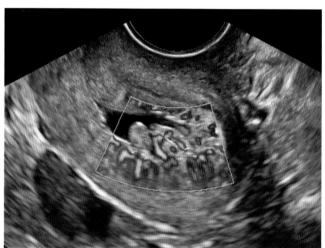

Fig. 2.30: B-mode with power Doppler image of two cervical polyps with feeding vessels.

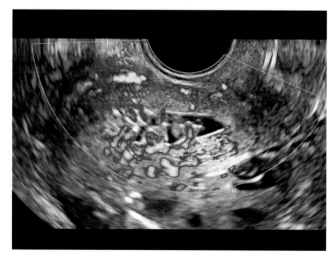

Fig. 2.29: Sonohysterography with power Doppler showing multiple polyps with single feeding vessel for each.

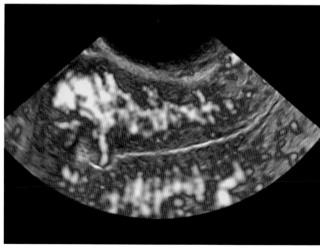

Fig. 2.31A: B-mode image of a polyp with power Doppler showing single feeding vessel with no branching.

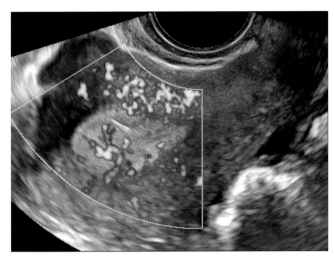

Fig. 2.31B: B-mode image of a polyp with power Doppler showing single feeding vessel with abundant branching.

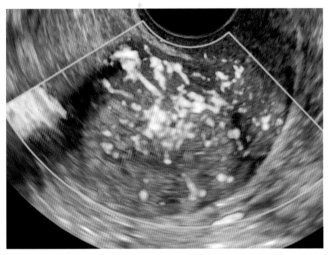

Fig. 2.32: B-mode with high-definition (HD) flow image of the thickened hypervascular endometrium with abundant and heterogeneously distributed vascularity suggestive of malignancy. It is also seen extending into the myometrium suggesting tumor extension into the myometrium.

the diagnosis of polyps. According to another study, the single feeding vessel (pedicle artery has a sensitivity of 76.4%, specificity of 95.3%, PPV of 81.3%, and NPV of 91.3% for the diagnosis of polyps).[5] Large polyps also have characteristic single feeding vessel, whereas hyperplastic endometrium shows uniformly distributed multiple vessels, as discussed earlier and malignant endometrial growth shows heterogeneously distributed, increased vascular density (Fig. 2.32), with vessels of asymmetrical caliber.

Apart from Doppler, sonohysterography is a useful investigation for diagnosis and differential diagnosis of endometrial lesions. It is a simple and painless procedure,

and does not require any analgesia or anesthesia. It can be used with Doppler or with 3D ultrasound. One can use a dedicated sonohysterography catheter for the procedure but we prefer to use Foley's catheter 6–8 Fr (external diameter 1.6 mm and internal diameter 1.1 mm). The catheter is introduced into the cervix, with the balloon in the cervical canal. Balloon is distended with 1.5–2 mL of normal saline or distilled water. After fixing the balloon, 5–7 mL of normal saline is slowly introduced in the endometrial cavity with 10–20 mL syringe. While filling the endometrial cavity with saline, the speculum and anterior retractor used earlier to visualize the cervix and facilitate the introduction of the probe are removed from the vagina and the probe is introduced to observe the endometrial cavity, as it is being filled up with saline. As the saline fills up and the endometrial cavity distends, the solid lesions of the endometrium can be clearly visualized in the endometrial cavity. Once the cavity is distended and the lesion is visualized, either a B-mode sweep in sagittal and axial planes can be taken and stored or a 3D volume of the uterus can be taken. One can also use Doppler after endometrial cavity is filled with saline for differential diagnosis of endometrial lesions.

Endometrial Fibroids

Fibroids are benign neoplasms originating in the myometrium. But some of these distort the endometrium and some may be pedunculated and grow in the endometrium. Though discussion about the fibroids will be further done in the chapter dedicated on the subject, its discussion here is relevant because these fibroids may mimic polyps and the differential diagnosis may be difficult. Intraendometrial fibroids also have the same morphology as the other fibroids. This means these are also hypoechoic to the myometrium. In the periovulatory phase, the endometrium is typically hypoechoic to the myometrium and the fibroids may be isoechoic to this and difficult to diagnose except for abnormal endometrial contour. Doppler can be a diagnostic in these cases as fibroids typically show peripheral vascularity (Fig. 2.33). Though on B-mode also, these fibroids can be seen in the secretory phase of the menstrual cycle that is hyperechoic and acts as a contrast for hypoechoic fibroid (Fig. 2.34).

Fibroid Polyp

This is a confusing and very loosely used term. Large polyps are often termed as fibroid polyps. Though true fibroid polyp on pathology may have a combination of myometrial and endometrial tissue and may be difficult to

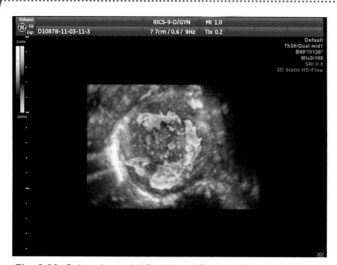

Fig. 2.33: Subendometrial fibroid on 3D power Doppler showing peripheral ring of vascularity.

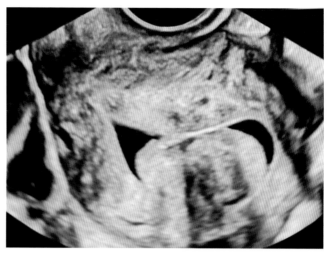

Fig. 2.35: B-mode ultrasound with sonohysterography showing a large solid sessile lesion protruding in the endometrial cavity possibly fibroid polyp.

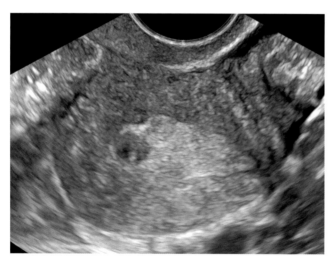

Fig. 2.34: Subendometrial fundal fibroid on B-mode ultrasound image seen as a round hypoechoic lesion against hyperechoic secretory endometrium.

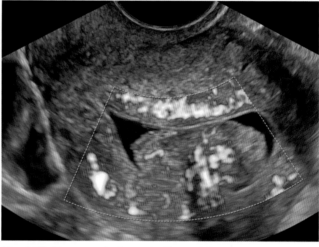

Fig. 2.36: The same lesion as in Figure 2.35 with power Doppler, showing the feeder extending through myometrium.

correctly diagnose on imaging. A typical fibroid polyp on B-mode or on 3D sectional planes may show broad base and a continuity of the myometrial interface may be seen toward the polyp wall (Fig. 2.35). It has a heterogeneous echogenicity. Unlike fibroid, this lesion typically shows feeding pedicle but usually this pedicle has multiple vessels. Abundant branching may be seen and this may be mistaken for atypia in the lesion. Tracing these feeding vessels, these show continuity from the myometrial radial vessels rather than from the spiral vessels, that are feeders to endometrium (Fig. 2.36).

Endometrial Synechiae

These are typically avascular lesions of the endometrium. It is known that synechiae occur as a result of surgical insult or inflammation finally leading to fibrosis. Patients present with severe oligomenorrhea or amenorrhea. These appear as soft tissue strands across the endometrium on B-mode ultrasound, but are often not seen on ultrasound, instead only appear as a thin fundus. Their echogenicity may vary depending on the firmness, thickness, or calcifications of the synechiae. Sonohysterography may be a more helpful investigation in these cases (Fig. 2.37).

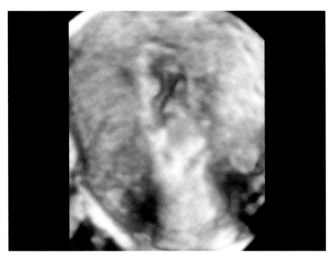

Fig. 2.37: 3D ultrasound image of the coronal image of the endometrium showing grossly contracted endometrial cavity due to synechiae.

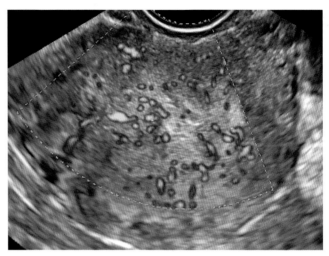

Fig. 2.39: Thick endometrium with heterogeneous echogenicity and irregular junctional zone with blood vessels of irregular caliber as seen on power Doppler suggest endometrial malignancy.

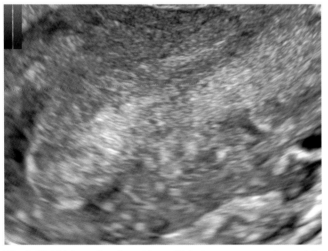

Fig. 2.38: Thickened endometrium with heterogeneous echogenicity on B-mode ultrasound may lead to suspicion of endometrial malignancy.

Endometrial Malignancies

Endometrial malignancy is the fourth most common malignancy in United States.[6] Its incidence in Asian countries and New Zealand is 1.5–2.5 times higher than that in European countries.[7] The increased rates of endometrial cancer may be related to obesity, failing fertility, and increased lifespan.[8] Endometrial malignancy may present with varied menstrual disturbances. Endometrial malignancy on ultrasound may have variable appearance depending on its stage. But still heterogeneous echogenicity is a consistent finding (Fig. 2.38). Depending on the extent, the disease there may be focal or diffuse thickening of the endometrium. Endometrial thickness of more than 15 mm in premenopausal women as mentioned in literature and more than 5 mm in a postmenopausal patient with bleeding disorders may be suspected of having endometrial malignancy. Endometrial thickness of less than 4 mm has a 100% NPV for endometrial cancer.[9] Interestingly, the endometrial echogenicity varies according to the stage and grade of the disease. Stage 1A cancers are hyperechoic or isoechoic, whereas Stage 1B and above are having mixed echogenicity or are hypoechoic. Well- or moderately differentiated (grade 1–2) tumors are hyperechoic, compared to grade 3 and more widespread lesions that are hypoechoic or heterogeneous.[10] Though irregular endometrial surface is another diagnostic criteria for the diagnosis of endometrial malignancy (Fig. 2.39), and this can be best appreciated by sonohysterography. But if malignancy is suspected either clinically or on ultrasound, sonohysterography is not preferred for the risk of its peritoneal spread and seeding.[11] At times, fluid may be seen in the endometrial cavity. When the endometrial malignancy grows beyond the endometrial margins, it leads to irregularity of the subendometrial halo. Irregular endometrial margin has a positive likelihood of 10 for endometrial malignancy.[12]

On Doppler, it typically shows heterogeneously distributed dense vascularity with low-resistance flow is seen in the premenopausal women with endometrial malignancy but in early endometrial carcinoma in perimenopausal women moderate-intratumoral resistance may be seen (Fig. 2.40A). The vascular pattern is of multifocal origin, dispersed vessels or single vessel with abundant

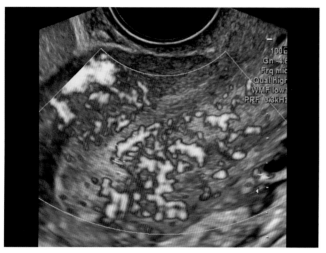

Fig. 2.40A: Heterogeneously distributed dense vascularity with irregular vascular caliber in a heterogeneously thickened endometrium—endometrial malignancy.

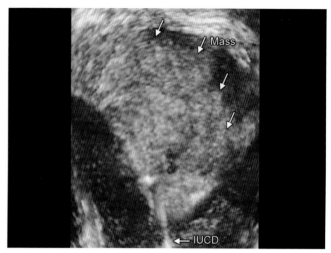

Fig. 2.41A: 3D ultrasound image of the uterus in coronal plane with hyperechogenicity extending into the myometrium, totally obliterating the junctional zone, and has irregular margins—endometrial malignancy with myometrial extension. (IUCD: Intrauterine contraceptive device)

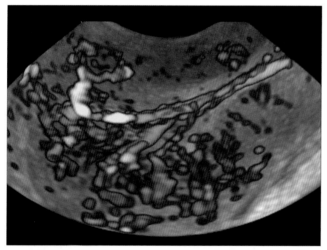

Fig. 2.40B: 3D power Doppler showing single vessel with abundant vascular branching in heterogeneously thickened endometrium—endometrial malignancy.

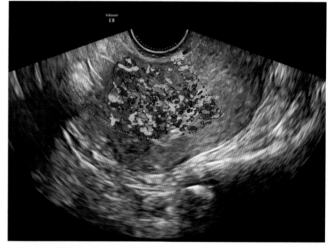

Fig. 2.41B: In the same lesion on sagittal plane, the tumoral vascular pattern is seen penetrating into the myometrium.

branching (Fig. 2.40B). In patients with endometrial malignancy, the uterine artery resistance is also low with uterine artery PI less than 1.45 and radial artery PI less than 1.06.[13] Typically the malignant neoangiogenesis shows chaotic vascular branching pattern with microaneurysms, arteriovenous shunts, elongation, and coiling (Fig. 2.40B). These are appreciated best on the 3D power Doppler (PD) angiography.

Combining morphological and 3D PD criteria sensitivity for endometrial carcinoma is 91.67%.[14] 3D ultrasound also plays an important role in diagnosing the extension of the endometrial carcinoma into myometrium (Fig. 2.41A). 3D

ultrasound can calculate the tumor volume accurately and increasing volume of the endometrium suggests higher grade of endometrial carcinoma and also myometrial invasion.[15] Volume larger than 25 mL has a high chance of pelvic node involvement at surgery. 3D hysterosonography with transverse plane picture may also show bladder or rectal infiltration. 3D PD is efficient for diagnosis of deep invasion with sensitivity 100%, specificity 94.44%, PPV 83.33%, and NPV 100%. The tumoral vascular pattern is seen penetrating into the myometrium (Fig. 2.41B). Higher stages of tumor shows lower resistance index, higher velocity, and higher microvessel density (VI).[16]

CONCLUSION

Transvaginal ultrasound is the modality of choice for assessment of the endometrium and diagnosis of endometrial pathologies. Doppler is an essential addition for the differential diagnosis of these pathologies. 3D plays an important role for demonstration of endometrial lesions. 3D PD especially is of importance for diagnosis, assessing the extent and follow-up of malignant lesions.

REFERENCES

1. Tsuda H, Kawabata M, Kawabata K, et al. Comparison between transabdominal and transvaginal ultrasonography for identifying endometrial malignancies. Gynecol Obstet Invest. 1995;40(4):271-3.
2. Leone FPG, Timmerman D, Bourne T, et al. Terms definitions and measurements to describe the sonographic features of the endometrium and intrauterine lesions: a consensus opinion from the International Endometrial Tumour Analysis (IETA) group. Ultrasound Obstet Gynecol. 2010;35:103-12.
3. Kurjak A, Kupesic S. Transvaginal colour Doppler and pelvic tumour vascularity: Lessons learned and future challenges. Ultrasound Obstet Gynecol. 1995;6:1-15.
4. Richman TS, Viscomi GN, Cherney AD, et al. Fallopian tubal patency assessment by ultrasound following fluid injection. Radiology. 1984;152:507-10.
5. Timmerman D, Verguts J, Konstantinovic ML, et al. The pedicle artery sign based on sonography with colour Doppler imaging can replace second-stage tests in women with abnormal vaginal bleeding. Ultrasound Obstet Gynecol. 2003;22(2):166-71.
6. Duong LM, Wilson RJ, Ajani UA, et al. Trends in endometrial cancer incidence rates in United States. 1999-2006. J Womens Health. 2011;20(8):1157-63.
7. Blakely T, Shaw C, Atkinson J, et al. Social inequalities or inequalities in cancer incidence? Repeated consensus-cancer cohort studies, New Zealand 1981-1986 to 2001-2004. Cancer Causes Control. 2011;22(9):1307-18.
8. Lambe M, Wigertz A, Garmo H, et al. Impaired glucose metabolism and diabetes and the risk of breast, endometrial and ovarian cancer. Cancer Causes Control. 2011;22(8):1163-71.
9. Karlsson B, Granberg S, Wikland M, et al. Transvaginal ultrasonography of the endometrium in women with postmenopausal bleeding—a Nordic multicenter study. Am J Obstet Gynecol. 1995;172(5):1488-94.
10. Epstein E, Van Holsbeke C, Mascilini F, et al. Gray-Scale and colour Doppler ultrasound characteristics of endometrial cancer in relation to stage, grade and tumour size. Ultrasound Obstet Gynecol. 2011;38(5):586-93.
11. Amant F, Moerman P, Neven P, et al. Endometrial cancer. Lancet. 2005;366(9484):491-505.
12. Epstein E, Valentine L. Gray-scale ultrasound morphology in presence or absence of intrauterine fluid and vascularity as assessed by colour Doppler for discrimination between benign and malignant endometrium in women with postmenopausal bleeding. Ultrasound Obstet Gynecol. 2006;28(1):89-95.
13. Bezircioglu I, Baloglu A, Cetinkaya B, et al. The diagnostic value of Doppler ultrasonography in distinguishing the endometrial malignancies in women with postmenopausal bleeding. Arch Gynecol Obstet. 2012;285(5):1369-74.
14. Kurjak A, Kupesic S. Three dimensional ultrasound and power Doppler in assessment of uterine and ovarian angiogenesis: a prospective study. Croatian Medical J. 1999;40(3):51-8.
15. Alcazar JL, Jurado M. Three dimensional ultrasound for assessing women with gynecological cancer: a systematic review. Gynecol Oncol. 2011;20(3):340-6.
16. Kupesic S, Kurjak A, Zodan T. Staging of endometrial carcinoma by 3D power Doppler. Gynecol Perinatol. 1999;8(1):1-5.

Doppler in Myometrial Lesions

INTRODUCTION

Uterus, a central landmark organ in the pelvis, is also a pivotal organ of female reproductive system. Myometrium—the muscle layer of the uterus forms the major bulk of the uterus mass. It protects the endometrial cavity and is surrounded by the serosa. It defines the margins of uterus and therefore its integrity confirms that the uterus is normal. Any mass lesion in the uterus changes the contour of the uterus and therefore the smooth pear shape is distorted.

The innermost layer of the myometrium is known as endometrial–myometrial junctional zone (JZ). This layer is structurally and functionally different from the rest of the myometrium. Myometrium is normally homogeneously hypoechoic and serosal surface is smooth and regular. Distortion of the shape or change in echogenicity suggests myometrial lesion.

SCAN ROUTES AND MODALITIES

Myometrial evaluation on ultrasound (US) can be done by transabdominal route or transvaginal route. Actually both are supplementary to each other. Transabdominal scan is of use to define the extent and margins of the myometrium. It is especially required in cases with large uterus or in cases in which due to space-occupying lesions like fibroid, the uterus is pushed upwards and its superior margin cannot be accessed by transvaginal scan. Whereas, the detailed morphology of the myometrium can be better studied by transvaginal scan due to proximity of probe to the uterus and better resolution due to high-frequency probe. Uterus is evaluated in sagittal and transverse planes on B-mode US. Coronal plane of the uterus may be best evaluated by 3D US. For assessment of the vascular changes, Doppler is

the modality of choice. Uterus is evaluated in a systematic manner on transvaginal scan.

METHOD OF ASSESSMENT OF THE UTERUS

Patient is first asked to empty the bladder and is placed in lithotomy position on the gynecological couch in the same way as for per speculum or per vaginal examination. US jelly is put on the head of the transvaginal probe and then the probe is covered with the condom, not to allow any air between the probe and the condom. A small amount of jelly is then placed over the condom on the probe head and the probe is gently slided into the patient's vagina. In case of difficulty in introduction or patient's resistance to introduction of the probe, she is advised to take deep long breaths with open mouth, i.e. deep inspirations and long complete expirations. Counseling the patient before examination and explaining the whole procedure and adequate privacy helps to eliminate the anxiety and resistance. Probe is introduced in the longitudinal position, with indicator on the probe facing the patient's anterior aspect (Fig. 3.1).

The indicator on the probe matches the logo on the screen. This means that if the indicator on the screen is on the left side of the screen, the structures anteriorly placed are on the left side of the screen (Fig. 3.2). Now, this longitudinal axis of the patient normally corresponds to the long axis of the uterus. That means the uterus must be seen in the sagittal plane on this view. It may be anteverted or retroverted. When anteverted, the uterine fundus will be directed toward the indicator on the screen and urinary bladder will also be seen on the same side of the screen, and when retroverted, fundus will be on the opposite side of the indicator and the urinary bladder (Figs. 3A and B).

If the uterus is not seen in this view, it means that the uterus is deviated towards one side. When it is deviated, it would indicate that either it is pulled on the side of the pathology like adhesions or is pushed away by the pathology, which is on the opposite side, say a mass.

Once the midsagittal plane of the uterus is seen, span the probe from one side to another, without rotating it, for the anatomical survey of the uterus in longitudinal axis. The spanning should extend from one side of the uterus across the midsagittal plane to the other side, till the uterus goes out of vision on either side. Then the probe is realigned in the midsagittal plane of the uterus and then rotate the probe 90° anticlockwise. This maneuver will give transverse view of the uterus with the right side of the patient on right side of the screen (Fig. 3.4). In this transverse position also, the whole uterus is evaluated from the fundus to the cervix by moving the probe up and down (anteriorly and posteriorly) in the vagina. This survey should give a complete idea about the anatomy of the uterus and the exact location of any fibroids, etc. Any localized lesion if seen in the uterus, its location in all three planes (sagittal, axial, and coronal) must be confirmed. This understanding of the orientation of the image and the uterus and the probe movement is essential to correctly diagnose the location of the lesions in the myometrium.

Myometrial lesions like fibroids and adenomyosis are among the most common uterine pathologies and still these are the ones that bring most surprises on surgery as

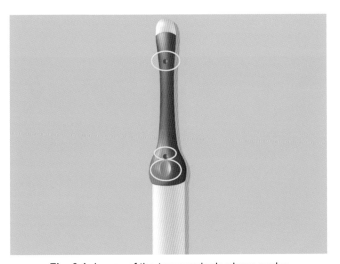

Fig. 3.1: Image of the transvaginal volume probe sowing the markers.

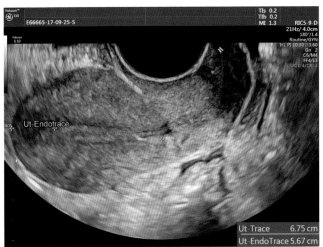

Fig. 3.3A: Midsagittal section of the uterus showing anteverted anteflexed uterus.

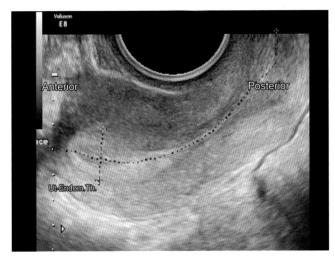

Fig. 3.2: Midsagittal section of the uterus on B-mode on transvaginal scan indicating anterior and posterior aspect of the patient.

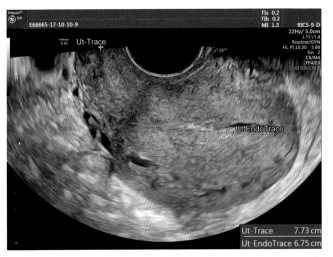

Fig. 3.3B: Midsagittal section of the uterus showing retroverted retroflexed uterus.

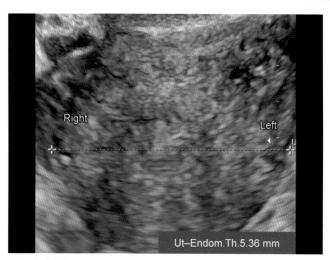

Fig. 3.4: Transverse section of the uterus with right and left side of the patient marked on the image.

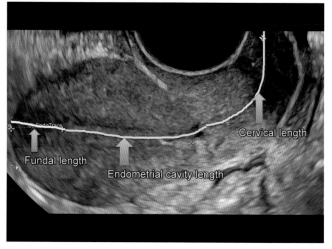

Fig. 3.5: Longitudinal measurements of the uterus on midsagittal section of the uterus, measured according to morphological uterus sonographic assessment (MUSA).

these are most inaccurately reported. The inaccuracy is because of random terms used for the description of US image and nonspecific terms used for localization. It is for this that a consensus was formed to describe the myometrial appearance or lesions and was termed as morphological uterus sonographic assessment (MUSA).

Morphological Uterus Sonographic Assessment[1]

It accurately describes the measurement techniques, specifies on the terms used for various US pictures, clearly defines the reporting formats, and also helps to identify reliable characters of benignity.

Measurements

The length of the uterus is measured as length of the three different segments. *Fundal length* is the distance from the fundal serosa to the fundal end of the endometrial cavity, in the line that is in continuity with the endometrial cavity. The second segment is the *length of the endometrial cavity* measured as a trace from fundal tip of the endometrium to the internal os. The third segment is the *cervical length*, length from the internal os to external os, measured as a trace (Fig. 3.5).

The *anteroposterior (AP) diameter* is measured in this same midsagittal plane as the longest diameter on the uterus body, perpendicular to the endometrial cavity (Fig. 3.6). The probe is then rotated for the transverse section (90° anticlockwise) to achieve the transverse section of the uterus. The broadest distance on this section, side-to-side is the *transverse diameter* (Fig. 3.7). The uterine volume is calculated as total length ×

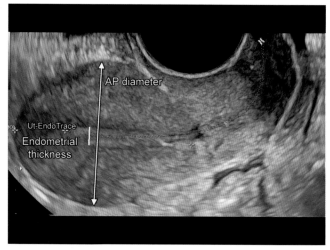

Fig. 3.6: Anteroposterior (AP) diameter and endometrial thickness of the uterus on midsagittal section of the uterus, measured according to morphological uterus sonographic assessment (MUSA).

width × AP diameter × 0.523. The thickness of the *anterior and posterior myometrial walls* may be measured separately in cases where these appear unequal or asymmetrical. This is measured as the longest distance from outer margin of endometrium to the serosa, perpendicular to the central line of the endometrium, both anteriorly and posteriorly (Fig. 3.8). The *endometrial thickness* is also measured on this same plane, at the level where the endometrium is thickest and measured from outer margin of the endometrium to outer margin of the endometrium (anterior and posterior), perpendicular to the central line of the endometrium (Fig. 3.6). *JZ thickness* is the measurement of the thickness of the hypoechoic zone in the most proximity of the outer hyperechoic margin of the

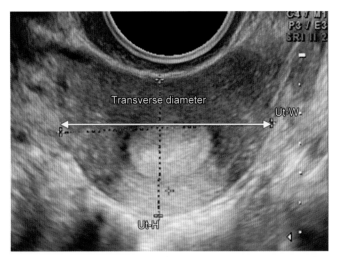

Fig. 3.7: Transverse diameter of the uterus on transverse section of the uterus, measured according to morphological uterus sonographic assessment (MUSA).

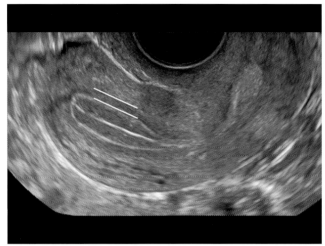

Fig. 3.9: Junctional zone measurement of the uterus on midsagittal section of the uterus, measured according to morphological uterus sonographic assessment (MUSA).

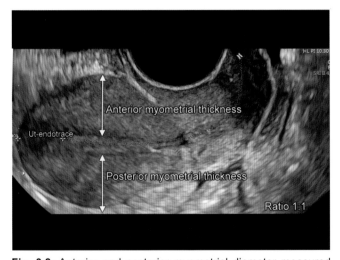

Fig. 3.8: Anterior and posterior myometrial diameter measured on midsagittal section of the uterus, measured according to morphological uterus sonographic assessment (MUSA).

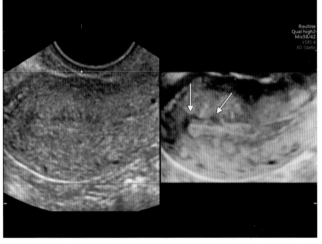

Fig. 3.10: B-mode and volume contrast imaging in the A plane (VCI-A) of the midsagittal section of the uterus, demonstrating clear delineation of the junctional zone on VCI-A.

endometrium, perpendicular to the endometrial outer margin and, if regular, it is measured as shown in the Figure 3.9. JZ is best assessed on 3D US with VCI (volume contrast imaging) (Fig. 3.10). If it is irregular, the maximum and the minimum thickness of the JZ are measured and are also important to mention the location and extent of the irregularity.

Description: Terminology used According to MUSA

Junctional zone qualitatively is described as regular, irregular (Fig. 3.11), interrupted (Fig. 3.12), or inaccessible (Fig. 3.13). The interruption of the JZ may be because of

cystic areas, hyperechogenic-dots, buds, or hyperechoic lines (Figs. 3.14A and B). JZ may be interrupted due to focal lesions/contractions. When the entire JZ cannot be identified, it is nonaccessible. But it may also be mentioned as inaccessible when it may not be clearly seen due to poor visibility, in obese patients or when uterus is deep.

If it is irregular, its thickness is measured at the thickest area of the JZ (Fig. 3.15). When JZ is interrupted or irregular, severity of irregularity is documented as a ratio of thickness of the thickest part of the JZ and thickness of the entire myometrium measured at the same level, in the same image, and in the same plane (Fig. 3.16). Magnitude of a JZ irregularity is expressed as the difference between the

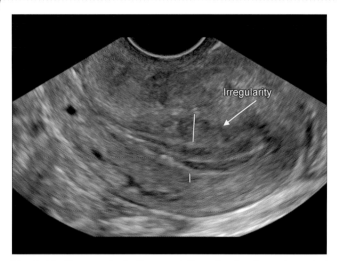

Fig. 3.11: Transvaginal ultrasound B-mode showing retroverted retroflexed uterus, midsagittal section of the uterus with irregular endometrial–myometrial junction on the posterior aspect.

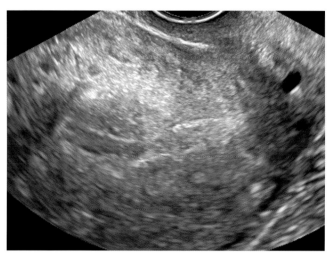

Fig. 3.13: Transvaginal ultrasound B-mode showing anteverted anteflexed uterus, midsagittal section of the uterus with inaccessible endometrial-myometrial junction on the anterior aspect.

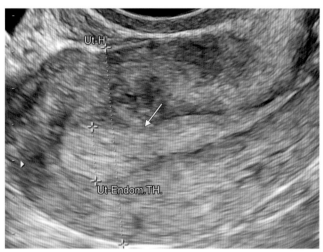

Fig. 3.12: Transvaginal ultrasound B-mode showing anteverted anteflexed uterus, midsagittal section of the uterus with interrupted endometrial–myometrial junction on the anterior aspect.

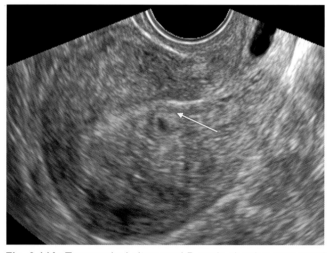

Fig. 3.14A: Transvaginal ultrasound B-mode showing anteverted anteflexed uterus with interruption of the junctional zone because of cystic areas.

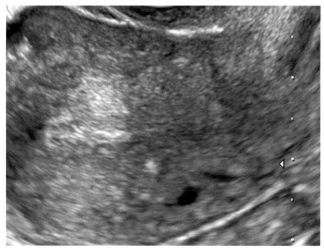

Fig. 3.14B: Transvaginal ultrasound B-mode showing anteverted anteflexed uterus with interruption of the junctional zone because of hyperechoic islands.

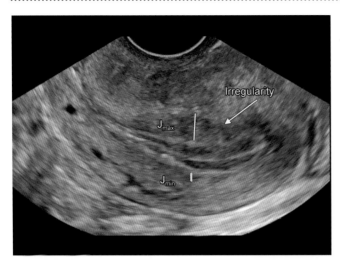

Fig. 3.15: Transvaginal ultrasound B-mode showing retroverted retroflexed uterus with irregularity of the junctional zone. The white line shows maximum thickness and yellow line shows minimum thickness of the junctional zone.

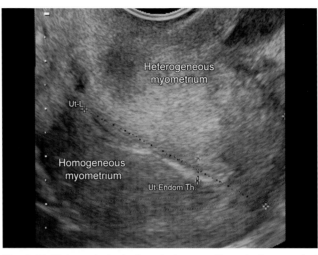

Fig. 3.17: Retroverted retroflexed uterus on B-mode, transvaginal ultrasound showing heterogeneous and thick posterior myometrium and homogeneous normal anterior myometrium.

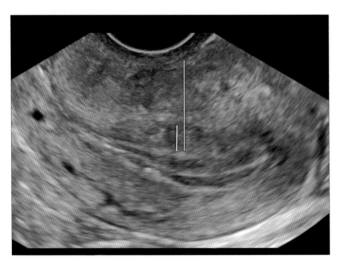

Fig. 3.16: Transvaginal ultrasound B-mode showing retroverted retroflexed uterus with irregularity of the junctional zone. The white line shows maximum thickness of the junctional zone and yellow line shows thickness of the posterior myometrium.

maximum and minimum JZ thickness: $(JZ_{dif}) = JZ_{max} - JZ_{min}$ (Fig. 3.15).

It is essential to mention that the irregularity/interruption involves anterior wall, posterior wall, right lateral wall, left lateral walls, or fundus. Extent of the irregularity can be subjectively described as less than 50% or more than 50%, for the uterus as a whole or for each location.

MYOMETRIAL DESCRIPTION

Myometrium is described homogeneous or hetero-geneous in echotexture/echogenicity (Fig. 3.17 and

Flowchart 3.1: Description of myometrium.

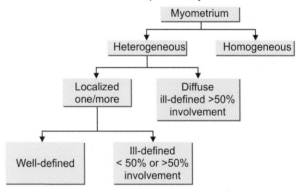

Flowchart 3.1). Heterogenicity may be due to cystic areas, hyperechogenicities, or shadowing (Figs. 3.18A and B). Heterogenicity may be localized (one/more areas) (Fig. 3.19A) or diffuse (Fig. 3.19B).

When the lesion is a localized one, it is essential to mention whether it is well-defined (Fig. 3.20) or ill-defined (Fig. 3.19A). Its location is described as anterior, posterior, fundal, right lateral, or left lateral and it involves upper, mid or lower body, or cervix. If the lesion is diffuse, it is described as a global heterogenicity/global involvement of the uterus by the lesion. The size of the lesion is measured as three orthogonal diameters. The longest diameter is measured in the longest plane, the AP diameter is the longest diameter perpendicular to this and the transverse diameter is measured as longest side-to-side diameter on a transverse plane that is achieved by only 90° rotation of the probe (Fig. 3.21). The

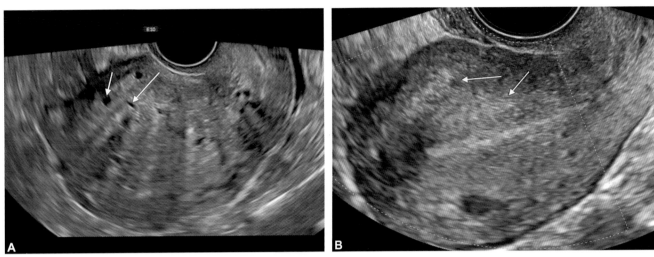

Figs. 3.18A and B: (A) B-mode ultrasound image of the uterus showing anechoic cystic areas of myometrial cysts marked by arrows; (B) Hyperechoic lines marked by arrows.

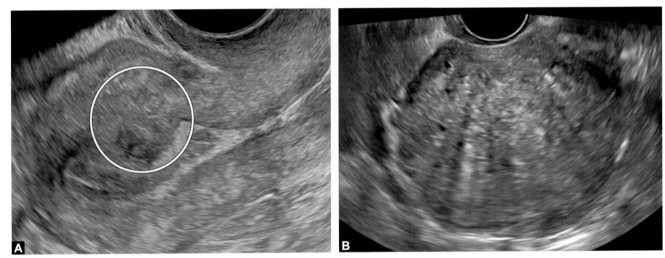

Figs. 3.19A and B: (A) Anteverted anteflexed uterus on B-mode on transvaginal scan with localized area of heterogeneous myometrium as marked by the circle, though the margins are ill-defined; and (B) Generalized heterogenicity of the myometrium.

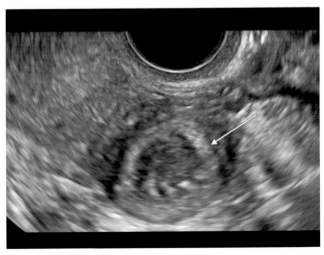

Fig. 3.20: A well-defined localized lesion is seen in the posterior wall of the uterus as marked by the arrow.

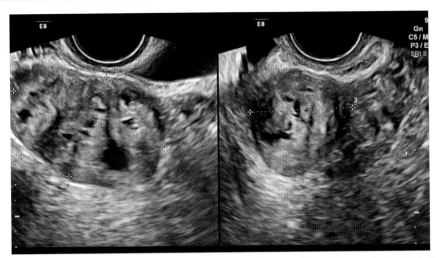

Fig. 3.21: Measurements of the localized myometrial lesion (fibroid), the long and the anteroposterior (AP) diameter measured on long section and transverse diameter on transverse section of the lesion.

site of the lesion is described as anterior, posterior, right or left lateral or fundal and then whether it is involving upper, middle, or lower part of the corpus or cervix is mentioned. Since myometrium is a thick layer of the uterus, most lesions will not involve its entire thickness. Therefore, it is essential to mention, how much thickness of the myometrium is affected by the lesion and also whether it is peripheral layer of the myometrium or central layer of the myometrium that is involved. These lesions are therefore classified according to PALM-COEIN classification.[2] For the exact localization of the lesion and also to get the guidance about the route of surgery, *minimum distance* of the lesion from endometrium (*inner lesion-free margin*) or minimum distance from serosa (outer lesion free margin) must also be mentioned (Fig. 3.22).

Description of the lesion includes its shape (round, oval, lobulated, irregular), rim/margins (ill-defined, hypoechoic, hyperechoic) and its echogenicity (homogeneous or heterogeneous). Most lesions in the myometrium cast an acoustic shadow and that must also be mentioned. These may be fan shaped (alternate hyper- and hypoechoic bands) (Fig. 3.23A) with or without edge shadows (Fig. 3.23B). Amount of shadowing is described as slight, moderate, or strong. The hyper-/hypoechogenicity of the lesion is described as follows:

- *Level of echogenicity*: It is compared to that of normal myometrium:
  - Very hypoechogenic (−−)
  - Hypoechogenic (−)
  - Isoechogenic
  - Hyperechogenic (+)
  - Very hypogenic (++)
  - Detailed description on the echogenicity is required.

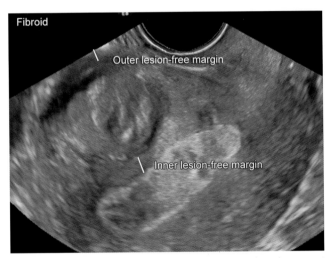

Fig. 3.22: Transvaginal ultrasound B-mode showing anteverted anteflexed uterus with anterior intramural fibroid showing outer and inner lesion-free margins.

When the lesion is diffuse, penetration of the diffuse lesions is described as a ratio between the maximum thickness of the lesion to the total uterine wall thickness and extent as more than or less than 50% of the total uterus body length. Anterior/posterior/lateral/fundal wall involvement is to be mentioned like localized lesion.

Myometrial Heterogenicities

Myometrial echogenicity is called to be heterogeneous either in presence of localized lesion or in presence of myometrial cysts (*see* Fig. 3.18A), hyperechoic islands (Fig. 3.24), hyperechogenic lines (*see* Fig. 3.18B)/dots. These are most often found in the adenomyosis, but may be seen

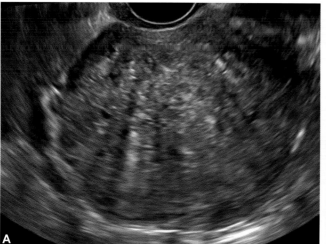 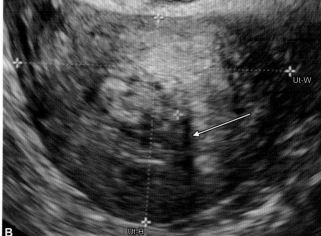

Figs. 3.23A and B: (A) Fan-shaped acoustic shadowing; and (B) Edge shadows as indicated by the arrow.

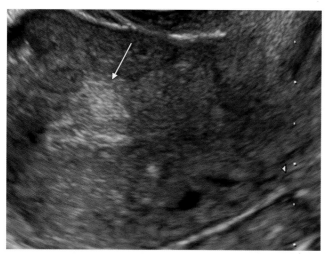

Fig. 3.24: Transvaginal ultrasound B-mode showing anteverted anteflexed uterus with hyperechoic localized area—hyperechoic island as marked by the arrow.

in certain chronic inflammations, postsurgical, vascular abnormalities, etc.

Myometrial Cysts

These are anechoic well-defined and mostly rounded lesions. The contents may be anechoic, may have low-level echogenicities, ground–glass echogenicities, or mixed echogenicities. One must mention number of cysts, locations, and largest diameters of the largest cyst. When these are distributed widely, walls that are involved and the upper, middle, or lower third of the body and whether it is involving more than/less than 50% of the myometrium. If multiple small cysts aggregate, it makes anechoic lacunae that may be irregular in shape.

Hyperechoic Islands

These are regular, irregular, or ill-defined hyperechoic areas. Same as for cysts, it is essential to mention the number of hyperechoic islands, size of the largest, and location of each. These are most commonly due to endometrial growth in the myometrium in patients with adenomyosis.

Hyperechoic Lines and Buds

Hyperechoic lines and buds are seen, leading to irregularity or interruption of the JZ. These hyperechoic lines and buds are different from hyperechoic spots. These lines and buds are in continuity with the endometrium and are perpendicular to endometrium or not, needs to be mentioned. These lines and buds affect anterior, posterior, right or left lateral or fundal JZ and what is the extent of the irregular or interrupted endometrium needs to be mentioned. If these are countable their number needs to be mentioned.

The vascularity study gives more information on these lesions, but it is very essential to evaluate the myometrium on B-mode and adequately analyze it before vascularity studies are done.

DOPPLER STUDIES

The distribution of the vascularity is described as uniform, if the entire lesion has uniformly distributed vascularity or nonuniform, if it shows heterogeneous distribution of blood vessels in the lesion (Figs. 3.25A and B). According to MUSA, the vascularity of the myometrial lesions can be scored as *Score:* 1—no color, 2—minimal vascularity, 3—moderate vascularity, and 4—abundant vascularity (Figs. 3.26A to D). Scoring is done, taking into consideration, the most vascular

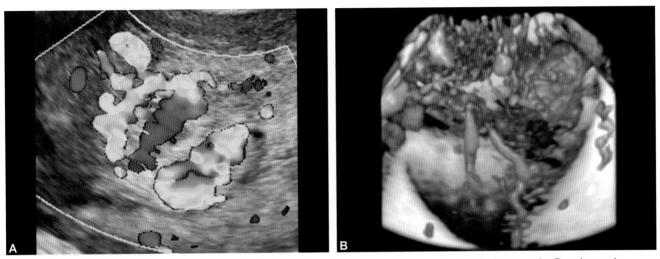

Figs. 3.25A and B: (A) Homogeneous distribution of the blood vessels in the myometrial lesion on color Doppler; and (B) Heterogeneous distribution of the blood vessels in the lesion on 3D power Doppler.

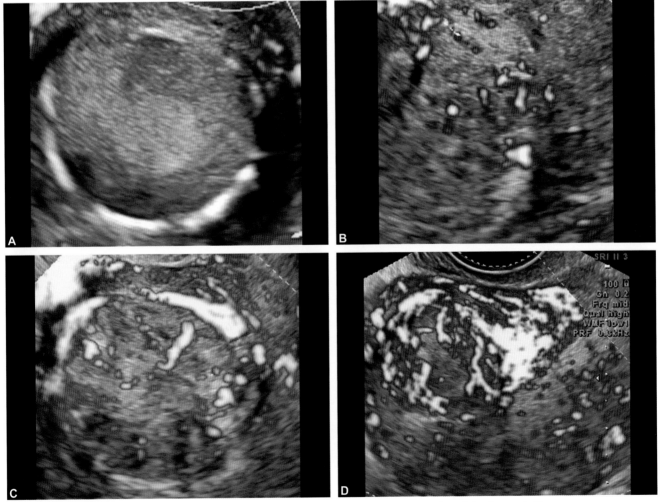

Figs. 3.26A to D: Vascular score of 1 to 4, as *Score*: 1—no color, 2—minimal vascularity, 3—moderate vascularity, and 4—abundant vascularity.

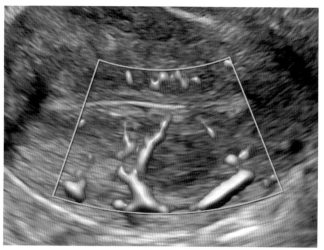

Fig. 3.27A: Circumferential vascularity in a fibroid as seen on high-definition (HD) flow.

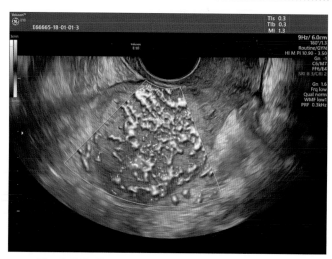

Fig. 3.27C: Translesional vascularity in adenomyosis as seen on high-definition (HD) flow.

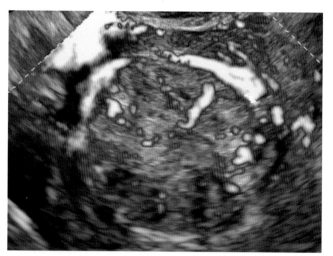

Fig. 3.27B: Circumferential and intralesional vascularity in a fibroid as seen on power Doppler.

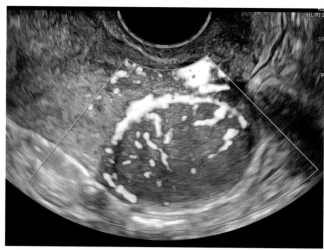

Fig. 3.28A: All vessels in the lesion showing almost equal diameter on high-definition (HD) flow.

area of a lesion. In lesions that show heterogeneous vascular distribution, do mention what percentage of the solid component is vascular. Commonly found myometrial lesions may show circumferential (Fig. 3.27A), intralesional, both (Fig. 3.27B) or translesional (Fig. 3.27C) vascularity. Circumferential is a peripheral vascularity of a lesion (like seen in a fibroid). The vessels that are seen in the lesion are intralesional vessels. Lesions, like degenerated fibroids, may show both circumferential and intralesional vascularity. Lesions like adenomyosis will show vessels traversing perpendicular to the uterine cavity/serosa crossing the lesion. These are described as translesional vessels.

Further description about the vessels that can be studied by Doppler is the number of vessels (single/multiple),

diameter of vessels as compared to normal myometrial vessels (large/small), whether all vessels in the lesion have an equal diameter (Fig. 3.28A) or they vary in diameter. It is essential to specifically mention whether the variability in diameter is seen in individual vessels also or is seen in different vessels. This may be reported as abnormal tortuous vessels, irregular caliber, when individual vessel shows variability in caliber (Fig. 3.28B).

The branching pattern of the vessels is especially different in benign and malignant lesions and so documenting the regular/irregular branching pattern is important. Branching pattern of vessels in malignant lesions are typically described as lack of hierarchy in branching, varying branching angles, chaotic vessel pattern, and this will be

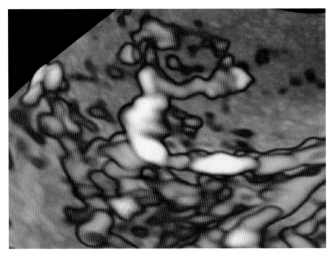

Fig. 3.28B: Abnormal tortuous vessels, irregular caliber, when individual vessel shows variability in caliber as seen on power Doppler.

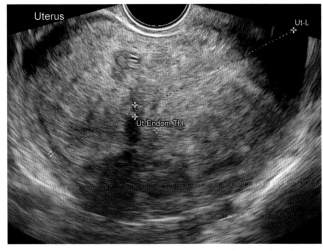

Fig. 3.29: Heterogeneous myometrial echogenicity of adenomyosis as seen on B-mode transvaginal ultrasound.

BOX 3.1: Reporting details of myometrial lesion.

The reporting should include:
- Size
- Symmetry of myometrial walls
- Echogenicity
- Junctional zone—regular, irregular, and ill-defined
- Extent and magnitude of irregularity
- *Lesion*: Well-defined/ill-defined, number, location, size, maximum diameter, echogenicity of the lesion (cysts, hyperechoic islands, buds, lines, spots, shadowing)
- *Mapping* of lesions
- *Vascularity*—pattern, score, branching pattern, number of vessels, diameter
- *If the lesion is present, is it relevant to the symptoms*

---

described in detail in chapter dedicated to gynecological malignancies (Box 3.1).

Keeping into consideration the descriptive terms discussed, let us now look into the US presentation of common myometrial lesions, with special consideration on their Doppler findings.

Myometrial lesions commonly seen are fibroids, adenomyosis, adenomyomas, and leiomyosarcomas. Fibroids and adenomyosis are among the most common pathologies found in patients presenting with various gynecological complaints and also with infertility.

Adenomyosis

Adenomyosis is an ectopic growth of endometrium into the myometrium, and is common in multiparous women. But it is seen in women with a history of any obstetric event

or any surgical procedure disturbing the endometrium. Pathologically, adenomyosis is defined as endometrial glands and stroma in the myometrium of half of one low-power field beneath the endomyometrial junction. Adenomyosis is often an incidental finding on US. But these patients may present with menorrhagia, metrorrhagia, pelvic pain, dysmenorrhea, and dyspareunia. Patients with adenomyosis often present with infertility and one of the major causes for this is inadequate endometrial receptivity. This may be due to physical compression effect due to thickened endometrium, but may also be due to inadequate development of estrogen receptors due to altered vascularity. Pathologies, like leiomyomas (6–28%), and endometrial hyperplasia may coexist with adenomyosis. On clinical examination, the uterus feels bulky and is tender on palpation.

On Ultrasound

Depending on the severity of the adenomyosis the uterus may or may not appear bulky. It may cause asymmetrical thickening of myometrium. Adenomyosis may be diffuse and focal.[3]

The affected myometrium shows a coarse heterogeneous echogenicity. Heterogeneous echogenicity has a sensitivity of 88% for diagnosis of adenomyosis[3] (Fig. 3.29).

Typically the myometrium shows alteration in the echogenicity depending on the phase of the menstrual cycle. Adenomyosis being an invasive lesion has indistinct margins.

The endometrial tissue that proliferates inside the myometrium tends to bleed on progesterone withdrawal during menstrual cycle. This gives the uterus a typically speckled appearance resembling "salt and pepper" (hyperechoic areas and hypoechoic areas)[4] (Fig. 3.30). Adenomyosis presents with alternate hyper- and hypoechoic zones, typically described as "rain in forest" or a "vanishing blind" appearance of the myometrium (Fig. 3.31). Anechoic irregular cystic spaces of 5–7 mm in diameter will disrupt the homogeneous echo pattern of the myometrium (Fig. 3.32). These are myometrial cysts. Myometrial cysts have 98% specificity and 78% accuracy for diagnosis of adenomyosis. The myometrial cysts typically have hyperechoic margins. This probably is the active endometrial tissue. These echogenic flecks seen at the endometrial–myometrial junction are thought to be collapsed myometrial cysts. Hyperechoic areas in myometrium may be due to fresh bleed or collapsed endometrial cavities. In some cases, hyperechoic spots or areas are also seen in the subendometrial myometrium and these may be islands of active endometrial tissue. These may be named as endometrial buds. Fan-shaped acoustic shadowing is typical of adenomyosis (Fig. 3.33).

Junctional zone is irregular or interrupted and in severe cases may also be inaccessible. High-resolution US now can show the endometrial strands extending into the myometrium, interrupting the JZ (Figs. 3.34A to C).

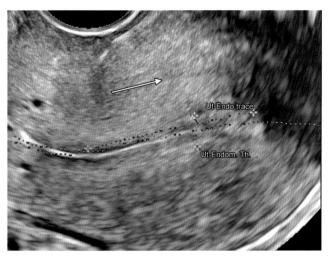

Fig. 3.30: "Salt and pepper" appearance of adenomyosis as seen on transvaginal B-mode ultrasound of the uterus, marked by arrow.

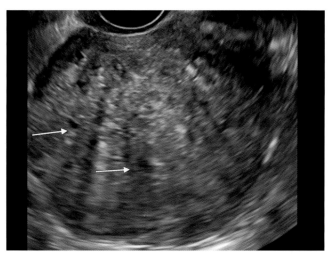

Fig. 3.32: Myometrial cysts (as marked by arrows) are seen in the heterogeneous adenomyotic myometrium.

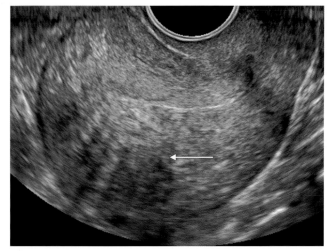

Fig. 3.31: "Rain in forest" or "vanishing blind" appearance of adenomyosis as seen on transvaginal B-mode ultrasound of the uterus, marked by arrow.

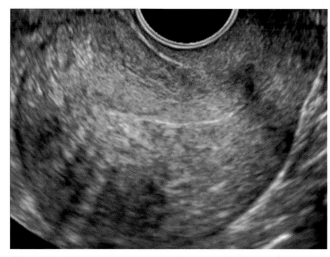

Fig. 3.33: "Fan-shaped acoustic shadowing" of adenomyosis as seen on transvaginal B-mode ultrasound of the uterus.

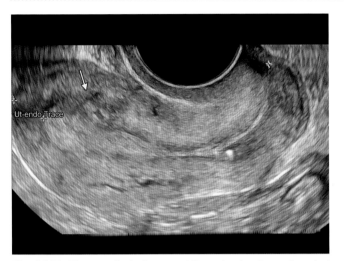

Fig. 3.34A: Transvaginal ultrasound B-mode showing anteverted anteflexed uterus, midsagittal section of the uterus with irregular endometrial–myometrial junction on the anterior aspect (arrow).

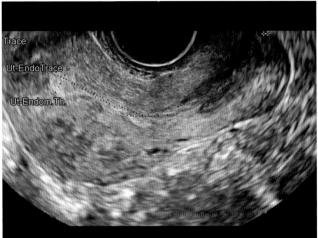

Fig. 3.34C: Transvaginal ultrasound B-mode showing anteverted anteflexed uterus, midsagittal section of the uterus with inaccessible endometrial–myometrial junction.

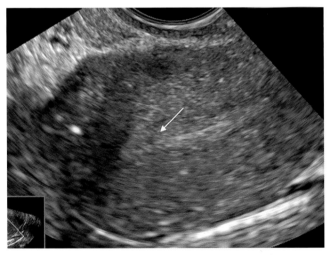

Fig. 3.34B: Transvaginal ultrasound B-mode showing anteverted anteflexed uterus, midsagittal section of the uterus with interrupted endometrial–myometrial junction on the anterior aspect due to endometrial strands extending into myometrium (arrow).

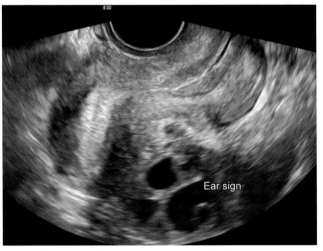

Fig. 3.35: Transvaginal ultrasound B-mode showing anteverted anteflexed uterus, midsagittal section of the uterus with question mark sign.

Adenomyotic uteri may commonly show an abnormal curvature of the fundal endometrial cavity, in a direction opposite to the normal direction of the fundus (Fig. 3.35). This is described as 'question mark sign' of the uterus.[5]

The more difficult situation is the adenomyoma. This is a localized adenomyosis, with heterogeneous echogenicity and less defined margins, and so is difficult to differentiate from degenerated fibroid as this also has heterogeneous echogenicity. But the main differentiating point between the adenomyoma and the fibroid is the capsular vascularity that is seen in the fibroid, is never seen in adenomyoma (Fig. 3.36). Like generalized adenomyosis, it alters its echogenicity with the phase of the cycle, which is never

the case in fibroid. Still one more important differentiating point is obliteration of the JZ in adenomyoma, unlike fibroid and absence of edge shadows. On US, adenomyoma can be diagnosed by the presence of an inhomogeneous circumscribed area in the myometrium with indistinct margins and intralesional vascularity with fan-shaped acoustic shadows (Box 3.2).

On Color Doppler

On color Doppler, affected myometrium shows markedly increased vascularity with vascular dilatation (Fig. 3.37). These vessels have resistance index (RI) of 0.56 ± 0.12. Diameter of these vessels is larger than those of normal myometrium.[6]

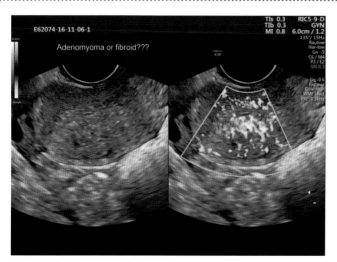

Fig. 3.36: Absence of circumferential vascularity and only intralesional vascularity in adenomyoma seen as a localized ill-defined lesion on B-mode.

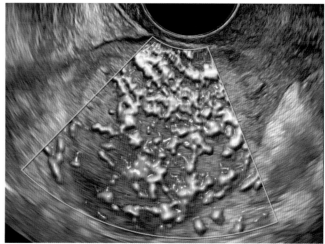

Fig. 3.37: High-definition (HD) flow showing translesional vascularity with nonparallel arrangement and increased diameter of the blood vessels (than the normal spiral vessels) in adenomyosis.

BOX 3.2: Ultrasound features of adenomyosis.

- Generalized/localized thickening of myometrial wall
- Asymmetrical thickening of anterior and posterior myometrial wall
- *Heterogeneous myometrium:* Salt and pepper appearance
- "Rain in forest" or "vanishing blind" appearance
- Fan-shaped acoustic shadowing
- Irregularity and interruption of endometrial-myometrial junctional zone
- Echogenic flecks, lines, and buds at junctional zone
- Myometrial cysts
- Endometrial strands penetrating into the myometrium
- Question mark sign
- Translesional vascularity
- Vessels with diameter larger than that of normal spiral vessels
- Abnormal orientation of myometrial vessels (chaotic arrangement)

Vascularity in adenomyosis is a penetrating type—translesional in distribution. Decreased uterine artery resistance and increased velocity is also noted.

Though *sonohysterography* is not a routine investigation for adenomyosis, if done by chance, it shows contrast (negative or positive), percolating into the myometrium.

Endometrial strands extending into myometrium are also seen on *3D US*. When seen on *3D power Doppler* also a vascular fibroid shows circumferentially arranged blood vessels, while in adenomyoma, the vascular arrangement is radial or penetrating (Figs. 38A and B). It is the JZ assessment that was not adequately possible with B-mode US always. That is why magnetic resonance imaging (MRI) was considered as an imaging modality for adenomyosis. Difference in the JZ thickness at two different places around the endometrium of more than 4 mm or a JZ thickness of 12 mm has 88% sensitivity and 85% accuracy for the diagnosis of adenomyosis.[7]

Three-dimensional transvaginal sonographic (TVS) markers:[7,8] JZ difference more than 4 mm and JZ infiltration and distortion have been proved as highly sensitive markers for the diagnosis of adenomyosis (Fig. 3.39).

Elastography

Elastography is a modality of US that measures tissue strain. This is useful for differentiating myometrial lesions, though it is more commonly used for differentiating benign from malignant lesions in breast, liver, and other organs. Elastography may be qualitative or quantitative. Qualitative elastography subjectively compares the stiffness/firmness of various tissues; whereas, quantitative elastography may measure the firmness objectively.

The tissues with different firmness are seen in different colors of the light spectrum. Blue side of this spectrum demonstrates hard or firm tissues and red side of the spectrum demonstrates soft tissues. For example, bowel appears red or yellow and myometrium shows uniform blue color. Fibroids are firmer (blue) than the myometrium and adenomyosis is softer (green). Elastography-based diagnosis is in excellent agreement with MRI[9] (Fig. 3.40).

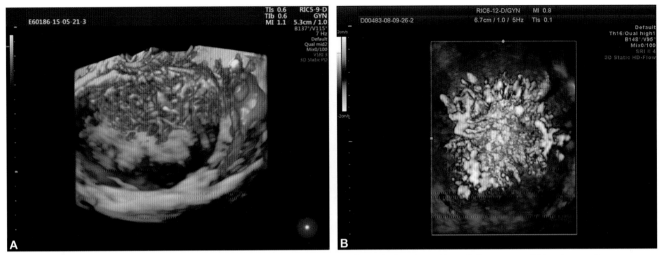

Figs. 3.38A and B: (A) 3D power Doppler showing vascular fibroid with circumferentially arranged blood vessels; (B) Adenomyoma showing penetrating vascular pattern.

Fibroids

Fibroids are found in 20–40% of women of more than 30 years of age and are more common in nulliparous. These are mostly an incidental finding, but may sometimes present with dysmenorrhea, menorrhagia, infertility, and pregnancy-related problems.

Fibroids affect fertility because of:
- Distortion of endometrial cavity due to submucous fibroid.
- Pressure of the fibroid and stretching of endometrium overlying it causing atrophy of endometrial glands and stroma due to submucous or large intramural fibroids.

Buttram et al. have shown in their study that fertility is chiefly affected by submucous fibroids due to altered uterine contractility, deranged cytokine profile, abnormal vascularization, and chronic endometrial inflammation.[10,11] These are benign tumors of myometrial and fibrous tissue origin, arising from the smooth muscle of uterine fundus and corpus. Fibroids are known to have a genetic basis and also have been shown to have a familial distribution or a hereditary transmission. Loss of tumor suppressor genes may be one of the causes. Estrogen and progesterone appear to promote the growth of fibroids as these have more estrogen and progesterone receptors as compared to normal myometrial tissue. Insulin-like growth factor may also affect the growth of the fibroid.

Fibroids may be seen in a variety of locations in the uterus. Depending on their location in relation to myometrium, endometrium or serosa, these are classified

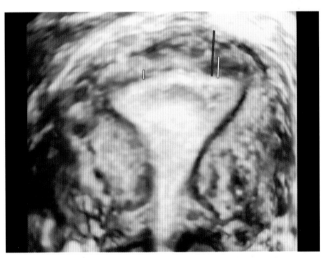

Fig. 3.39: Irregularity of the junctional zone in adenomyosis as seen on 3D ultrasound with the white line showing J_{max} and yellow line showing J_{min}. Red line indicates myometrial thickness.

as subendometrial and subserosal and intramural fibroids.
Subserosal and intramural fibroids were further classified as:
- *Type 0*: Pedunculated subserosal fibroid
- *Type 1*: Involvement of less than 50% of the outer uterine wall
- *Type 2*: More than 50% of the myometrial wall
- *Type 3*: Fibroids extending from mucosa to serosa.

Submucosal fibroids were further classified as:[12]
- Type 0, if they are pedunculated and 100% in the cavity (Fig. 3.41A)
- Type 1, if the fibroid is more than 50% in endometrial cavity (Fig. 3.41B)

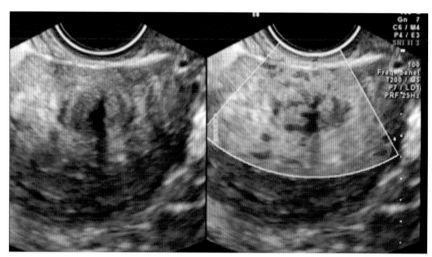

Fig. 3.40: Elastography showing blue-colored fibroid indicating its firm consistency.

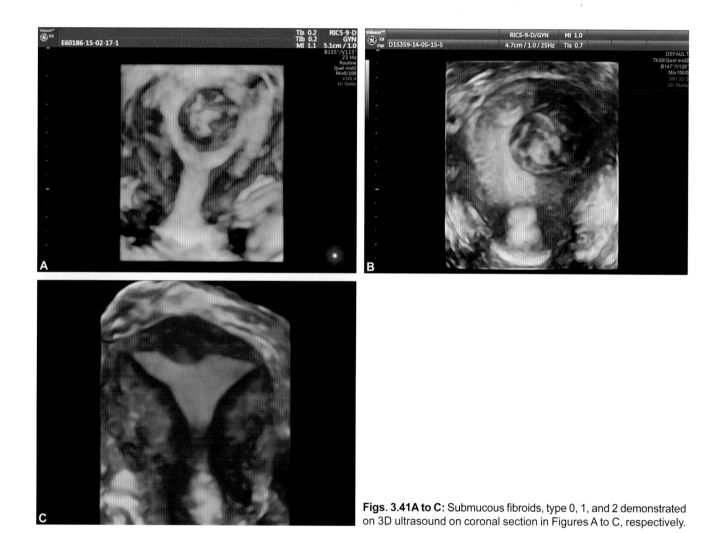

Figs. 3.41A to C: Submucous fibroids, type 0, 1, and 2 demonstrated on 3D ultrasound on coronal section in Figures A to C, respectively.

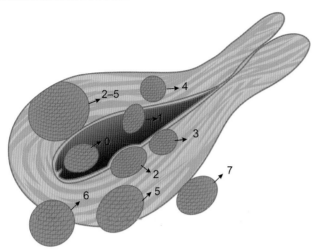

Fig. 3.42: Diagrammatic demonstration of types of fibroid according to FIGO (International Federation of Gynecology and Obstetrics) classification.

TABLE 3.1: Types of fibroid according to FIGO (International Federation of Gynecology and Obstetrics) classification.		
SM–Submucosal	0	Pedunculated intracavitary
	1	<50% intramural
	2	≥50% intramural
O–Other	3	Contacts endometrium; 100% intramural
	4	Intramural
	5	Subserosal ≥50% intramural
	6	Subserosal <50% intramural
	7	Subserosal pedunculated
	8	Other (specify, e.g. cervical, parasitic
Hybrid leiomyomas (impact both endometrium and serosa)	Two numbers are listed separated by a hyphen. By convention, the first refers to the relationship with the endometrium while the second refers to the relationship to the serosa. One example is below:	
	2–5	Submucosal and subserosal, each with less than half the diameter in the endometrial and peritoneal cavities, respectively.

- Type 2, if less than 50% is protruding in the endometrial cavity (Fig. 3.41C).

According to the new FIGO (International Federation of Gynecology and Obstetrics) classification, fibroids are classified into eight types[2] (Fig. 3.42 and Table 3.1).

On Ultrasound

On US, fibroid appears as a well-defined, hypoechoic, homogeneous, round/oval, solid lesions, with peripheral

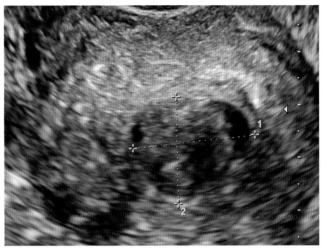

Fig. 3.43: Round well-defined isoechoic lesion is seen in the myometrium with hypoechoic margins—fibroid on B-mode transvaginal ultrasound.

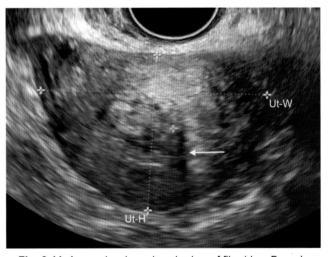

Fig. 3.44: Arrow showing edge shadow of fibroid on B-mode transvaginal ultrasound.

hypoechoic rim due to displacement of myometrial fibers (Fig. 3.43). When large and especially subserosal or intramural, these distort the serosal surface, whereas when subendometrial, these distort the endometrial cavity. Fibroids typically show edge shadows along with the linear stripes like fan-shaped acoustic shadowing (Fig. 3.44). Echogenicity increases with increasing amount of fibrous tissue and vascularity.

Degeneration in fibroids leads to heterogenicity of texture and may become hyperechoic (Fig. 3.45). Cystic degeneration leads to anechoic spaces in the fibroid (Fig. 3.46). Red degeneration is the most common form of degeneration in fibroids with pregnancy. Though red degeneration is not easily diagnosed on US. When the

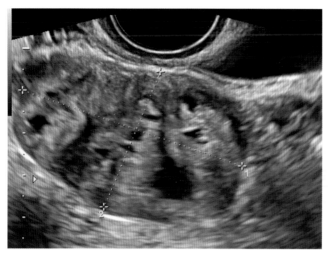

Fig. 3.45: Degenerated fibroid showing heterogeneous echogenicity.

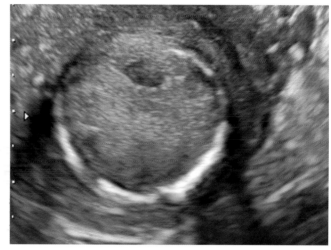

Fig. 3.47: B-mode transvaginal ultrasound showing fibroid with a calcified rim.

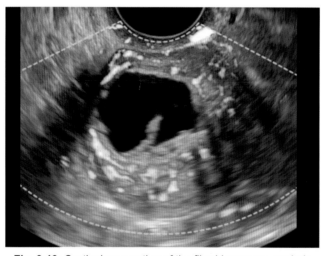

Fig. 3.46: Cystic degeneration of the fibroid seen as anechoic center with high-definition (HD) flow showing circumferential flow.

BOX 3.3: Fibroid mapping.

The correct location of the fibroid can be defined by:
- Its position in the uterus—involving upper, middle, or lower part of the body of the uterus or the cervix
- Involving anterior, posterior, or right/left lateral walls
- Its position/penetration according to the FIGO classification
- Its size—preferably three orthogonal diameters
- Its distance from the endometrium or from the serosa to which ever wall it is closer.

(FIGO: International Federation of Gynecology and Obstetrics)

BOX 3.4: Reporting of the fibroids.

Fibroids reporting should include:
- Homogeneous/heterogeneous
- Well-defined
- Number
- Location, size, site, penetration
- Mapping
- Vascularity—circumferential, equal diameter, homogeneous/heterogeneous distribution
- Red, hyaline, cystic/myxoid, or hydropic degeneration
- It is important to have a standard report format for any scan that first describes the ultrasound features of a lesion/organ and then derives the diagnosis

---

fibroid undergoes an acute degeneration, patient may present with marked pain, sometimes vomiting and fever and the fibroid shows increase in size. Calcification may be seen in fibroids as hyperechoic (++) areas with posterior shadowing (Fig. 3.47). When uterine artery embolization is done for fibroids, air may be seen in the fibroids as hyperechoic areas with comet shadows.

Correct localization of the fibroid on imaging is essential for better planning of the surgery (Box 3.3). That is why fibroid mapping is an essential part of reporting a fibroid (Box 3.4). This is especially important when there are multiple fibroids. Mapping can be correctly done by survey of the uterus in longitudinal and transverse axis by sweeping across the entire uterus in sagittal and transverse planes on B-mode and also by the use of 3D for assessing the correct location on the coronal plane. The mapping report of the fibroids consists of clear documentation of location of the fibroid (which wall), topography (upper, middle or lower third), size, FIGO type, echogenicity, inner and outer free margin and vascularity of the fibroid along with hand drawn diagram of sagittal, transverse and coronal plane of the uterus showing fibroid location and size of each fibroid. In cases with multiple fibroids, when the endometrium is also grossly distorted, establishing the correct location of these fibroids may be difficult and then the endometrial line may be traced from the cervical canal to cephalad.

On Doppler

Peripheral vascularity is typical of a fibroid (*see* Fig. 3.27A). These vessels are vessels of displaced muscle fibers and therefore show a RI of 0.54 ± 0.08,[13] similar to that of normal myometrial vessels. Resistance is higher in submucosal fibroids and deep intramural fibroids compared to subserosal fibroids but lower compared to submucosal fibroids. This variability is because of the compression effect of the muscle fibers on the fibroid and therefore on the surrounding vessels. Fibroids with degeneration show intralesional vascularity with low-resistance flow and a vascular score of 2–3 (*see* Fig. 3.27B). In addition to the peripheral vascularity, amount of vascularity decides the activity or growth potential of a fibroid. Malignant change leading to leiomyosarcoma shows a resistance as low as 0.37 ± 0.03 RI, with rapid growth in size and disruption of well-defined margins (Fig. 3.48). But resistance indices of vessels cannot be used as only evidence for malignant change, because it is equally low in degenerating fibroid also. In fact even on B-mode US due to the heterogenicity

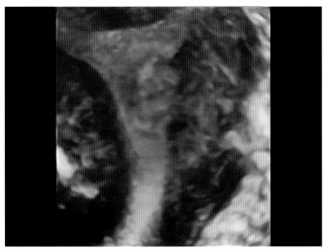

Fig. 3.48: 3D ultrasound of the uterus showing coronal section of the uterus, with a submucous fibroid showing ill-defined margin on its myometrial surface.

being a common finding in degenerating as well as malignant fibroid, it is not possible to confidently diagnose a leiomyosarcoma on B-mode or color Doppler. Uteri with fibroids also show higher uterine artery peak velocity and lower RI (mean: 0.74 ± 0.09).[13]

Volume Ultrasound

Volume US is especially useful in fibroids to find the relationship of fibroids to the endometrium and assess the distortion or invasion of the endometrium with the fibroid as it can evaluate the lesion in three orthogonal planes. Sonohysterography with saline combined with 3D US may demonstrate the distortion of the endometrial cavity by submucosal fibroids better.[14,15]

Three-dimensional power Doppler indices—VI, FI, and VFI are especially useful for follow-up of fibroids in patients who are on gonadotropin-releasing hormone agonist (GnRha) therapy, menopausal or pregnant.

Diffuse Leiomyomatosis

Diffuse leiomyomatosis is a rare condition in which there is diffuse and uniform involvement of entire myometrium by multiple fibroids.

Fibroids are also seen arising from the cervix and show similar appearances as fibroid in the uterus.

Disseminated Peritoneal Leiomyomatosis

This is a very rare condition. There are several nodules of smooth muscle seen scattered through out the peritoneum. It may occur due to seeding during surgeries, especially laparoscopic morcellation of fibroids. Multiple lesions may distort the pelvic anatomy and therefore lead to symptoms, but may also occur spontaneously at times. It is associated with elevated estrogen levels. According to another hypothesis, it is also thought to be due to metaplasia of subperitoneal mesenchymal cells.[16] Diameter of the lesions may vary from 0.1 cm to 10 cm. These lesions appear to have estrogen and progesterone receptors and also luteinizing hormone (LH) receptors.[17,18] It is for this reason that these lesions may grow due to hormonal stimulation.

Benign Metastasizing Leiomyoma

In the uterus, it appears like a typical fibroid, but similar lesion may be seen in the lungs and may lead to deterioration of lung function. Being hormonal dependent, oophorectomy may treat the condition. Lung lesions are also seen in another fibroid like composition called lymphangioleiomyomatosis and this is more serious condition, and has a genetic origin.

CONCLUSION

The most common myometrial lesions are adenomyosis and fibroid. Though on B-mode US, these have certain overlapping features, Doppler is diagnostic for these, due to typical intralesional and peripheral vascularity, respectively.

REFERENCES

1. Van den Bosch T, Dueholm M, Leone FP, et al. Terms, definitions and measurements to describe sonographic features of myometrium and uterine masses: a consensus opinion from the Morphological Uterus Sonographic Assessment (MUSA) group. Ultrasound Obstet Gynecol. 2015;46(3):284-98.
2. Munro MG, Critchley HOD, Broder MS, et al. FIGO classification system (PALM-COEIN) for causes of abnormal uterine bleeding in nongravid women of reproductive age. Int J Gynecol Obstet. 2011;113(1):3-13.
3. Raine-Fenning N, Jayaprakasan K, Deb S. Three-dimensional ultrasonographic characteristics of endometriomata. Ultrasound Obstet Gynecol. 2008;31(6):718-24.
4. Aleem F, Pennisi J, Zeitoum K, et al. The role of color Doppler in diagnosis of endometriomas. Ultrasound Obstet Gynecol. 1995;5:51-4.
5. Di Donato N, Bertoldo V, Montanari G, et al. Question mark form of uterus: a simple sonographic sign associated with presence of adenomyosis. Ultrasound Obstet Gynecol. 2015;46(1):126-8.
6. Perrot N, Frey I, Mergui JL, et al. Picture of the month. Adenomyosis: power Doppler findings. Ultrasound Obstet Gynecol. 2001;17(2):177-8.
7. Exacoustos C, Brienza L, Di Giovanni A, et al. Adenomyosis: three-dimensional sonographic findings of the junctional zone and correlation with histology. Ultrasound Obstet Gynecol. 2011;37:471-9.
8. Kupesic S, Kurjak A, Pasalic L, et al. The value of transvaginal colour Doppler in the assessment of pelvic inflammatory disease. Ultrasound Med Biol. 1995;21(6):733-8.
9. Stoelinga B, Hehenkamp WJK, Brolmann HAM, et al. Real-time elastography for assessment of uterine disorders. Ultrasound Obstet Gynecol. 2014;43:218-26.
10. Buttram VC Jr, Reiter R. Uterine leiomyomata: etiology, symptomatology and management. Fertil Steril. 1981;36:433-45.
11. Taylor E, Gomel V. The uterus and fertility. Fertil Steril. 2008;89:1-16.
12. Wamsteker K, de Blok S. Resection of intrauterine fibroids. In: Lewis BV, Magos AL (Eds). Endometrial Ablation. Edinburgh, UK: Churchill Livingstone; 1993.
13. Kurjak A, Kupesic S, Miric D. The assessment of benign uterine tumour vascularization by transvaginal colour Doppler. Ultrasound Med Biol. 1992;18:645-9.
14. Balen FG, Allen CM, Gardener JE, et al. 3 dimensional reconstruction of ultrasound images of the uterine cavity. Br J Radiol. 1993;66(787):588-91.
15. Weinraub Z, Maymon R, Shulman A, et al. Three dimensional saline contrast hysterosonography and surface rendering of uterine cavity pathology. Ultrasound Obstet Gynecol. 1996;8(4):277-82.
16. Drake A, Dhundee J, Buckley CH, et al. Disseminated leiomyomatosis peritonealis in association with oestrogen secreting ovarian fibrothecoma. BJOG. 2001;108(6):661-4.
17. Akkersdjik GJ, Fli PK, Giard RW, et al. Malignant leiomyomatosis peritonealis disseminata. Am J Obstet Gynecol. 1990;163(2):591-3.
18. Butnor KJ, Burchette JL, Robboy SJ. Progesterone receptor activity in leiomyomatosis peritonealis disseminate. Int J Gynecol Pathol. 1999;18(3):259-64.

Role of Doppler in Diagnosing Gynecological Malignancies

INTRODUCTION

Malignancies of female reproductive organs are referred to as gynecological malignancies. These consist of malignancies of uterus body—endometrium and myometrium, malignancy of cervix, ovarian malignancies, tubal malignancies, vaginal and vulval malignancies. Though we shall also include the malignancies related to trophoblastic tissue in this chapter.

Ultrasound (US) is the modality of choice for the assessment of the pelvic organs, and transvaginal is the preferred route for assessment of female reproductive system. Though it is essential that the patient assessment should be started with the transabdominal scan. This allows the understanding of anatomy that may be grossly disturbed in cases of large tumors. Moreover, malignancies of reproductive organs are often associated with metastasis in peritoneum, abdominal organs, and retroperitoneal tissue, the assessment of which is not possible without abdominal scan. Several studies have shown that using B-mode US with Doppler significantly increases the detection and diagnosis of malignancies than B-mode alone.[1]

ANGIOGENESIS IN MALIGNANCIES

Like other tissues in the body, vascular endothelium also has an ability to regenerate and spread through other tissues to perfuse them. Formation of these blood vessels is called angiogenesis. The angiogenesis in the growing tissues like tumors is different from the angiogenesis in the normal tissues and this has been observed before more than 100 years.[2] Experiments in 1960s showed that in absence of vascular response of the surrounding host tissue can restrict the tumor growth.[3,4] It was proposed by Judah Folkman

that once a tumor has occurred, increase in the tumor cell population is preceded by an increase in new capillaries that sprouted towards early growth of the tumor.[5] Several other authors also have potentiated that the new vessel growth (angiogenesis) is essential for tumor growth.[6,7] As the tumor grows and the cells of the tumor in its center become hypoxic, it initiates angiogenesis and this is called *angiogenic switch*. The activity of this is dependent on the angiogenetic inhibitors and stimulators and both primary tumor and the distant metastasis are involved in complex regulation by angiogenic and antiangiogenetic factors. Folkman et al. documented that tumor produces vascular endothelial growth factor (VEGF).[8] The regulation of VEGF expression by hypoxia is mediated by family of hypoxia inducible transcription factors (HIF) that increases the transcription of VEGF gene.[9] The diagnosis of malignancy based on Doppler is therefore dependent on the observation of this neoangiogenesis initiated by VEGF and other angiogenetic factors.

The tumor vascularity develops from the host vasculature of surrounding tissues, but its organization is absolutely different than the parent vasculature. Tumor vasculature may be peripheral or central.

Any tumor has four regions of different perfusion rates in a tumor: (1) avascular (necrotic) region, (2) seminecrotic or ischemic region, (3) stabilized microcirculation, and (4) advancing front—tumor hyperemia.

But whatever the distribution, the malignant vessels have some particular characteristics:[10]
- Variable caliber of the vessels
- Elongation and coiling
- Nonhierarchical vascular network, vascular rings, and sinusoids

- Abnormal precapillary architecture with dichotomous branching and no decrease in diameter of higher order branching
- Incomplete vascular wall with gaps in endothelium.

Another study has also shown the difference between the normal and the tumor vessels is that tumor vessels are dilated, saccular and tortuous, and may also contain tumor cells in the endothelial lining of the vessel wall.[11] The blood in tumor vessels may flow from one venule to another venule and also through arteriovenous shunts. But only 20–80% of the vascular bed is perfused in the tumor at any particular given time.[12] The number of vessels developed per unit volume of tumor is called tumor vascularity and the number of flowing blood elements is tumor flow. The tumor flows in the same tumor may vary at different times.

It is these vascular characteristics that can be studied and documented by Doppler and 3D power Doppler (PD).[13] It has been suggested by the multitude of data that, apart from the conventional chemotherapy, controlling the angiogenesis can serve as a complementary treatment for malignancies.[6,14,15] The decrease in the vascularity may occur much faster than the decrease in the size of the tumor and this can be used to assess the control of the disease. These studies can be very effectively carried out by 3D PD studies.

Doppler studies of the tumor vessels and the evaluation of their resistance indices are important for diagnosis of malignant tumors. Blood vessels in malignant tumors have decreased resistance as compared to benign tumors. This is because of absence of muscularis in the tumor vessels that make them more distensible and lead to low-resistance flow. The variable caliber of the tumor vessels also lead to variable resistance and velocity in these vessels. Some vessels may have very low velocity and these may be difficult to be picked up on color or PD.[16] The sensitivity of the PD imaging is 14 dB greater than the standard Doppler imaging.[17] US contrast can be used to potentiate these Doppler signals and plays an important role to study the tumor vessels and to differentiate between benign and malignant tumors.[18] The small blood vessels can also be demonstrated better the use of ultrasound contrast and by activating the contrast mode on the scanner.

UTERINE MALIGNANCIES

Sarcoma

These are malignant myometrial lesions found in perimenopausal patients. These consist of 1–3% of all genital tract tumors and 3–7.4% of malignant tumors of uterine body. These lesions present like fibroids. Patients may have dysmenorrhea, menorrhagia, and pelvic pain.

On Ultrasound

It usually shows a single large tumor, often heterogeneous in echogenicity with anechoic areas due to necrotic areas, but may be hypoechoic or isoechoic. Typical fan-shaped acoustic shadow seen in a benign fibroid is not seen in these malignant tumors (Fig. 4.1A). It may show irregular margins, but in early stages—the margins may still be regular like in a fibroid. Unlike fibroids, these lesions have a rapid growth rate.

Doppler shows peripheral vascularity with marked internal vascularity. These vessels have a typical chaotic pattern, with variable caliber, and randomly dispersed vessels (Fig. 4.1B). On pulse Doppler, it typically shows low-resistance high-velocity flow. Like most malignant tumors, the resistance index (RI) is less than 0.42 (Fig. 4.1C). The velocities may be as high as 42 cm/s that is even more than the normal uterine artery velocity. Though it is important to mention here that even the degenerated fibroids would show heterogeneous echogenicity and high-internal vascularity with low-resistance flow. On US, therefore, it is not possible to confidently diagnose or differentiate sarcoma from a degenerated fibroid.

Endometrial Carcinoma

This is most common gynecological malignancy. Patients with endometrial malignancy present with menorrhagia, metrorrhagia, postmenopausal bleeding, and/or foul-

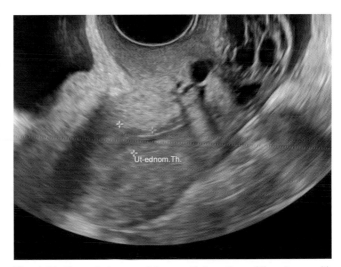

Fig. 4.1A: B-mode image of the sagittal section of the uterus with large multiloculated cystic lesion seen posterior to the lower part of the body of the uterus.

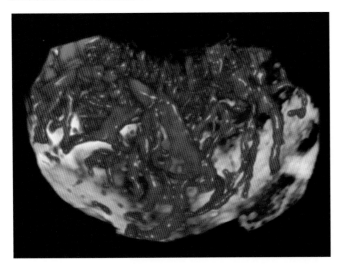

Fig. 4.1B: The same lesion as in Figure 4.1A shows markedly increased vascularity, with abundant branching and asymmetrical caliber suggesting the possibility of malignancy.

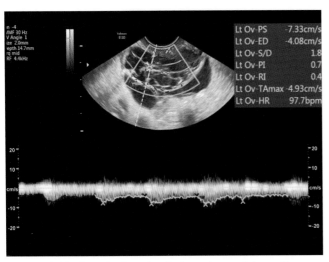

Fig. 4.1C: On color Doppler, it shows low resistance flow.

smelling blood-stained vaginal discharge. The symptoms usually appear early during the disease and therefore these malignancies are often diagnosed early.

This tumor may have various cell types and accordingly may be classified as adenocarcinoma, papillary serous, clear cell, or mucinous carcinoma. But 90% of the patients with endometrial malignancies have adenocarcinoma. Moreover on US, it is not possible to confirm the histopathology.

On Ultrasound

The endometrium is thickened on B-mode US. The endometrial thickness in literature is mentioned to be considered as suspicious of malignancy when it is more

than 15 mm in thickness in premenopausal and more than 5 mm in thickness in postmenopausal age group. But it is important to mention here that only increased thickness of the endometrium cannot be considered a specific parameter to diagnose endometrial malignancy. In normal patients also in mid-luteal phase, especially in conception cycles the endometrial thickness may reach up to 15 mm. Endometrial volume of more than 13 mL increases the possibility of endometrial malignancy.[19] Most reliable assessment of the volume of the US can be done by 3D US[20] (Figs. 4.2A and B). Though it is the heterogenicity of the endometrium that is a more relevant US feature than the thickness, which may raise the suspicion of endometrial malignancy (Fig. 4.3). The heterogenicity may involve the entire endometrium or may be focal depending on the extent of the disease. Anechoic areas may be seen in the endometrium, and this may be due to intracavitary fluid or may be because of blood collection in the endometrial cavity. Endometrial surface may appear irregular and is best appreciated on sonohysterography. If the lesion extends toward the myometrium, the endometrial–myometrial junction may appear interrupted and the heterogeneous echogenicity may extend into the myometrium (Fig. 4.4). Interruption of the endometrial–myometrial junction has a positive likelihood ratio of 10 for endometrial malignancy. Distance between lower end of the mass and the external os, if it is less than 2 cm, it indicates cervical invasion (Fig. 4.5). 3D with transverse plane picture may demonstrate bladder or rectal infiltration. 3D US may be of help for better definition of the extent of the lesion by the use of volume contrast imaging (VCI) and even for more precise volume calculation by VOCAL (Virtual Organ Computer-aided Analysis) (Figs. 4.2A and B). Volume calculation of the tumor can be used for prediction of extension of the tumor into the myometrium or in the cervix. Increasing volume size of the endometrium suggests myometrial invasion. If the total volume measurement of the mass is more than 50% of the total uterine volume measurement, it indicates myometrial involvement. 3D US has been found to be effective to assess myometrial invasion. This is because of better assessment of the endometrial–myometrial junction by 3D US and also its better ability to estimate maximum penetration of the tumor in the myometrium.[21,22] Larger endometrial volume can be associated with lymph node metastasis also. Volume larger than 25 mL has high chances of pelvic node involvement at surgery.[23]

Doppler studies typically show increased vascularity with low-resistance flow. Larger the tumor and more the

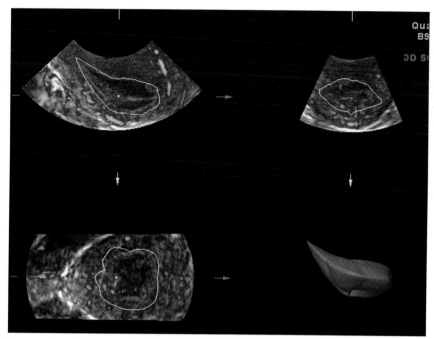

Fig. 4.2A: 3D power Doppler acquired volume of the uterus with VOCAL (virtual organ computer-aided analysis) calculated endometrial volume.

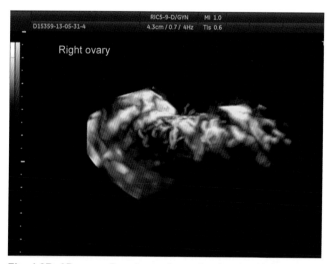

Fig. 4.2B: 3D power Doppler angiography showing high-vascular density of the endometrium with heterogeneous distribution.

Fig. 4.3: Thickened endometrium with heterogeneous echogenicity raising a suspicion of endometrial malignancy.

tumor invasion, lesser is the resistance. RI of the range of 0.34–0.39 is seen with grade 3, stage II tumors with more than half myometrial invasion and lymphovascular emboli. Lymph node involvement further decreases this RI to 0.3. 3D PD can potentially detect the lesions that require aggressive intervention. The vessels show sacculations and irregular caliber (Fig. 4.6). The vascularity is heterogeneously distributed. Vascularity score is usually 3–4. It is markedly

increased in the growing part of the tumor and is absent in the necrotic part of the tumor. This vascular pattern extends with the tumor in the myometrium in case the tumor extends into the myometrium[24] (Fig. 4.7). Vascularization index of the endometrial carcinoma can be associated with tumor grade.[23]

Endometrial polyps may also undergo malignant change. In these cases, the polyp surface shows irregular margins

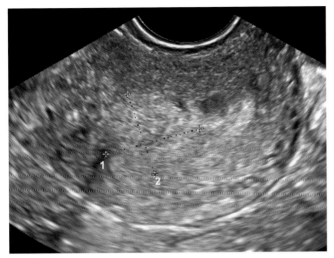

Fig. 4.4: Thick heterogeneous endometrium with ill-defined junctional zone.

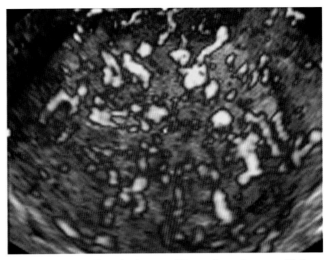

Fig. 4.6: Power Doppler image of the malignant mass with the vessels show sacculations and irregular caliber.

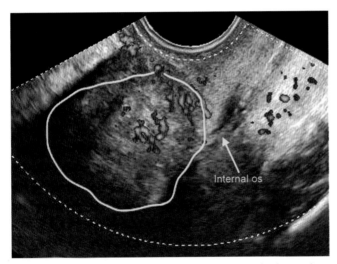

Fig. 4.5: Endometrial mass lesion extending up to the internal os, suggesting its extension into the cervix.

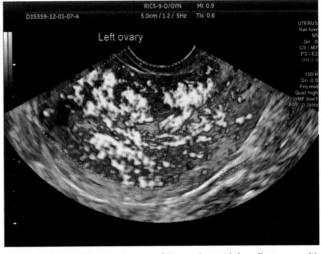

Fig. 4.7: Power Doppler image of the endometrial malignancy with extension in the endometrium shows extension of the malignant vascular pattern into the myometrium. There is markedly increased vascular density and the vessels show irregular caliber and chaotic arrangement.

and heterogeneous echogenicity. The central feeding vessel shows abundant branching with vessels showing irregular caliber and low-resistance flow (Figs. 4.8A to C).

Cervical Carcinoma

Cervical carcinoma is more common than endometrial carcinoma in developing countries and especially in lower socioeconomical group. Human papilloma virus (HPV) is believed to be causative for the same. Patients with cervical carcinoma may present with intermenstrual spotting or bleeding, vaginal discharge, and may also complain of postcoital bleeding. Cervical cancer may extend into the uterine body or may extend anteriorly into bladder and posteriorly up to rectum. This may lead to symptoms like pain, melena, and hematuria. Pap smear is an effective screening test for early diagnosis of cervical cancer. Cervical carcinoma histologically may be adenocarcinoma or squamous cell carcinoma.

Cervical malignancies can be diagnosed by B-mode US, Doppler, 3D US, 3D PD, and magnetic resonance imaging (MRI). Though the later is chiefly of importance for assessing the spread of the tumor and staging of the disease.

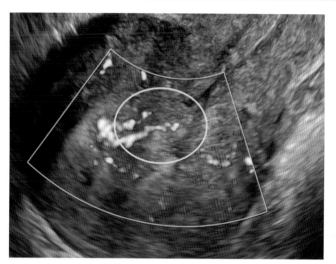

Fig. 4.8A: B-mode with high-definition (HD) flow showing a not very well-defined oval solid lesion showing a single feeding vessel in early proliferative phase.

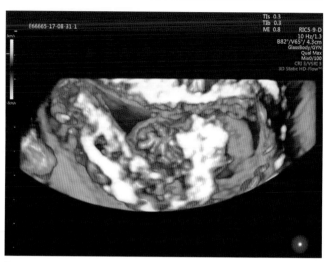

Fig. 4.8C: 3D power Doppler of the same lesion shows abundant vascularity with abundant branching raising the suspicion of malignancy in the polyp.

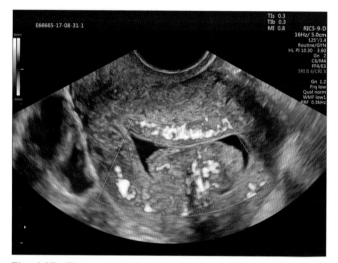

Fig. 4.8B: The same lesion on sonohysterography shows well-defined oval mass with fluid in endometrial cavity and high-definition (HD) flow shows unifocal multiple vessels feeding it with several branches.

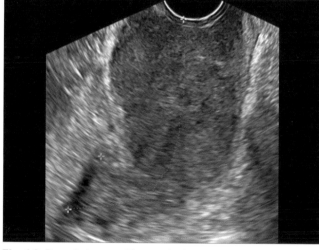

Fig. 4.9: B-mode image of the cervix showing marked enlargement and loss of normal anatomical planes with homogeneous hypoechogenicity and a small uterine body.

On Ultrasound

Cervical carcinoma presents on US as an isoechoic (adenocarcinoma) or hypoechoic (squamous cell carcinoma) (Fig. 4.9) solid mass lesion. Anteroposterior diameter of the cervix to the anteroposterior diameter of the corpus, normally is 0.71. If it reaches more than 1, it is definitely indicative of malignancy.

The mass lesion may be endophytic or exophytic. There may also be pericervical canal—diamond-shaped tumors. It has irregular margins and has heterogeneous echogenicity.

But when the lesions are isoechoic, these may be difficult to identify.

Endophytic lesions are usually small and then their exact location can be described by the distance from the internal os and from the cervical canal or serosa. Stromal infiltration can be assessed by checking the thickness of the tumor-free cervical stroma around the margin of the tumor (Fig. 4.10). When exophytic, it is more likely to disrupt the tissue planes and involve the surrounding structures especially the parametrium, bladder/urethra, and rectum (Fig. 4.11). When infiltration in the surrounding tissue

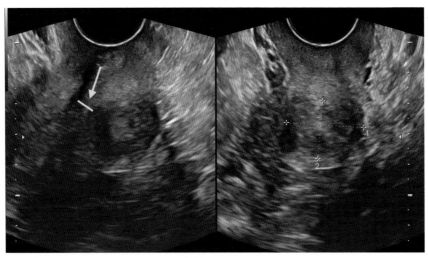

Fig. 4.10: A B-mode transvaginal ultrasound image showing a heterogeneous well-defined cervical mass. The image on the left shows the tumor-free wall measurement of the cervix and the image on the right shows the tumor measurement in two orthogonal planes.

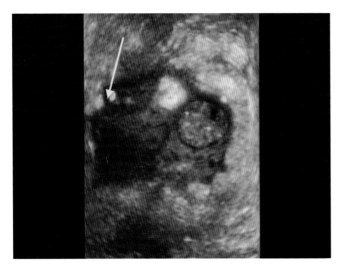

Fig. 4.11: A coronal plane image of the cervical mass showing irregular margins and disruption of the tissue planes (arrow). The tumor is seen extending into both parametria and also anteriorly infiltrating through the vaginal wall and posteriorly infiltrating into rectal wall.

layers is present, it can be diagnosed by extension of heterogeneous echogenicity in the surrounding structures and disruption of the tissue planes. Mobility of the surrounding tissues in relation to the mass can be best appreciated by in and out movement of the probe to check the mobility of the structures. 3D US is the modality of choice for the volume assessment of the tumor mass. Large tumors may extend up to the lateral pelvic wall. When the lesion extends in the parametrium, there is a high risk of involvement of the ureters and therefore assessment of

the kidneys is required by transabdominal scan for back pressure changes and hydronephrosis. Lymph gland enlargement may be seen along the iliac vessels. 3D US has been used for staging of cervical carcinoma based on multiplanar imaging. Concordance of 3D US and pathology for assessing parametrial, rectal, and bladder involvement was 93%, 93%, and 100%, respectively.[25]

Doppler shows increased vascularity with vessels showing irregular caliber, abundant branching, and low-resistance flow (Fig. 4.12). The resistance is lower with larger tumors. The abnormal vascular pattern is seen extending up to the total extension of the tumor. Doppler reveals four types of vascular pattern in early stage cervical carcinomas—(1) localized, (2) peripheral, (3) scattered, and (4) single vessel type. Though no significant difference in 3D PD blood flow parameters is seen in cervical carcinoma depending on the tumor grade, tumor diameter, and histological type.[26]

VAGINAL MALIGNANCY

Vaginal malignant masses may be primary (20%) or secondary (80%). Secondary may occur in vagina by local spread from cervical or vulval malignancies or by hematogenous or lymphatic spread.

Primary Vaginal Carcinoma

These are very rare tumors consisting of hardly 1-2% of all gynecological cancers. Histopathologically, these malignancies may be squamous cell carcinoma (not

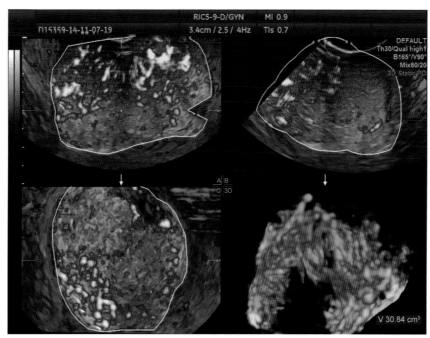

Fig. 4.12: 3D power Doppler image of the cervical mass showing markedly increased vascularity with vessels showing irregular caliber, abundant branching. The vascular pattern is seen extending beyond the cervix in the tumor extension.

common), clear cell carcinoma, melanoma, sarcoma botryoides, and leiomyosarcoma. Patients with these tumors present with postcoital bleed, painless vaginal bleeding, vaginal discharge, and pelvic pain. If the tumor extends into bladder or bowel, the patient may also have dysuria, hematuria, urgency, painful defecation, and constipation.

On Ultrasound

These tumors appear as solid hypoechoic or heterogeneous masses, when seen on transvaginal or transrectal scan. Gel vaginosonography may improve the visibility of these lesions. The tumors are highly vascular with score of 3–4. The vessels are seen perpendicular to the vaginal wall. Like other malignancies, the vessels typically show irregular caliber and dichotomous branching pattern. When the lesion extends into the surrounding tissues, along with the extension of the hypoechoic mass in these structures, extension of the vascular pattern is also seen into these extensions.

Adnexal Lesions

Adnexal malignancies chiefly consists of ovarian malignant lesions. Tubal malignancies are not very common and if advanced, not possible to differentiate from the ovarian lesions. As for ovarian lesions also, except for a few lesions that have typical B mode appearances, it is not possible to give histopathological diagnosis on B-mode alone, Though it has been established that complex lesions with cystic and solid components, irregular margins and heterogeneous echogenicity are more likely to be malignant. In a multicentric European study, color Doppler evaluation was more accurate in diagnosis of adnexal malignancies compared to gray-scale US.[27] 3D US has significantly improved the prediction of malignancy as compared to 2D US.[28] Better recognition of ovarian lesion, accurate characterization of surface features, determination of the extent of tumor infiltration, and clear depiction of the tumor volume are the advantages of 3D US.[29]

The sensitivity of risk of malignancy index (RMI) for ovarian malignancy was found to be 88% in one study and that for 3D PD was 75% but both used together, showed sensitivity of 99%.[30] For the reliability of the 3D PD, standardization of the PD pulse repetition frequency (PRF) (0.6) and gains is essential. Another study has shown that 3D PD studies had 100% PPV (positive-predictive value) and 95% NPV (negative-predictive value) for diagnosis of ovarian cancers.[31] As compared to 2D US with Doppler, 3D PD decreases the false-positive rates[32] and increases the sensitivity for the diagnosis of adnexal lesion.[32,33] Qualitative analysis of the tumor vascular architecture by

3D PD increases the sensitivity and specificity of the ovarian malignancy diagnosis to 100% and 76%, respectively.[34] 3D PD with volume histogram for quantitative assessment of the global vascularity of the tumor can differentiate between the benign and malignant tumor and can also predict tumor prognosis.[35-37] Another study documented that VI and FI may become good predictors for tumor neovascularization and can replace qualitative and semiquantitative 3D PD evaluation.[37] In a study by Alcazar et al., logistic regression has shown that only the central blood flow in the solid component of the tumor and ascites are independent predictors and both features correlated in 98.6% of patients of adnexal malignancy. Absence of both features was detected in 82.1% of benign tumors.[38] A virtual spherical sampling has been used to assess the vascularity in a localized vascular area. The vascularity was more in malignant as compared to benign tumors[39,40] (Box 4.1).[41]

BOX 4.1: 3D power Doppler criteria for malignant adnexal lesions (Figs. 4.13A and B).[41]

- Loss of tree-like branching pattern of vessels
- Sacculations of arteries and veins
- Focal narrowing of arteries
- Internal shifts in velocity within arterial lumen
- Beach ball finding of increased and disorganized peripheral flow around the malignant mass
- Increased flow to center of the solid lesion
- Crowding of vascularity
- "Start and stop" arteries—arteries that stop abruptly without branching

---

Contrast-enhanced 3D PD has shown 100% sensitivity, 93.9% specificity, 85.7% PPV, and 100% NPV for the diagnosis of ovarian malignant lesions.

Malignant Ovarian Tumors

- *Epithelial tumors*: These may be serous, mucinous, endometrioid, clear cell, Brenner tumor, and undifferentiated tumors and may be borderline or malignant tumors.
- *Germ cell tumors*: Immature teratomas, dysgerminomas, yolk sac tumors, and choriocarcinoma
- *Sex cord or stromal tumors*: Granulosa cell tumor, Sertoli–Leydig cell tumor
- Metastatic tumors.

Epithelial Tumors

Serous epithelial tumors: About 30–50% of these may be malignant. These may be often multilocular and may be bilateral. Septae are thick and irregular in malignant tumors. These tumors may show multiple papillae and solid projections. Solid projections may sometimes be so large that the entire mass may appear solid looking. Fluid part of these tumors show internal echogenicities (Fig. 4.14A). These tumors may show microcalcifications or psammoma bodies. Psammoma bodies are concentric, lamellated, and calcified solid components of the tumor, less echogenic than calcification, and do not show acoustic shadowing. Ascites may be seen.

On Doppler, low-resistance vascularity is identified in the walls, septae, and in the solid projections (Fig. 4.14B).

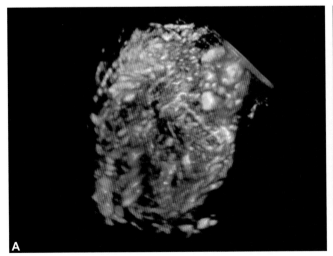 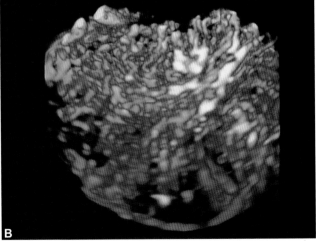

Figs. 4.13A and B: 3D power Doppler angiography of two different ovarian lesions showing sacculations and narrowing of the vessels with loss of tree-like branching pattern and disorganized flow around the malignant mass.

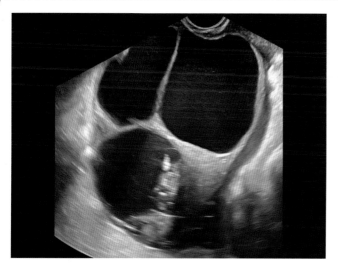

Fig. 4.14A: B-mode ultrasound image of a multiloculated solid mass and low level echoes in the fluid.

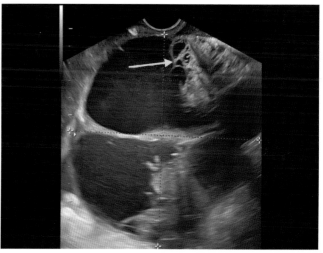

Fig. 4.15A: Multilocular solid lesion with cluster of locules: an ultrasound appearance commonly seen in borderline tumors.

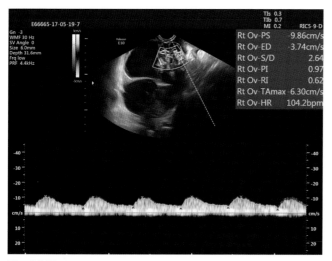

Fig. 4.14B: Pulsed Doppler shows low-resistance flow in this lesion. Both the features together strongly suggest the malignant nature of the lesion.

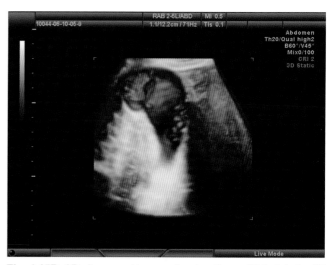

Fig. 4.15B: 3D ultrasound image showing the multilobulated solid component in a multiloculated tumor.

Mucinous epithelial tumors: These are multilocular tumors with rigid and bright septae and internal echogenicities. Borderline tumors may show cluster of tiny locules in the solid component of the tumor. These are very tiny cysts and may require 6–12 MHz frquency probe and transvaginal scan with an optimized image to visualize them. These cysts are typically seen in borderline tumors and not in benign or malignant lesions, localized to one area (Figs. 4.15A and B), but tiny locules may give hyperechogenicity. Multiple papillarities and even some solid projections may be seen (Fig. 4.15B). Low-resistance flow is seen in the walls, septae, solid projections, and papillarities. Ascites with internal echogenicities may also be present.

Germ Cell Tumors

Malignant germ cell tumors have mixed cell types, with increased alpha fetoprotein and human chorionic gonadotropin (hCG).

On ultrasound—chiefly unilateral lesions may be solid, lobulated, but may also show heterogencous echogenicity, with high-score vascularity in solid areas and septae.

Dysgerminoma: This is a malignant tumor of young age (2nd–3rd decade), commonly found in patients with primary amenorrhea or may be associated with gonadal dysgenesis of gonadoblastoma. But dysgerminoma may often be diagnosed during pregnancy. On US, these are well-defined solid masses with smooth or lobulated outer margins (Fig. 4.16), with moderate-to-high vascularity seen on Doppler.

Sex Cord–Stromal Tumors

Granulosa cell tumor: This is the most common hormone producing ovarian tumor seen in postmenopausal women more commonly and in prepubertal females (5%) less commonly. These are estrogen-secreting tumors and lead to endometrial hyperplasia and occasionally endometrial carcinoma. These are large tumors with low-malignant potential.

On US, these appear as solid tumors with or without multiple well-defined cystic areas giving a moth-eaten appearance. The solid part of the tumor has heterogeneous echogenicity and high vascularity.

Sertoli and Sertoli–Leydig cell tumors: These tumors of varying malignant potential, also known as androblastomas, consist of sertoli cells, leydig cells, and fibroblasts. These tumors are more commonly seen in young women. Depending on which cell type is dominating, these may show androgenic, estrogenic, or progestogenic manifestations. These tumors also may have solid or multilocular solid appearance, with moderate-to-high vascularity (Fig. 4.17).

Leydig cell tumor: This is an androgen producing tumor of postmenopausal age, typically small (mean diameter of 2.4 cm) and solid with high vascularity.

Actually, if summarized, all the malignant ovarian tumors share a similar appearance with solid and cystic components, with or without septae, solid components consisting of papillarities or solid projections and typical malignant vascular pattern. Therefore based on US alone, it is almost impossible to confirm a histopathological diagnosis.

Metastatic Ovarian Tumors

Based on US features, ovarian metastatic tumors can be divided into two categories:
1. *Category A*: Solid tumors that metastasize from breast, stomach, uterus, and lymphoma.[42]
2. *Category B*: Mostly multilocular solid or multilocular tumors, but sometimes solid also, metastasized from colon, rectum, appendix, and biliary tract.

These tumors are often bilateral. Solid tumors are homogeneous, unless necrosis leads to heterogenicity. These have well-defined margins. Multicystic tumors may have several loculi and in necrotic tumors, septae may be fragmented. The fluid may be anechoic or may have low-

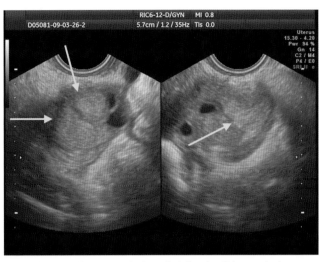

Fig. 4.16: A mildly hyperechoic well-defined solid mass lesion seen in the ovary in two orthogonal planes. In the image on the left side, the image shows a septum like shadow creating an appearance of septated solid tumor—commonly seen in dysgerminoma.

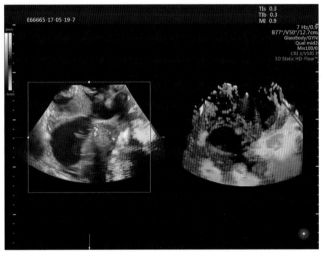

Fig. 4.17: Multilocular solid tumor on B mode with vascularity seen on 3D high-definition (HD) flow. The features indicate malignancy.

level echoes. These tumors do not always have well-defined margins.

On Doppler, these lesions show low-resistance and high-velocity flow. "Lead vessel" with tree-like branching pattern is the typical vascular morphology of solid metastatic tumors (Fig. 4.18). Krukenberg tumors are also solid metastatic tumors and show similar vascular morphology.[43]

TUBAL MALIGNANCIES

Malignancy of the fallopian tubes is very rare and may comprise of only about 0.18–1.6% of all gynecological malignancies. Though when diagnosed in advanced stage, it may be difficult to differentiate from ovarian malignancies. Histopathologically, these may be serous adenocarcinoma (80%), endometrioid carcinoma, clear cell carcinoma, and mucinous or undifferentiated carcinomas. These tumors commonly occur in the distal third of the tube and present with vaginal discharge, bleeding, abdominal pain, at times intermittent and colicky, and pelvic mass are more commonly found in females with a history of infertility or chronic pelvic infection.

On Ultrasound

These tumors may appear solid hypo- to isoechoic, ovoid- or sausage-shaped mass, at times with internal anechoic areas, with moderate-to-high vascularity, with vessels oriented perpendicular to the mass (Figs. 4.19A to C). At times, the tube may be distended with fluid and may show mass protruding

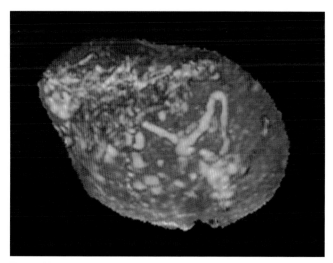

Fig. 4.18: 3D power Doppler ultrasound on glass body rendering is showing a single feeding vessel with abundant branching and also chaotic arrangement—a metastatic ovarian tumor.

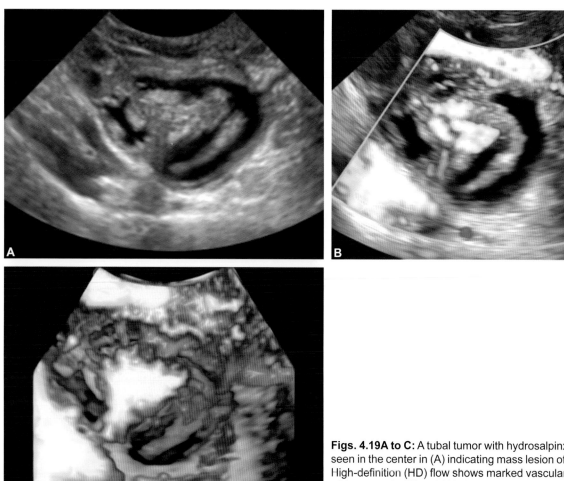

Figs. 4.19A to C: A tubal tumor with hydrosalpinx and a solid tumor seen in the center in (A) indicating mass lesion of the fallopian tube. High-definition (HD) flow shows marked vascularity in the solid part of the tumor in (B) and (C) shows 3D ultrasound with pulse Doppler showing typical malignant pattern of vascularity—fallopian tube malignant tumor.

in the hydrosalpinx lumen. Free fluid may be seen in the pelvis or fluid may also be seen in the endometrial cavity. Ovary if seen separately, diagnosis may be more confident.

GESTATIONAL TROPHOBLASTIC NEOPLASIA

In patients with complete mole, the possibility of development of choriocarcinoma or invasive mole increases and this can be diagnosed by persistently high beta-hCG levels after evacuation of the mole. 20% of all complete mole patients may have this risk. Though gestational trophoblastic neoplasia (GTN) may also arise after normal pregnancy, miscarriage, or ectopic pregnancy. This group of tumors includes more common, choriocarcinoma and invasive mole; and less common, placental site trophoblastic tumor (PSTT) and epithelioid trophoblastic tumor (ETT). These may be malignant or potentially malignant. The malignant ones have a tendency to metastasize into vagina or lung. Patients present with high–beta-hCG levels, vaginal bleeding, hyperthyroidism, and pelvic pain. The history and clinical presentation are so typical that biopsy is usually not required for confirmation of diagnosis.

Invasive Mole

When hydropic villi invade into the myometrium, it is invasive mole. On US, it appears as ill-defined solid mass in the myometrium with multiple fluid-filled anechoic areas (Fig. 4.20). These lesions show high score of vascularity with low-resistance flow (RI: 0.4–0.45). Dilated vessels may also be seen in the surrounding myometrium. The neoangiogenesis of the mass lesion shows arteriovenous shunts and therefore turbulent flows. Ovaries show multi-loculated cystic lesions with thin septae (theca lutein cysts).

The positive response to treatment may be indicated by decreasing size and vascularity of the lesion.

Choriocarcinoma

This tumor usually follows a molar or a nonmolar pregnancy, invades into the myometrium, consists of cytotrophoblast and syncytiotrophoblast and has a high-malignant potential.

On Ultrasound

These tumors present as ill-defined solid mass lesions with heterogeneous echogenicity consisting of solid components and anechoic areas (Fig. 4.21A) that consist of vascular channels and cystic areas secondary to hemorrhage and

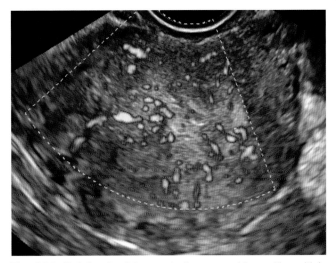

Fig. 4.20: Ill-defined solid mass in the myometrium with multiple fluid filled anechoic areas as seen on transvaginal ultrasound with power Doppler showing blood vessels with irregular caliber.

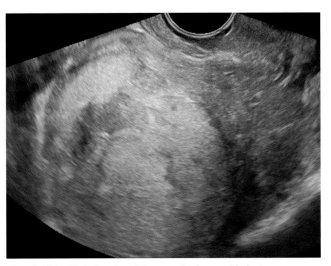

Fig. 4.21A: Ill-defined solid mass lesions with heterogeneous echogenicity consisting of solid components and anechoic areas seen on transvaginal B-mode scan.

necrosis. These tumors are highly vascular and on Doppler show moderate-to-high vascularity (score 3–4), with vessels of irregular caliber, arteriovenous shunts, and vascular lakes (Fig. 4.21B). The uterine artery also shows low-resistance flow. In more widespread tumor, there may be enlargement of the uterus also, with entire myometrium showing heterogeneous echogenicity. The tumor, if it extends into the parametrium, may show similar echogenicity and Doppler findings till the extension of the tumor. Theca lutein cysts are also seen in ovaries as multiloculated cystic lesions with thin septae.

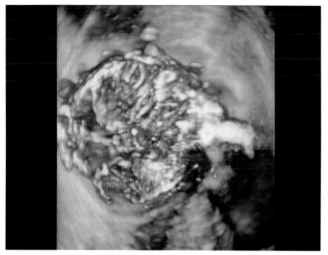

Fig. 4.21B: Doppler shows moderate-to-high vascularity (score 3–4), with vessels of irregular caliber, arteriovenous shunts, and vascular lakes.

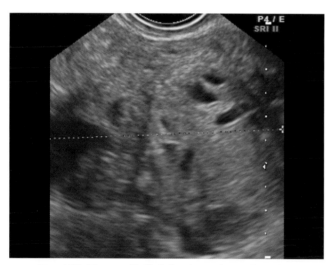

Fig. 4.22: Tumor with ill-defined margins and multiple small cystic spaces of variable route.

Placental Site Trophoblastic Tumor and Epithelioid Trophoblastic Tumor

These tumors arise from intermediate cells of extravillous trophoblast of nonmolar pregnancy and secrete low levels of hCG but high levels of human placental lactogen (HPL).

These tumors have indistinct margins and show multiple cystic spaces (Fig. 4.22). The vascularity is low and the amount of vascularity represents its sensitivity to chemotherapy.

CONCLUSION

Ultrasound is a modality of choice for assessment of gynecological tumors. Transvaginal is the preferred route for more detailed assessment of these tumors. Doppler plays an important role to assess the vascularity of the tumor. Low-resistance and high-velocity flow with vascularity score of 3–4 are the features almost consistently found in all adnexal malignancies. 3D PD especially helps to study the vascular branching pattern, caliber variability, arteriovenous malformations, and venous lakes, all diagnostic of malignancy, thus increasing the sensitivity, specificity, and positive predictive value of 3D PD for diagnosis of malignant tumors.

REFERENCES

1. Kinkel K, Hricak H, Lu Y, et al. US characterization of ovarian masses: A meta-analysis. Radiology. 2000;217:803-11.
2. Warren BA. The vascular morphology of tumours. In: Peterson HI (Ed). Tumour blood circulation: Angiogenesis, vascular morphology, and blood flow of experimental human tumours. Boca Raton, Florida: CRC Press; 1979. pp. 1-47.
3. Folkman J, Long DM, Becker FF. Growth and metastasis of tumor in organ culture. Cancer. 1963;16:453-67.
4. Folkman J, Cole P, Zimmerman S. Tumor behavior in isolated perfused organs: In vitro growth and metastasis of biopsy material in rabbit thyroid and canine intestinal segment. Ann Surg. 1966;164:491-502.
5. Folkman J. What is the evidence that tumours are angiogenesis dependent? J Natl Cancer Inst. 1990;82(1):4-6.
6. Auerbach R. Angiogenesis-inducing factors: A review. In: Pick E (Ed). Lymphokines. London: Academic Press; 1981. pp. 69-88.
7. Rak JW, St Croix BD, Kerbel RS. Consequences of angiogenesis for tumor progression, metastasis and cancer therapy. Anticancer Drugs. 1995;6(1):3-18.
8. Folkman J, Klagsbrun M. Angiogenic factors. Science. 1987;235(4787):442-7.
9. Pugh CW, Ratcliffe PJ. Regulation of angiogenesis by hypoxia. Role of HIF system. Nat Med. 2003;9(6):677-84.
10. Kurjak A, Kupesic S, Breyer B. The assessment of ovarian tumor angiogenesis by three-dimensional power Doppler. In: Kurjak A (Ed). Three-dimensional power Doppler in obstetrics and gynecology. Nashville, TN 37205, USA: The Parthenon Publishing Group; 2000.
11. Jain RK, Ward-Harley K. Tumor blood flow characterization, modifications and role in hyperthermia. Trans Sonics Ultrasonics. 1984;31:504-9.
12. Vaupel P, Kallinowski F, Okunieff P. Blood flow oxygen and nutrient supply, and metabolic microenvironment of human tumors: A review. Cancer Res. 1989;49(23):6449-65.

13. Kurjak A, Kupesic S, Breyer B, et al. The assessment of ovarian tumor angiogenesis: what does three-dimensional power Doppler add? Ultrasound Obstet Gynecol. 1998;12(2):136-46.

14. Folkman J, Merler E, Abernathy C, et al. Isolation of a tumor factor responsible for angiogenesis. J Exp Med. 1971;133(2):275-88.

15. Hanahan D, Folkman J. Parameters and emerging mechanisms of the angiogenetic switch during tumorigenesis. Cell. 1996;86:353-4.

16. Rubin JM, Bude RO, Carsson PL, et al. Power Doppler US: A potentially useful alternative to mean frequency-based color Doppler US. Radiology. 1994;190(3):853-6.

17. Burns PN. Harmonic imaging with ultrasound contrast agents. Clin Radiol. 1996;1:50-5.

18. Kupesic S, Kurjak A. Contrast enhanced three-dimensional power Doppler sonography for the differentiation of adnexal masses. Obstet Gynecol. 2000;96(3):452-8.

19. Gruboeck K, Jurkovic D, Lawton F, et al. The diagnostic value of endometrial thickness and volume measurements by three-dimensional ultrasound in patients with postmenopausal bleeding. Ultrasound Obstet Gynecol. 1996;8:272-6.

20. Alcaözar JL, Merce LT, Garcia-Manero M, et al. Endometrial volume and vascularity measurements by transvaginal three-dimensional ultrasonography and power Doppler angiography in stimulated and tumoral endometria: an inter-observer reproducibility study. J Ultrasound Med. 2005;24:1091-8.

21. Bonilla-Musoles F, Raga F, Osborne NG, et al. Three-dimensional hysterosonography for the study of endometrial tumours: comparison with conventional transvaginal sonography, hysterosalpingography, and hysteroscopy. Gynecol Oncol. 1997;65:245-52.

22. Su MT, Su RM, Yue CT, et al. Three-dimensional transvaginal ultrasound provides clearer delineation of myometrial invasion in a patient with endometrial cancer and uterine leiomyoma. Ultrasound Obstet Gynecol. 2003;22:434-6.

23. Saarelainen SK, Vuento MH, Kirkinen P, et al. Preoperative assessment of endometrial carcinoma by three-dimensional power Doppler angiography. Ultrasound Obstet Gynecol. 2012;39:466-72.

24. Kupesic S, Kurjak A, Zodan T. Staging of the endometrial carcinoma by three-dimensional power Doppler ultrasound. Gynaecol Perinatol. 1999;14:139-43.

25. Ghi T, Giunchi S, Kuleva M, et al. Three-dimensional transvaginal sonography in local staging of cervical carcinoma: description of a novel technique. Ultrasound Obstet Gynecol. 2007;30:778-82.

26. Testa AC, Ferrandina G, Distefano M, et al. Color Doppler velocimetry and three-dimensional color power angiography of cervical carcinoma. Ultrasound Obstet Gynecol. 2004;24:445-52.

27. Kinkel K, Hricak H, Lu Y, et al. US characterization of ovarian masses: A meta-analysis. Radiology. 2000;217:803-11.

28. Geomini PM, Coppus SF, Kluivers KB, et al. Is Three-dimensional ultrasonography of additional value in the assessment of adnexal masses? Gynecol Oncol. 2007;106(1):153-9.

29. Riccabona M, Nelson TR, Pretorius DH. Three-dimensional ultrasound: Accuracy of distance and volume measurements. Ultrasound Obstet Gynecol. 1996;7(6):429-34.

30. Mansour GM, El-Lamie I, El-Sayed H, et al. Adnexal mass vascularity assessed by three-dimensional power Doppler: Does it add to the risk of malignancy index in prediction of ovarian malignancy? Four hundred-case study. Int J Gynecol Cancer. 2009;19(5):867-72.

31. Chase DM, Crade M, Basu T, et al. Preoperative diagnosis of ovarian malignancy: Preliminary results of the use of three-dimensional vascular ultrasound. Int J Gynecol Cancer. 2009;19(3):354-60.

32. Kurjak A, Kupesic S, Anic T, et al. Three-dimensional ultrasound and power Doppler improve the diagnosis of ovarian lesions. Gynecol Oncol. 2000;76:28-32.

33. Kurjak A, Kupesic S, Sparac V, et al. Three-dimensional ultrasonographic and power Doppler characterization of ovarian lesions. Ultrasound Obstet Gynecol. 2000;16:365-71.

34. Breyer B, Kurjak A. Tumor vascularization Doppler measurements and chaos: what to do? Ultrasound Obstet Gynecol. 1995;5(3):209-10.

35. Fleischer AC, Pairleitner H. Transvaginal Doppler assesses ovarian flow. Diag Imag. 1998;9:47.

36. Fleischer AC, Pairleitner H. 3D transvaginal color Doppler sonography: current and potential applications. Med Imag Int. 1999;9:10-13.

37. Pairleitner H, Steiner H, Hasenoehrl G, et al. Three-dimensional power Doppler sonography: Imaging and quantifying blood flow and vascularization. Ultrasound Obstet Gynecol. 1999;14(2):139-43.

38. Alcazar JL, Royo P, Pineda L, et al. Which parameters could be useful for predicting malignancy in solid adnexal masses? Donald School J Ultrasound Obstet Gynecol. 2009;3(1):1-5.

39. Jokubkiene L, Sladkevicius P, Valentin L. Does three-dimensional power Doppler Ultrasound help in discrimination between benign and malignant ovarian masses? Ultrasound Obstet Gynecol. 2007;29:215-25.

40. Kudla MJ, Timor-Tritsch IE, Hope JM, et al. Spherical tissue sampling in 3-dimensional power Doppler angiography: a new approach for evaluation of ovarian tumors. J Ultrasound Med. 2008;27:425-33.

41. Crade M. Tissue block ultrasound and ovarian cancer—a pictorial presentation of findings. Donald School J Ultrasound Obstet Gynecol. 2009;3(1):41-7.

42. Testa AC. Imaging in gynecological disease: Ultrasound features of metastases in the ovaries differ depending on the origin of the primary tumour. Ultrasound Obstet Gyencol. 2007;29:505-11.

43. Testa AC, Mancari R, Di Legge A, et al. The 'lead-vessel': a vascular ultrasound feature of metastasis in theories. Ultrasound Obstet Gyencol. 2008;31:218-21.

Doppler for Differential Diagnosis of Adnexal Lesions

INTRODUCTION

Uterus, ovaries, and tubes are the pelvic organs that consist of female genital tract. Adnexa comprises of ovaries, fallopian tubes, and ligaments. International Ovarian Tumor Analysis (IOTA)[1] is the most systematic consensus for differential diagnosis of ovarian lesions and also for calculating the risk of malignancy. Though as the scope of this chapter is to discuss the role of color Doppler for differential diagnosis adnexal lesions, we shall not discuss IOTA in detail, but we shall take it as a reference wherever relevant.

OVARY

Ovary is an organ that changes its morphology several times during the menstrual cycle. Cystic structures with different morphologies appear and disappear. And this is absolutely physiological, when these are follicle, corpus luteum luteinized unruptured follicle or a follicular cyst. But there may be pathological cysts also appearing in the ovary. It is therefore very important to differentiate between the physiological and pathological cysts in the ovaries. Of course majority of the ovarian lesions are chiefly cystic with or without solid components, but these may also be solid masses. So let us start with the physiological cystic structures and then let us discuss, what are the pathological cystic structures that simulate those structures and how to differentiate those.

It is known that the ovary at the start of the menstrual cycle has multiple small follicles—antral follicles. These follicles grow as the cycle progresses and then one or two follicles grow to dominance (>10 mm). Dominant follicle

may progress to maturity and may rupture. After rupture, it converts into corpus luteum. And then if the cycle is not a conception cycle, the corpus luteum gradually regresses.

The follicle is a round cystic [unilocular cystic (IOTA)] structure with thin walls and anechoic contents with no solid components or internal echogenicities (Fig. 5.1). It is seen in the proliferative phase of the menstrual cycle. A mature follicle (18–24 mm in diameter) normally shows perifollicular vascularity covering two-thirds to three-fourths of its circumference with low-resistance flow[2] (Fig. 5.2). The low-resistance flow in the perifollicular vessels can be correlated with the rising estrogen levels. Lesions that appear similar to follicle, thin walled, anechoic contents with no internal echogenicities or solid components, may be simple cyst or a follicular cyst. On B-mode ultrasound

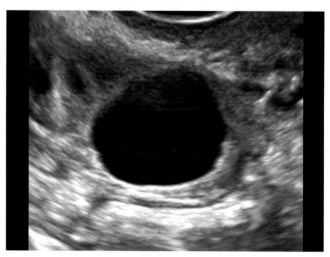

Fig. 5.1: B-mode ultrasound image of unilocular cyst with clear contents and thin walls.

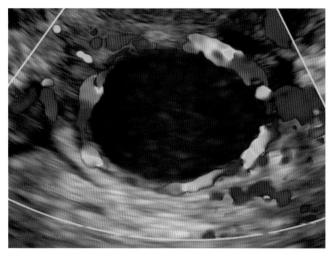

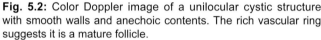

Fig. 5.2: Color Doppler image of a unilocular cystic structure with smooth walls and anechoic contents. The rich vascular ring suggests it is a mature follicle.

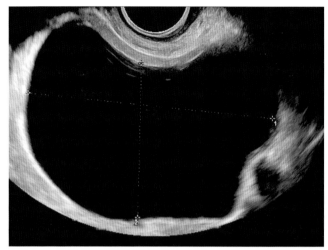

Fig. 5.3: Large intraovarian unilocular cyst—follicular cyst.

TABLE 5.1: Differential diagnosis of clear, nonseptated ovarian cystic lesions—(unilocular cystic lesions).

Feature	Follicle	Follicular cyst	Simple cyst
Size	Up to 24 mm	25 mm or larger	>25 mm, often >50 mm
Phase of cycle	Proliferative	Late proliferative or secretory	Any phase of the cycle
Vascularity	Low resistance ring of color	Scanty, high resistance	No flow
Natural course	Convert into corpus luteum	Regresses	Persists

follicle cannot be differentiated from simple cyst or follicular cyst. Simple cysts in the ovaries can be of any size but typically these are hormonally inactive and do not show any vascularity around. Unlike follicles, these cysts do not change the morphology or disappear even in luteal phase of the cycle. Another lesion that has a similar appearance is popularly known as a follicular cyst. When a follicle keeps on growing beyond 25 mm in diameter, it is usually called follicular cyst (Fig. 5.3). A follicle that gradually loses its sensitivity to follicle-stimulating hormone (FSH), the estrogen production is reduced from the granulosa cells of the same. This is when this follicular structure is known as follicular cyst. As is known that the perifollicular vascularity with the low-resistance flow of the follicle is correlated with estrogen production, the decreased estrogen production, evidently reflects as higher perifollicular flow resistance. Follicular cyst is a physiological cyst and has a tendency to regress in the course of time (4–6 weeks) (Table 5.1).

At this point, it is important to differentiate the ovarian from extraovarian lesions. The sliding organ sign[3] or the Timor-Tritsch sign differentiates between the ovarian and extraovarian lesions. On the scanner screen when the ovary and the lesion are seen adjacent to each other, the probe is pushed in and out pressing and de-pressing on the point of apposition of the lesion and the ovary (Fig. 5.4). If this maneuver separates the lesion from the ovary the lesion is extraovarian, but if this is not possible, the lesion may be intraovarian or extraovarian but adherent to the ovary. If the rim or a beak of ovarian tissue (Figs. 5.5A and B) is seen around the lesion, it is intraovarian, if not it is extraovarian but adherent to the ovary.

The extraovarian lesion that may mimic the ultrasound morphology of the follicle is paraovarian cyst (Fig. 5.6). As a rule uncomplicated paraovarian cyst is never adherent to any of the surrounding structures or does not show any internal echogenicities. If it does, then infection or rarely a malignant change is suspected in the paraovarian cyst. It must be remembered that uncomplicated paraovarian cysts are always avascular. If the vascularity is seen around the paraovarian cyst, strong suspicion of infection or malignancy arises. Though when paraovarian cyst is suspected, rotation of the probe is a must before confirmation of diagnosis. If this cystic lesion changes shape (elongates) on rotation of the probe it may be hydrosalpinx, and not a paraovarian cyst. Hydrosalpinx will be discussed later in this chapter.

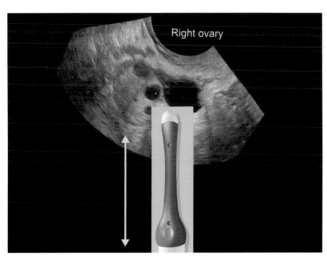

Fig. 5.4: Ultrasound image of a unilocular cystic lesion and closely placed ovary. The figure also shows positioning of the probe and the arrow shows the movement direction of the probe.

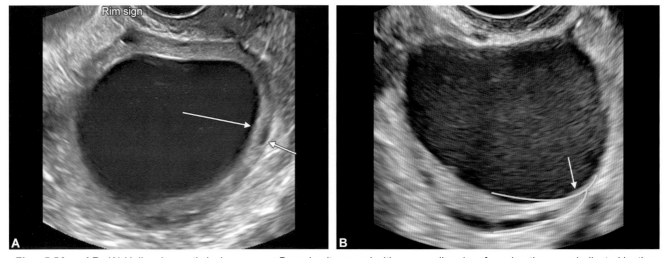

Figs. 5.5A and B: (A) Unilocular cystic lesion seen on B-mode ultrasound with surrounding rim of ovarian tissue as indicated by the arrows; (B) Unilocular cystic lesion with the beak of ovarian tissue outline by yellow line and marked by arrow.

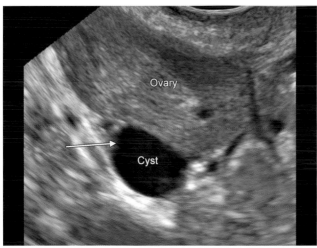

Fig. 5.6: Paraovarian cyst marked by arrow on the B-mode ultrasound image.

When multiple follicles have grown together, as it may happen in the patients on ovulation induction treatment, these may get placed close to each other, appear polygonal in shape and may also sometimes appear like a septated cystic lesion, with anechoic contents [multilocular cystic lesion (IOTA)]. On Doppler, blood flow is seen in the follicular walls, as seen in single follicle and this may be mistaken for multilocular cystic lesion with vascularity in septae (Fig. 5.7). Benign serous cystadenoma is an ovarian lesion that has very similar ultrasound morphology. Serous cystadenoma presents as multilocular cystic lesion in which the septae are thin and are typically avascular. Benign serous cystadenoma has walls, thinner than

3 mm in thickness, septae thinner than 3 mm, no internal echogenicities, no papillarities, and no solid projections[4] (Fig. 5.8). The vascularity is limited to the periphery and the resistance index (RI) of these vessels is always more than 0.5. Development of septal vascularity and internal echogenicities or papillarities may be the few earliest signs of conversion of this benign serous cystadenoma to malignant.

Very interestingly multiple nabothian cysts may appear like multiple follicles at times (Fig. 5.9). Of course confirming the organ of origin, will clear this confusion. Other extraovarian cystic lesion that has no internal echogenicities, but may have septae and mimic the above described lesions is peritoneal inclusion cyst (Fig. 5.10). It is extraovarian, irregular in shape, changes shape on probe pressure, has thin septae that are mobile, may have parietal papillae, appearing like papillarities and also may have one of the ovaries lying close to it, but typically shows no vascularity on Doppler. It typically has no floating bowel loops, unlike free fluid in pelvis (Fig. 5.11).

Unilocular or multilocular cystic structures may also show internal echogenicities. The physiological lesions in this group are corpus luteum, hemorrhagic cyst, and luteinized unruptured follicle. Corpus luteum is a thick-walled cystic structure with blood and blood products in the lumen. With the rupture of the follicle, the walls break and with that the vessels in the follicular wall rupture, resulting into hemorrhage (Fig. 5.12).

The lesions that appear similar on ultrasound are hemorrhagic cyst, luteinized unruptured follicle, and

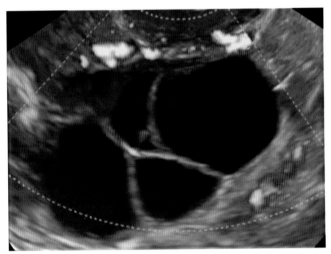

Fig. 5.7: Power Doppler ultrasound image showing multiple follicles mimicking multilocular cyst with blood flow in the follicular walls mimicking septal blood flow of multilocular lesion.

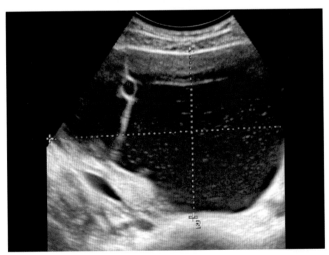

Fig. 5.8: Multilocular intraovarian cystic lesion with anechoic contents and thin septa—possibly benign serous cystadenoma.

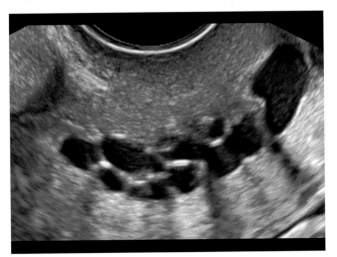

Fig. 5.9: B-mode ultrasound image showing multiple nabothian cysts.

endometriomas. Though infected simple cysts or infected paraovarian cysts may also appear similar to these lesions. These lesions have thick walls, at times shaggy. The contents have internal echogenicities, but no solid components or septae [unilocular cystic lesions with internal echogenicities (IOTA)]. Fibrin strands need to be differentiated from septae. On rotation of the probe, at some point of rotation, the concavity of the margins, also known as retraction sign, excludes the possibility of septum (Fig. 5.13). If a septum-like echogenicity on rotation of the probe shows concavity at least on one side it indicates that it is a retracted fibrin strand and is not a septum. These lesions may have debris. Solid projections need to be excluded in this group of lesions.

Debris can be differentiated form the solid components by in and out movement of the probe. This if leads to movement of the contents in relation to the cystic wall, it is debris, otherwise it is a solid component. More often, debris tends to settle dependent on gravity, whereas solid components have convex margins in the lumen (Figs. 5.14A and B).

Corpus luteum typically has thick, crenulated or shaggy isoechoic walls (Fig. 5.15). It is thought of first when this lesion is seen in the luteal phase of the cycle. Contents of the cyst show heterogeneous echogenicity with or without fibrin strands. This is described as a typical appearance of corpus luteum. But corpus luteum has variable appearances. The contents may have a fishnet appearance, ground-glass

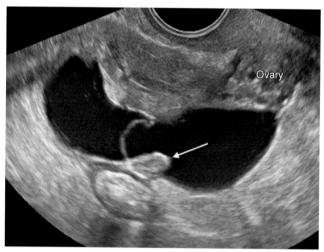

Fig. 5.10: Peritoneal inclusion cyst with curved septum, arrow showing parietal papilla and ovary is seen by the side of the cystic lesion.

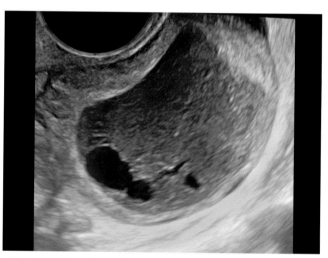

Fig. 5.12: B-mode image of corpus luteum with thick walls and hemorrhagic contents.

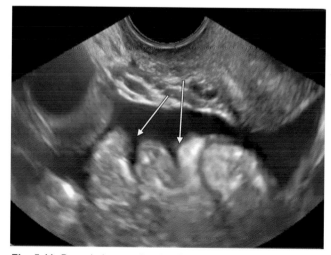

Fig. 5.11: B-mode image showing free fluid in pelvis with floating bowel loops as marked by the arrows.

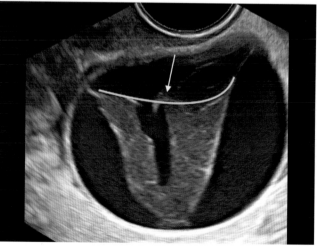

Fig. 5.13: B-mode image of retracted fibrin strand in a cystic lesion with hemorrhage inside.

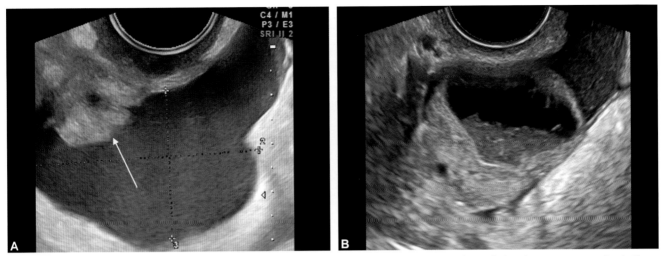

Figs. 5.14A and B: (A) B-mode image of a unilocular solid lesion with the solid component (arrow) showing convex margins in the lumen; (B) B-mode ultrasound image of a unilocular cystic lesion with echogenic debris settled posteriorly.

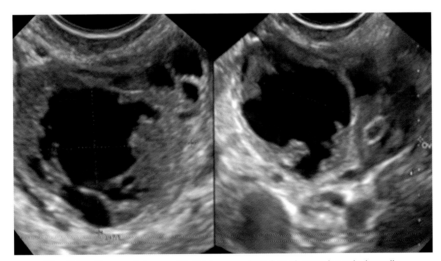

Fig. 5.15: Corpus luteum with thick, crenulated or shaggy isoechoic walls.

appearance (Figs. 5.16A and B) or may even show debris (Fig. 5.14B). The consistent feature of a healthy corpus luteum is low-resistance flow (RI < 0.5), with blood flows covering the corpus luteum almost completely (Fig. 5.17).

When such a lesion is seen in the proliferative phase, the possibility of hemorrhagic cyst is likely as the first possibility. As the name suggests it is a cyst containing blood, fresh or degenerated. It is usually a nonresolved hormonally inactive corpus luteum and therefore shows no flow or rarely very scanty and high resistance blood flow. Lace-like echo pattern (Fig. 5.18) is very typical of a hemorrhagic cyst but may show fibrin strands, ground-glass appearance or debris also, similar to corpus lutea. It changes its echogenicity over time due to fibrinolysis of the clot. Hemorrhagic cyst is a physiological cyst and has a tendency to regress and disappear in 4–6 weeks' time.[5]

The third intraovarian lesion in the same morphological group is luteinized unruptured follicle. It typically has thick but not shaggy walls. The walls of luteinized unruptured follicle are typically hyperechoic. Being an unruptured follicle the internal echogenicities are typically not like that of corpus luteum. There are no fibrin strands or fishnet appearance. It shows low level echogenicities (Fig. 5.19). On Doppler, the lesion shows peripheral vascularity with high resistance flow, with RI usually between 0.50 and 0.60.[6]

Endometrioma is an ovarian endometriosis. These may be bilateral and are typically tender on probe pressure. Endometriomas may have thick walls, often shaggy.

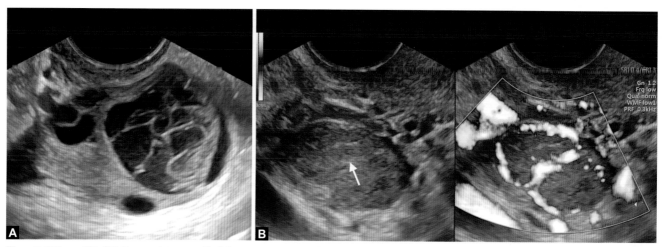

Figs. 5.16A and B: (A) Corpus luteum with fishnet appearance; (B) Corpus luteum with ground-glass appearance as marked by arrow.

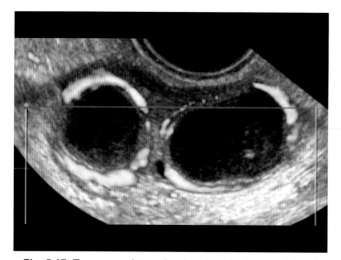

Fig. 5.17: Two corpus lutea showing ring of color—peripheral vascularity on high-definition flow.

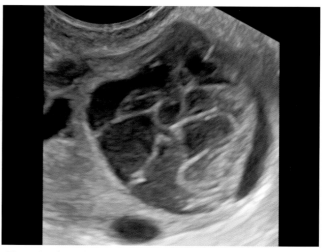

Fig. 5.18: Lace-like echo pattern of hemorrhagic cyst on B-mode ultrasound.

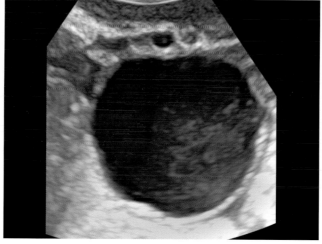

Fig. 5.19: Luteinized unruptured follicle—low level echogenicities.

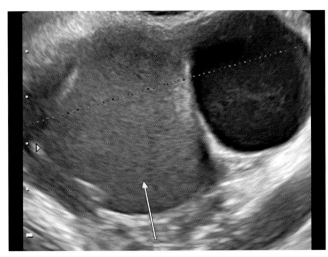

Fig. 5.20: Endometrioma on B-mode ultrasound with ground-glass echogenicities.

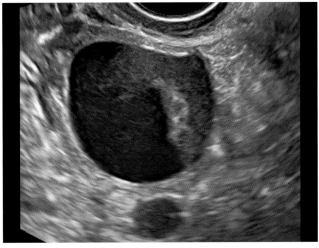

Fig. 5.22: Endometrioma showing fluid of different echogenicities—layering effect.

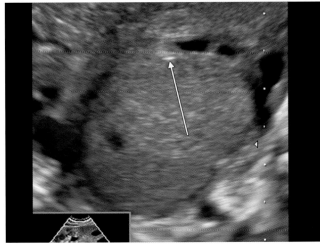

Fig. 5.21: Endometrioma with ground-glass echogenicity and hyperechoic flecks in the wall, marked by arrow.

Of course ground-glass is the appearance typically described for endometriomas (Fig. 5.20) and is due to thick chocolate sauce-like contents in the cyst, but interestingly at least 40% of endometriomas may not have a typical appearance. Hyperechoic flecks are typically seen in the walls and are thought to be due to hemosiderin or cholesterol deposits[7] (Fig. 5.21). Blood clots may appear like solid components at times. The degenerated blood products and fresh bleed from the endometrial lining in the cyst lead to layering effect (Fig. 5.22). This results in a vertical fluid level seen on longitudinal scan, that typically has echogenic fluid layer posteriorly and anechoic layer anteriorly.[8] Though this appearance may disappear on rotation of the probe or may also not be seen on transabdominal scan.

Dynamic examination is very important for the diagnosis of endometriomas. As described earlier, probe movement may cause pain, when pressed on the lesion. These lesions are often fixed or adherent to surrounding structures and show negative sliding organ sign. The probe movement in relation to the lesion also leads to movements in the chocolate sauce-like thick fluid content of the endometrioma, leading to acoustic streaming sign. Though acoustic streaming cannot discriminate reliably between endometriomas and other adnexal lesions.[9] Scattered vascularity at ovarian hilus with moderate vascular impedance has been described in endometriomas. The ovarian hilar RI varies between 0.40 and 0.56. It is higher during menstruation and in symptomatic patients.[10]

Avascular lesions indicate scarification and are less convenient for delivery of medication and therefore should be considered for surgical therapy.[11] Kurjak et al. have shown a sensitivity of 83.9%, specificity of 97.1%, positive predictive value (PPV) 82%, and negative predictive value (NPV) 97.5% of vaginal sonography for characterization of endometriomas. If cancer antigen (CA)-125 more than 35 IU/mL, it was added as a cut off to these parameters, the sensitivity and specificity reached 99.04% and 99.64%, and PPV and NPV reached 98.10% and 99.82%.[11] Similar results were also confirmed by several other workers.

Endometriomas typically show short coursed vessels. The vessels are seen approaching the lesion wall, but do not run long with the wall (Fig. 5.23). These vessels show variable resistance depending on the phase of the menstrual cycle. These vessels show low resistance vascularity (RI 0.4) in menstrual period but is high (RI 0.4–0.56) in preovulatory

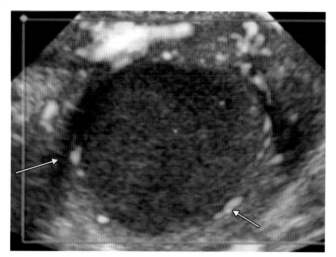

Fig. 5.23: High-definition flow showing short coursed vessels as marked by arrows.

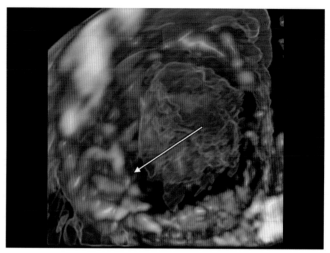

Fig. 5.24: 3D power Doppler image of endometrioma, showing criss-crossing of the vessels—bird's nest appearance.

TABLE 5.2: Ovarian lesions with thick walls and internal echogenicities.

Feature	Corpus luteum	Luteinized unruptured follicle (LUF)	Hemorrhagic cyst	Endometrioma
Walls	Thick, isoechoic, shaggy	Thick, hyperechoic	Thick, isoechoic shaggy	Thick, isoechoic shaggy, hyperechoic flecks
Contents	Fishnet, fibrin stands, ground glass, isoechoic, solid debris	Low level echoes	Fishnet, fibrin stands, ground glass, isoechoic, solid debris	Ground glass, fluid level, solid looking debris, fibrin strands, fishnet
Vascularity	Ring of color, low resistance	High resistance, not abundant	No vascularity	Short coursed vessels
Phase of cycle	Luteal	Luteal	Proliferative	Any phase

and secretory period. More vascular the lesion is, better is the response to medical line of treatment. 3D power Doppler shows a well-perfused lesion with regularly placed vessels with a short course, with minimal variability in diameter. This gives a "bird's nest" appearance[12] (Fig. 5.24).

When a patient with endometrioma gets pregnancy, there is a possibility that the endometrial lining in the cyst also undergo decidualization and in that case, the endometrial lining may get thickened and may also show solid projections. These projections show marked vascularity and may mimic malignancy (Table 5.2).

Ovarian ectopic though rare may present as similar lesions. This is a roundish mass with thick walls and gestational sac seen as an anechoic center. If it shows presence of yolk sac and/or fetal pole, it is easy to diagnose. When these are not seen, it appears very similar to corpus luteum both on B mode and also on Doppler due to its ring of vascularity with low resistance. It is the hyperechogenicity of the lesion walls, due to decidual reaction (Fig. 5.25),

along with the history of missed period and positive urine pregnancy test or high serum beta-human chorionic gonadotropin (hCG) levels that may be indicative. Tenderness on probe pressure, minimal free fluid and spotting or fainting attacks may be additional supportive signs. Indirect signs of ectopic pregnancy may be seen in uterus as a thickened endometrium with decidual reaction at times, but typically showing symmetrical thickness of endometrial leaves (Fig. 5.26). In an intrauterine pregnancy, the endometrial leaves have asymmetrical thickness. Apart from diagnosis, Doppler plays an important role in deciding the conservative or medical line of management and follow-up in cases of ectopic pregnancy.

Apart from these lesions, ovaries and adnexa may present with inflammatory lesions and neoplasms. Ovaries are also likely to undergo hyperstimulation and torsion or rarely torsion of the fallopian tube is also known.

The inflammatory lesions in the ovaries and adnexa may be acute or chronic.

Acute inflammation of the ovary acute oophoritis is almost always a consequence of acutely inflamed fallopian tube, acute salpingitis and/or pelvic inflammatory disease (PID). PID usually presents as free fluid in the pelvis that is usually anechoic but in presence of fulminant infection and pus formation, it may show low level echogenicities (Fig. 5.27). In case of this being blood the low level echogenicities in the fluid may also be seen with thin linear freely mobile echogenicities due to fibrin bands (Fig. 5.28). Though it is very important to mention here that some amount of free fluid in the pelvis is normal in periovulatory period of the menstrual cycle, that may be due to high estrogen levels or fresh rupture of the follicle. The fluid then may persist till the late luteal phase. Retrograde menstruation may also show fluid in the pelvis during early proliferative phase.

Acute PID though may present with systemic signs of inflammation and also with pain on probe pressure at the site of primary inflammation that may be ovary or the tube. Acute salpingitis, though is not always easy to diagnose, and close observation of the adnexal soft tissue band extending from the uterus to the ovary may aid in the diagnosis of the same (Fig. 5.29). Thickening of this band to more than 10 mm, when measured perpendicular to its long axis, may be the clue. This is due to thickening of the tubal walls in acute inflammation. Thickened tubes can also be

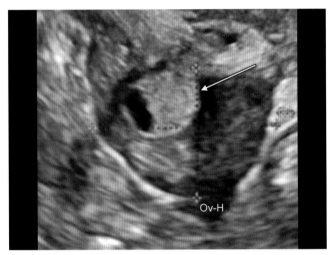

Fig. 5.25: B-mode ultrasound image of the ovary with ovarian ectopic pregnancy.

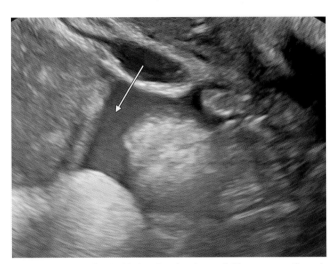

Fig. 5.27: Free fluid with low level echogenicities, suggestive of thick fluid may be pus.

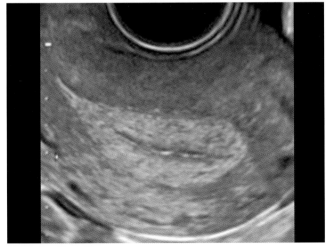

Fig. 5.26: B-mode image of the uterus, showing hyperechoic secretory endometrium with symmetrical leaves of endometrium.

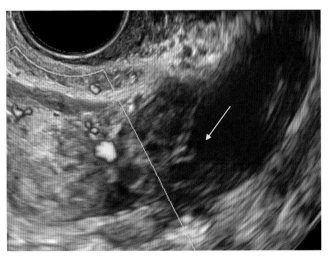

Fig. 5.28: Free fluid with low level echogenicities and also thin linear echogenicities—fibrin strands, suggesting blood in pelvis.

documented when there is free fluid around. This soft tissue band normally consists of tube, vessels, and ligaments and therefore normally shows vessels, running parallel to its long axis on color Doppler. In case of inflammation, color Doppler will show small vessels, in a direction, not parallel to the long axis of the adnexal soft tissue band (Figs. 5.30A and B). These vessels typically show RI less than 0.5, due to inflammatory neoangiogenesis.

Acute oophoritis leads to mild enlargement of the ovary due to edema, but this is difficult to document if the ovary was not measured earlier, or may also be because the size of the ovary changes in the different phases of the cycle due to development of follicles or corpus luteum or their regression. Though more reliable ultrasound sign may be hypoechoic ovarian stroma (in relation to normal myometrium) and in severe edema, follicles may be pushed to the periphery (Fig. 5.31). On color Doppler the stroma shows abundant vascularity with low-resistance flow (RI < 0.5) (Fig. 5.32). This can be differentiated from polycystic ovaries where the ovarian stroma shows abundant vascularity, by the fact that patients with polycystic ovaries typically show hyperechoic stroma.

Inflammation of the tube and marked thickening of the tubal walls may lead to tubal obstruction and collection of the tubal secretions in the tubal lumen, leading to hydrosalpinx. Hydrosalpinx may also be a result of involvement of the tubal fimbria in the inflammatory process and formation of adhesions. Hydrosalpinx may present differently on B-mode ultrasound, depending on its severity and acute or chronic nature. Especially in acute inflammations, it may have thick walls that may be appreciated on long axis as tubular lesions with anechoic fluid content and thick irregular walls, due to thickened haustra (Fig. 5.33). On transverse section this gives "cog wheel" appearance as the thickened haustra then appears like papillarities (Fig. 5.34). On color Doppler the walls show low resistance vascularity (RI < 0.5) (Fig. 5.35). With marked distention of the tubes due to hydrosalpinx, the tubes on transverse section may appear like an extraovarian cystic lesion that may need to be differentiated from paraovarian cyst. On rotation of the probe this leads to change in shape of the lesion. It may show a beak-like projection or may elongate to make a sausage-shaped lesion. This is typical of a hydrosalpinx (Fig. 5.36). Another typical ultrasound sign of

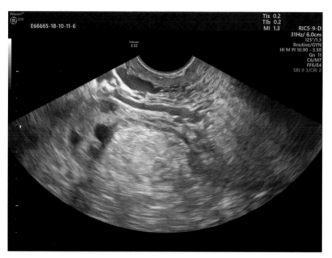

Fig. 5.29: B-mode ultrasound showing adnexal soft tissue band on transverse section.

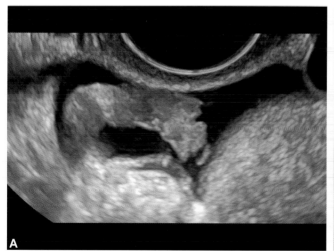

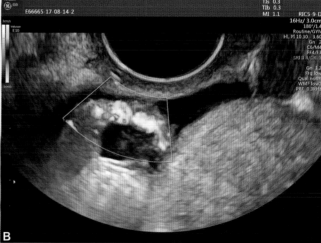

Figs. 5.30A and B: (A) B-mode ultrasound image showing free fluid in pelvis with thickened fallopian tube suggestive of acute salpingitis; (B) High-definition Doppler showing marked vascularity with blood vessels-oriented perpendicular to its long axis.

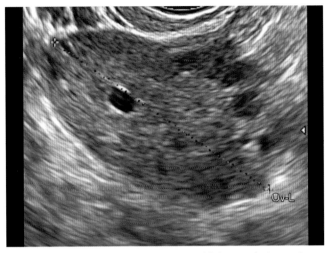

Fig. 5.31: B-mode ultrasound image with hypoechoic ovarian stroma.

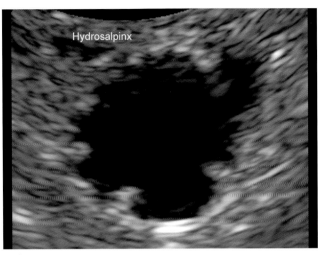

Fig. 5.34: Transverse section of hydrosalpinx—cog wheel appearance.

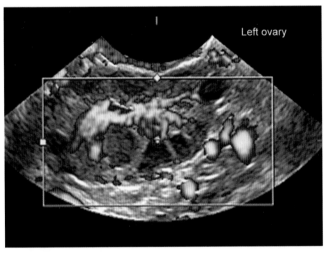

Fig. 5.32: Power Doppler showing hypervascularity in this ovary.

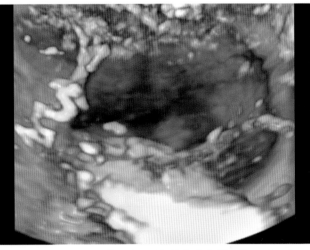

Fig. 5.35: 3D power Doppler with high-definition flow showing hypervascularity in an acute hydrosalpinx.

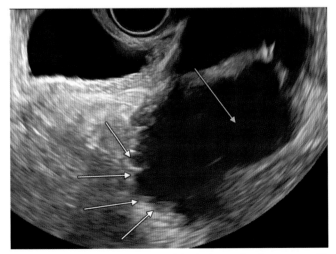

Fig. 5.33: Cystic lesion (hydrosalpinx) shown by the arrow with irregular margins as marked by white arrows due to thickened haustra.

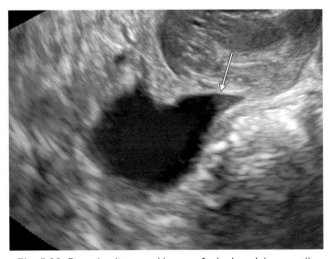

Fig. 5.36: B-mode ultrasound image of a hydrosalpinx—cystic lesion with beak-like projection as marked by arrow.

hydrosalpinx is incomplete septum (Fig. 5.37). Though the later two features may be seen in bowel loop. It is peristalsis seen in the bowel loop that can be used as a differentiating sign. The iliac vessels are large comparatively and also are seen as round structures on transverse section and elongate on rotation of the probe (Fig. 5.38). Doppler is the modality to differentiate the two. Though it is important to remember that with large hydrosalpinx, due to movement of the fluid in it sometimes, Doppler may show color and care must be taken not to misinterpret this as a vessel. Acute salpingitis is often associated with ascites.

Inflammations, involving both, fallopian tube and ovary, may lead to adhesion of the two and formation of tubo-ovarian mass (Fig. 5.39). The ovary and the tube may be identified separately but cannot be separated from each other. Whereas at times the inflammation may be more severe and the tubal and ovarian margins cannot be identified. There is disruption of the normal anatomical structure of both and this is a tubo-ovarian abscess (Fig. 5.40). Tubo-ovarian abscess is a complex mass with cystic and solid components with variable degree of vascularity seen on color or power Doppler. The resistance of these vessels may be variable. This depends on whether these are pre-existing vessels or are neoangiogenesis of inflammation and also depending on whether the inflammation is acute or chronic. Chronic inflammations are more commonly associated with adhesions and therefore it is important to establish the mobility of uterus, ovaries, and bowel in each case.

When endometrioma is present in the ovary or there is an evidence of endometriosis, the hydrosalpinx may be suspected due to the extension of endometriosis. Hydrosalpinx is considered a soft marker of endometriosis.[13] And hydrosalpinx may also be due to adhesions as a result of previous surgeries.

Ovarian hyperstimulation is a commonly found condition in today's era of assisted reproductive techniques (ARTs). Usually, it is as a result of high doses of gonadotropins used for ovulation induction, but rarely it is also seen as a result of hyper-response to clomiphene citrate stimulation. Development of multiple follicles, leading to longest ovarian diameter of more than 10 cm is considered as ovarian hyperstimulation. Hormonal derangement and overproduction of ovarian vasoactive substances from the enlarged ovaries with multiple follicles lead to a state of hyperpermeability with increased secretion of vascular endothelial growth factor (VEGF) leading to the manifestations of ovarian hyperstimulation syndrome (OHSS). It is especially feared of in patients with more

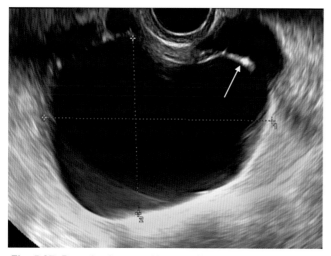

Fig. 5.37: B-mode ultrasound image of a large cystic lesion with incomplete septum—hydrosalpinx.

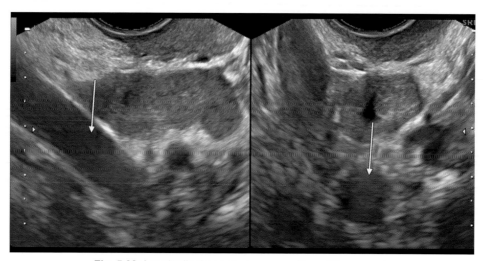

Fig. 5.38: Longitudinal and transverse section of iliac vessel.

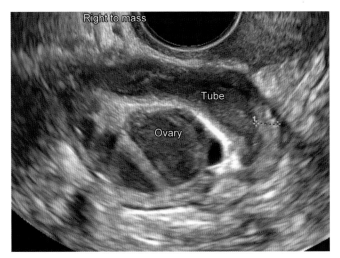

Fig. 5.39: B-mode ultrasound image of the tubo-ovarian mass.

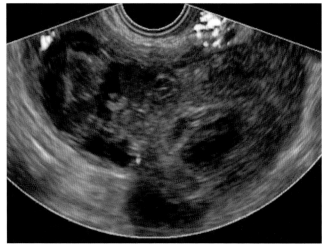

Fig. 5.40: Tubo-ovarian abscess—tubal and ovarian anatomy cannot be identified separately and the mass shows multiple cystic areas and septa.

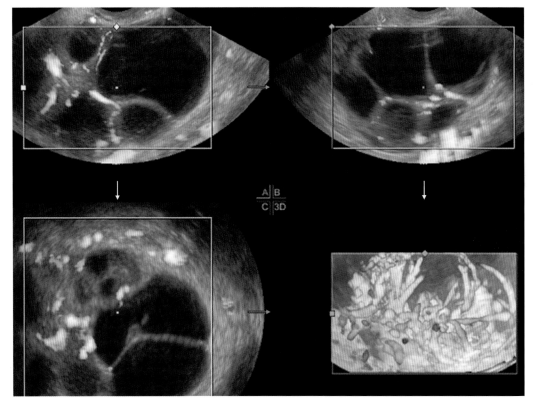

Fig. 5.41: 3D power Doppler with high-definition flow image of the hyperstimulated ovary showing marked vascularity.

number of antral follicles and especially with more ovarian stromal vascularity on the base line scan.[14] This indicates that a Doppler study of the ovaries on the baseline scan can be a useful tool to predict and therefore prevent OHSS. Patients having ovarian stromal RI less than 0.5, stromal peak systolic velocity (PSV) of more than 10 cm/sec[15] or ovarian stromal flow index (FI) more than 15[16] have higher risk of developing OHSS. Ovaries with multiple medium or small follicles on the pretrigger scan have a higher risk of OHSS. Longest ovarian diameter of more than 10 cm is a hyperstimulated ovary, either on pretrigger scan or in the luteal phase. These are hypervascular ovaries (Fig. 5.41), though there are no definite cut offs to define the vascular parameters in ovaries for OHSS.

Coasting is one of the modes of treatment in patients with hyperstimulated ovaries. Before the ovarian size decreases as a result of coasting, the vascularity decreases and this may be confirmed by increasing perifollicular RI and also by decrease in ovarian vascularization index (VI) and vascularization flow index (VFI). Though the Doppler studies are of importance in OHSS to confirm its regressing state and also to suspect or diagnose torsion. Ovaries in OHSS are large and therefore have a higher tendency to develop torsion. Patients with torsion have acute abdominal pain, nausea, vomiting, etc. that may be of help to clinically suspect torsion, though these are also present in patients with OHSS. Thus, sudden decrease in the vascular signals in the hyperstimulated ovary with the above mentioned symptoms may be of help in suspecting torsion. Patients with OHSS when are on treatment, supportive or definitive (gonadotropin-releasing hormone antagonist), decreasing vascularity in the form of increasing resistance or decreasing VI and VFI may be important parameters to assure the treatment is effective.

Ovarian Neoplasms

Ovarian neoplasms may be divided under four groups, depending on their origin:
1. Epithelial tumors
2. Germ cell tumors
3. Sex cord-stromal tumors
4. Metastatic tumors.

Epithelial Tumors

These are the most common group (about 85%) of tumors found in the ovaries. Their origin is mesothelium of the ovary (surface epithelium), invaginated in the stroma. The subcategories in this group are serous, mucinous, endometrioid, clear cell, Brenner's and undifferentiated tumors. These tumors may be benign, borderline or malignant.

- *Serous epithelial tumors (serous cystadenoma),* when benign, may be unilocular or multilocular. When multilocular, the locules are usually fewer. The septae are thin and smooth. These tumors have less than 3 papillae [solid projections arising from the wall or septum, that are <3 mm in height (IOTA)]. The contents are anechoic. Benign lesions do not show any solid projections and show minimal vascularity (score 1/2).[1]
  - *Serous cystadenofibroma*: These tumors have epithelial and fibrous stromal component. These tumors are rarely malignant. These tumors have a very typical ultrasound appearance. These cystic tumors have one or more papillary projection with acoustic shadowing (Fig. 5.42).

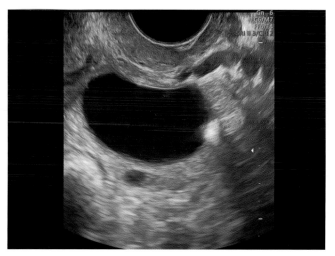

Fig. 5.42: Cystic lesion with a solid component with posterior shadow—possibly cystadenofibroma.

- *Brenner's tumors*: These also are most often benign. They may appear solid and may show dystrophic calcification with posterior shadowing (Fig. 5.43).
- *The borderline tumors* show thicker walls and septae. Septae may show irregularities and papillarities. These tumors may show psammoma bodies. These are concentric, lamellated, calcified looking structures (less dense than calcification with no posterior shadowing). The calcified areas may appear like microcalcifications (Fig. 5.44).
- *Malignant serous tumors* show more septae that are thick and irregular, and show papillarities, more than 3 in number. It may show solid projections with flow seen in the solid projections on Doppler, especially in malignant serous adenocarcinomas. The fluid in these complex lesions may have low level echogenicities and ascites may also be present (Fig. 5.45). Endometrioid and clear cell tumors are more often malignant and may also be associated with pelvic endometriosis. Endometrioid tumors also lead to endometrial growth and endometrial carcinoma in about 30% of the patients.
- *Mucinous epithelial tumors*:
  - *Benign mucinous cystadenoma*: These are large multilocular tumors with rigid bright septae. The cystic contents may have variable echogenicity. These tumors may show vascularity in the wall and septae and so are difficult to differentiate from the malignant serous tumors (Fig. 5.46).
  - *Borderline mucinous tumors*: These tumors typically show cluster of tiny locules, often in one part of the tumor. This may appear like a solid lesion with multiple small anechoic areas. This component of the tumor shows vascularity (Fig. 5.47).

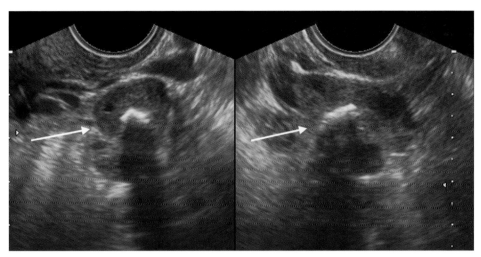

Fig. 5.43: Solid ovarian tumor with calcification and posterior shadowing—Brenner's tumor.

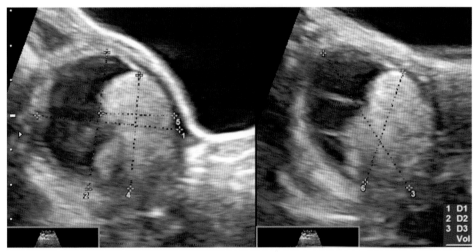

Fig. 5.44: Ovarian mass with cystic lesion with septa and solid echogenic projections—possibly serous borderline tumor.

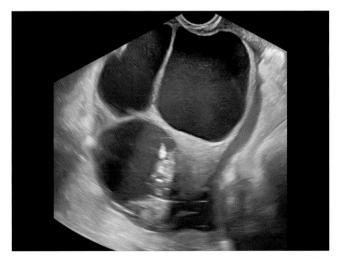

Fig. 5.45: Multiloculated ovarian tumor, cystic component showing fluid with low level echoes and solid component with ascites—malignant serous cystadenoma.

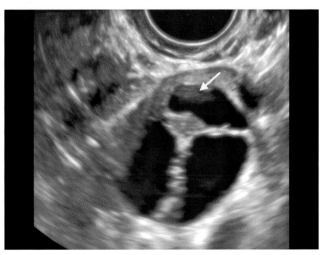

Fig. 5.46: Multilocular tumor with thick septa and tiny papillarities (arrow)—possibly benign mucinous cystadenoma.

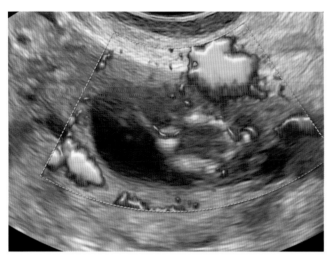

Fig. 5.47: Mucinous borderline tumor—complex tumor with septated cystic component, typically show cluster of tiny locules, often in one part of the tumor. This may appear like a solid lesion with multiple small anechoic areas. Power Doppler shows vascularity.

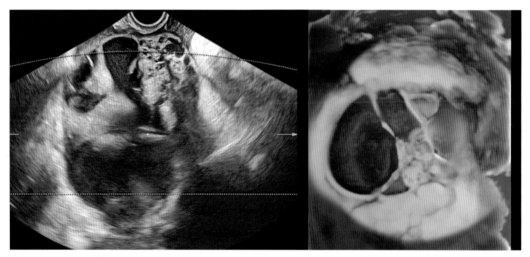

Fig. 5.48: Typical complex malignant ovarian tumor on B-mode and 3D ultrasound.

– *The malignant counter part* of these tumors may also show solid projections and vascularity with a score of 3–4. Like with malignant serous tumors, even the mucinous tumors, when malignant, may show ascites and the peritoneal fluid may also show low level echogenicities (Fig. 5.48).

Germ Cell Tumors

These tumors arise from primordial germ cells and are more often seen in young females. The tumors in this group may be dermoids (mature teratomas), immature teratomas, dysgerminoma, yolk sac tumor, and choriocarcinoma. The only benign tumor in this group is dermoid.

Dermoids: These are typically benign lesions with cystic and solid components. Since it is originated from totipotent cells, the contents of the lesion may vary. It may be fluid, fat, hair, bone, or any other tissues. On ultrasound, it therefore shows hypoechoic and echogenic components. The cyst may show bright scattered linear echoes or bright dots, due to hair (Fig. 5.49A). It may show bony or tooth-like components with posterior shadowing (Fig. 5.49B). Combination of hair and sebaceous material will show ball-like echogenic structures in the cyst (Fig. 5.49C). These cysts typically show echogenic fluid (fat floating over the fluid contents of the cyst) anteriorly and anechoic fluid posteriorly (Fig. 5.49D). This appearance may be described as fluid-fluid level. Dermoid may appear like solid looking round echogenic lesion of various sizes (Fig. 5.49E). Smaller lesions or hyperechogenic areas may show posterior shadowing. Larger lesions may appear like snow balls (Fig. 5.49F) and the posterior margins of the

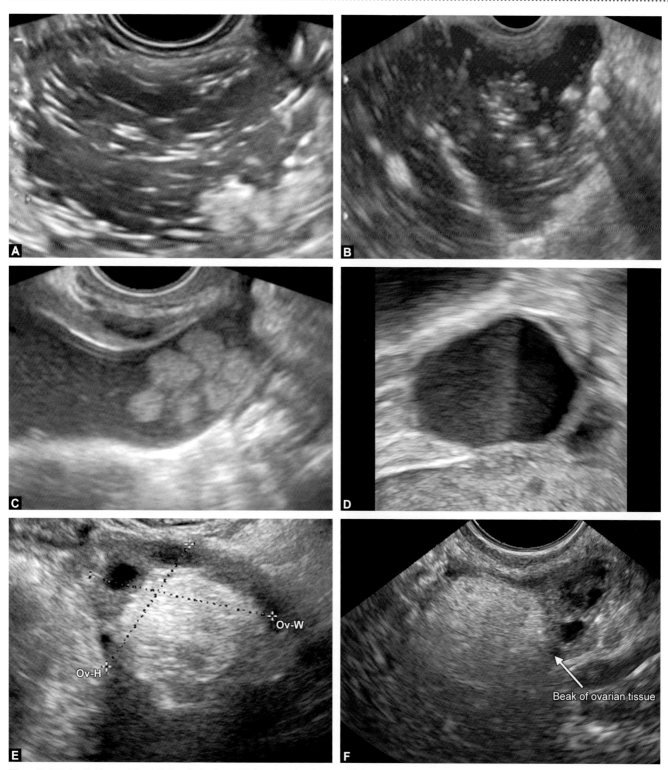

Figs. 5.49A to F: Dermoids. (A) Cystic lesion with low level echoes with hyperechoic lines and dots; (B) Cystic lesion with hyperechoic lines and teeth-like shadows with posterior shadowing; (C) Cystic lesion with hair balls; (D) Cystic lesion with fluid–fluid level, echogenic fluid anteriorly and anechoic fluid posteriorly; (E) Hyperechoic ovarian mass with and posterior shadowing; (F) Hyperechoic roundish mass with ill-defined posterior margins of the mass and beak sign of ovarian tissue (arrow).

same may not be identifiable. This is described as "tip of the iceberg sign". This may mimic bowel gas but the intraovarian origin of the lesion, confirmed by beak or rim of ovarian tissue (Fig. 5.49F), differentiates the two. Solid components of the dermoid are called Rokitansky's tubercles. At times a hair mesh (dermoid mesh) may be seen radiating out from this in dermoids. Dermoids are avascular or may show minimal vascularity. These are bilateral in about 10–15% of cases. Combination of transabdominal and transvaginal scans may be required for large dermoids. Torsions are common in ovaries with dermoids.

Malignant germ cell tumors: As is known that germ cell tumors arise from totipotent cells, even the malignant versions may have several cell types. These are usually unilateral. The most common in this group is dysgerminoma. These on ultrasound are solid tumors, smooth or lobulated. The

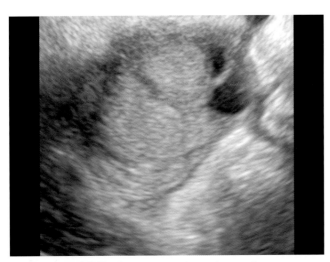

Fig. 5.50: Solid septated lesion—dysgerminoma.

solid mass often looks like it is septated (Fig. 5.50). Though often homogeneous, it may also show heterogeneous echogenicity. Doppler shows high vascularity. The yolk sac tumors may show high alpha-fetoprotein levels. Choriocarcinomas may show high hCG levels.

Sex Cord-stromal Tumors

These are typically solid tumors arising from ovarian stromal (theca and granulosa) cells and the tumors in this class are granulosa cell tumors, Sertoli-Leydig cell tumors, fibroma or fibrothecoma. These are the tumors usually of the postmenopausal age or prepubertal age.

- *Granulosa cell tumor* is typically estrogen-producing tumor. May cause endometrial hyperplasia, but in rare cases may also progress into endometrial carcinoma. It may be a cause of precocious puberty in prepubertal girls. Though usually slow growing, these have a malignant potential. These solid tumors on ultrasound have heterogeneous echogenicity and show anechoic areas in solid lesion (Swiss cheese appearance). Being malignant shows a vascular score of 3 or 4.
- *Sertoli and Sertoli-Leydig cell tumors*: Depending on the predominance of the cell type, these tumors may produce androgen, progesterone or estrogen. These are solid or multilocular tumors with solid components, with high vascularity. Leydig cell tumors though are usually small and can often be missed.
- *Fibroma and fibrothecoma*: These have similar ultrasound appearance. These are well-defined, round, oval or lobulated solid mass. Usually, these masses do not show cystic spaces, but some may. These tumors typically have an ultrasound appearance similar to that of a fibroid, including the edge shadows (Fig. 5.51). The

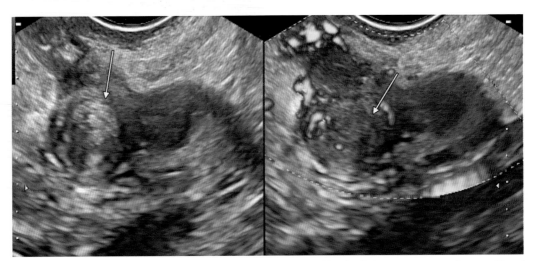

Fig. 5.51: Ovarian fibroma on B-mode showing isoechoic stroma with whorled appearance and power Doppler.

vascular pattern is also peripheral, like that in fibroids, but may be higher in fibrothecoma. When large fibromas may be associated with fluid in peritoneal, pleural and pericardial cavities, is called Meigs syndrome.

CONCLUSION

The physiological lesions and those arising out of physiology-related abnormalities can be confidently differentiated and diagnosed by the morphology and the vascular studies by Doppler. Doppler has a very important role In diagnosis and post-treatment follow-up of inflammatory lesions, OHSS, and ectopic pregnancies. Though certain neoplasms have typical appearance like serous cystadenoma, serous cystadenofibroma, dysgerminoma, fibromas, and borderline tumors, but for most others ultrasound even with Doppler cannot confidently diagnose the pathology. Though it is true that Doppler plays a very important role for assessing the growth potential or malignant nature of these lesions.

REFERENCES

1. Timmerman D, Valentin L, Bourne TH, et al. Terms, definitions and measurements to describe the sonographic features of adnexal tumours: a consensus opinion from international ovarian tumour analysis group. Ultrasound Obstet Gynecol. 2000;16:500-5.
2. Kupesic S, Kurjak. Uterine and ovarian perfusion during the periovulatory period assessed by transvaginal color Doppler. Fertil Steril. 1993;3:439-43.
3. Timor Tritsch IE. Sliding organs sign in gynecological ultrasound. Ultrasound Obstet Gynecol. 2016;46:124-7.
4. Campbell S. Ovarian cancer: role of ultrasound in pre-operative diagnosis and population screening. Ultrasound Obstet Gynecol. 2012;40:245-54.
5. Osmers R. Sonographic evaluation of ovarian masses and its therapeutic implications. Ultrasound Obstet Gynecol. 1996;8:217-22.
6. Kupesic S, Kurjak A. The assessment of normal and abnormal luteal function by transvaginal color Doppler sonography. Eur J Obstet Gynecol. 1997;72:83-7.
7. Patel MD, Feldstern VA, Chen DC, et al. Endometriomas: diagnostic performances of US. Radiology. 1999;210:739-45.
8. Asch E, Levine D. Variations in appearance of endometriomas. J Ultrasound Med. 2007;26(8):993-1002.
9. Van Holsbeke C, Zhang J, Van Bello V, et al. Acoustic streaming cannot discriminate reliably between endometriomas and other types of adnexal lesion: a multicenter study of 633 adnexal masses. Ultrasound Obstet Gynecol. 2010;35:349-53.
10. Alcazar JL. Transvaginal colour Doppler in patients with ovarian endometriomas and pelvic pain. Hum Reprod. 2001;16(12):2672-5.
11. Kurjak A, Kupesic S. Scoring system for prediction of ovarian endometriosis based on transvaginal colour and pulsed Doppler sonography. Fertil Steril. 1994;62(1):81-8.
12. N Raine-Fenning, Jayaprakasan K, Deb S. Three-dimensional ultrasonographic characteristics of endometriomata. Ultrasound Obstet Gynecol. 2008;31:718-24.
13. Okaro E, Condous G, Khalid A, et al. The use of ultrasound-based 'soft-markers' for the prediction of pelvic pathology in women with chronic pelvic pain-can we reduce the need for laparoscopy? BJOG. 2006;113(3):251-6.
14. Engmann L, P Sladkevicius, Agrawal R, et al. Value of ovarian stromal blood flow velocity measurement after pituitary suppression in the prediction of ovarian responsiveness and outcome of in vitro fertilization treatment. Fertil Steril. 1999;71(1):22-9.
15. Panchal S, Nagori C. Baseline scan and ultrasound diagnosis of PCOS. Donald School Journal of Ultrasound in Obstetrics and Gynecology. 2012;6(3):290-9.
16. Kupesic S, Kurjak A. Predictors of IVF outcome by three-dimensional ultrasound. Hum Reprod. 2002;17(4):950-5.

Understanding Reproductive Endocrinology by Doppler

INTRODUCTION

Female reproductive system in humans is a finely balanced highly dynamic hormonal system. Hormones behave differently in different phases of cycle and their action also changes with change in the environment (other hormones and biochemicals in circulation) and lead to changes in ovarian and uterine morphology and vascularity that can be effectively studied by B-mode ultrasound, Doppler, and to some extent by three-dimensional (3D) ultrasound and 3D power Doppler also. The vascular changes precede the morphological changes. Correlating the morphological and vascular changes with their physiological and hormonal basis can interpret the hormonal changes occurring during the menstrual cycle.

To understand the hormonal changes more clearly, and their ultrasound correlation also, we shall divide the discussion into three phases of the menstrual cycle. These are the phases when specific hormonal investigations are asked for. These phases are the early proliferative phase—days 2–3, and the scan done at that stage is called baseline scan. The second phase is the preovulatory phase, preovulatory, or pretrigger scan depending on the follicular maturity and the third is the mid-luteal phase—mid-luteal scan, that is about 8 days after ovulation.

The hormones of major interest on the baseline scan are:

- Androgen
- Anti-Müllerian hormone (AMH)
- Follicle-stimulating hormone (FSH)
- Luteinizing hormone (LH)
- Estrogen
- Progesterone.

Of course, other hormones like thyroid and prolactin also have an impact on fertility and it is insulin resistance (IR) that may also be of concern. Though, our ultrasound knowledge is still limited on interpreting the effects of thyroid and prolactin on the reproductive organs in different phases of menstrual cycle.

ANDROGEN

The menstrual cycle starts on 1st day of the menstruation. Recruitment of the follicles from preantral to primary antral starts in the late luteal phase of the previous cycle. Recruitment of the secondary antral follicles starts from day 1 of the menstrual cycle. The antral follicles of 2–9 mm in size are identifiable on ultrasound. Though with the more sensitive high end ultrasound scanners, follicles as small as 1 mm can also be identified by ultrasound. Recruitment of these follicles is a function of androgen, and antral follicle count (AFC) represents the functional ovarian reserve. Higher androgen level would lead to more follicles being converted from preantral to antral and so higher AFC.[1] It is for this reason that, patients with polycystic ovarian syndrome (PCOS), who have hyperandrogenemia, show higher AFC as compared to controls (Figs. 6.1A to C). Though low AFC cannot be directly correlated to low androgen level. Instead, it is a marker of poor ovarian reserve.

What Happens in Polycystic Ovarian Syndrome Patients?

High basal androgen levels in the PCOS patients lead to recruitment of more antral follicles. As follicles grow to a size of 6–7 mm, these develop FSH receptors and then may

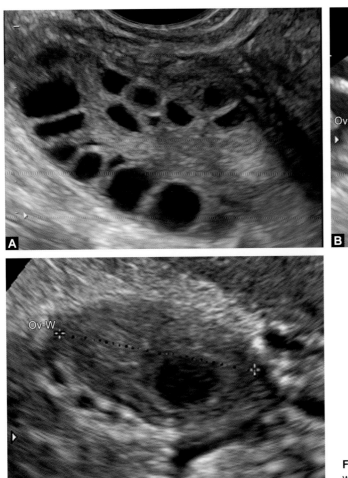

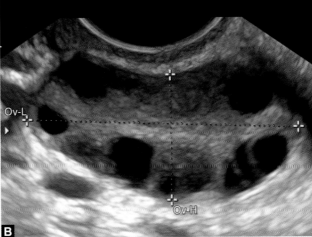

Figs. 6.1A to C: B-mode images of the ovary. (A) Polycystic ovary with multiple antral follicles; (B) Normal ovary; and (C) Low reserve ovary with only one follicle.

not grow beyond that size without FSH. The granulosa cells of these follicles produce low levels of estrogen. The excess androgen in the PCOS patients is also converted to estrogen by aromatization. Both these combinely lead to rise in estrogen levels even in the absence of a single dominant or mature follicle. Due to increasing estrogen levels, the FSH rise is dampened or may also be stopped in some cases, depending on the levels of estrogen. This prevents follicular growth but also stimulates LH secretion, which leads to follicular atresia of the follicles due to conversion of granulosa cells into theca cells (two-hormone two-cell theory).[2] Follicular atresia leads to anovulation and increase in the theca cell population that leads to increased stroma. *Thus, more androgen levels in PCOS patients are indicated by more antral follicles.* But it is interesting to know that this follicular excess is ultimately controlled by insulin. Obesity and IR may enhance follicular excess by dysregulation of AMH through pathway of hyperandrogenemia.[3] In turn, follicular excess causes excess estrogen, high LH, anovulation, and increased stroma. AFC and ovarian

volume showed significant correlation with AMH, total testosterone, and free androgen index.[3] The ovarian stromal volume total ovarian volume ratio was the most accurate predictor of both hyperandrogenemia (area under the curve, 0.915; p < 0.0001) and hirsutism (area under the curve, 0.891; p < 0.0001).[4] But androgen also leads to sensitizing of the follicles to FSH.

Moreover, androgen is responsible for smooth muscle tone. Uterine arteries have thick muscularis layer to allow the flexibility and dynamicity in its caliber during different phases of menstruation and also during pregnancy and labor. This layer consists of smooth muscle fibers and therefore, androgen leads to increased tone in these muscles and therefore, high resistance flow in uterine arteries in PCOS patients, during the whole cycle (Fig. 6.2).[5]

High androgen is reflected as:
- More antral follicles
- Increased uterine artery resistance
- Stromal predominance.

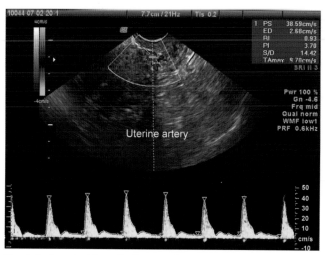

Fig. 6.2: Spectral Doppler image of the uterine artery flow waveform showing high resistance flow suggested by very low diastolic flow.

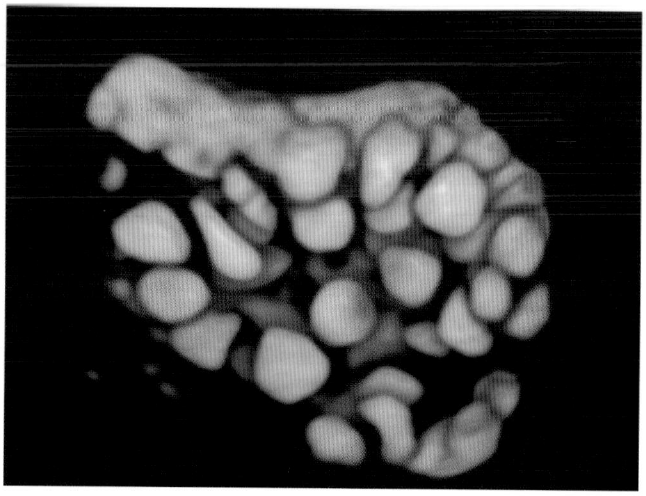

Fig. 6.3: Three-dimensional (3D) ultrasound image of the ovary showing multiple antral follicles on inversion mode rendering.

ANTI-MÜLLERIAN HORMONE

Biochemically, ovarian reserve can be assessed by AMH, FSH, and inhibin B.

Anti-Müllerian hormone is produced by granulosa cells of preantral and small antral follicles of between 2 mm and 6 mm, before they become sensitive to FSH. It is a regulator of recruitment of follicles. AMH has an advantage, that it can be tested in any phase of cycle, though threshold in late luteal phase may be different. This can be also explained and correlated with the fact that the number of follicles between 2 mm and 6 mm remains same almost throughout the cycle except when these follicles undergo atresia in the late luteal phase.

Serum AMH levels have been shown to strongly correlate with the number of antral follicles[6,7] and have appeared to be cycle independent.[8,9] The number of small antral follicles (2–6 mm) is significantly related to age and also, independent of age, to all endocrine ovarian reserve tests, suggesting that the number of small antral follicles represents the functional ovarian reserve.[10] Small AFC and AMH have similar predictive accuracy for high ovarian response with area under curve of 0.961 and 0.922, respectively. The sensitivity and specificity for prediction of high ovarian response were 89% and 92% for small AFC and 93% and 78% for AMH at the cutoff values of more than or equal to 16 pmol/L and more than or equal to 34.5 pmol/L, respectively.[11] The ROC curves do not suggest a clearly better predictive ability for AMH than for AFC, and the difference was not statistically significant (P¼.73). This implies that the best poor response predictor to date,

AFC,[11] has obtained company from a test that may have some crucial advantages. Sensitivity and specificity for AMH were 82% and 76%, respectively, and 82% and 80%, respectively for AFC. Comparison of the summary estimates and ROC curves for AMH and AFC showed no statistical difference in this study which shows that both AMH and AFC are accurate predictors of excessive response to ovarian hyperstimulation. Moreover, both tests appear to have clinical value.[12] In our study, we compared the efficacy of AFC and AMH in PCO and non-PCO group. This study also showed that correlation of AFC and follicles more than 12 mm on day of human chorionic gonadotropin (hCG) in PCO group is 0.56 and non-PCO group is 0.63 and for AMH and follicles more than 12 mm on day of hCG in PCO group is 0.42 and non-PCO group is 0.47. Correlation of AFC with number of ova retrieved on ovum pick-up (OPU) in PCO group is 0.44 and for non-PCO group is 0.50. The value for AMH is 0.39 in PCO and 0.43 for non-PCO group (significance of correlation at 0.01 level is required to be higher than 0.283).[13] In a meta-analysis by Broer et al., it has been shown that AMH has at least the same level of accuracy and clinical value for the prediction of poor response and nonpregnancy as AFC.[13,14]

Anti-Müllerian hormone can be closely correlated with AFC (Fig. 6.3) and can also be used as a test for ovarian reserve instead of AMH without compromising the accuracy and efficacy. It will be worth mentioning here that androgen is the cause and AMH is the effect of recruited antral follicles.

Antral follicle count and ovarian volume showed significant correlation with AMH. AFC and ovarian volume

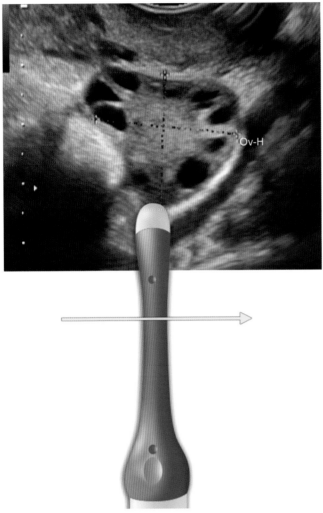

Fig. 6.4: B-mode ultrasound image of the ovary with the transvaginal volume probe. The blocked arrow demonstrates the movement direction of the probe.

provide direct measurements of ovarian reserve, while AMH, inhibin B, and estradiol are released from growing follicles and so their levels reflect the size of developing follicle cohort.[15]

This means that increased androgen may be recognized on ultrasound by more number of antral follicles. Antral follicles can be counted on B-mode as well as on 3D ultrasound. On B-mode by scrolling across the ovary and eyeballing, the number of antral follicles can be counted (Fig. 6.4). On 3D ultrasound, a software called Sono-AVC can be used to count the number of antral follicles (Fig. 6.4).

FOLLICLE-STIMULATING HORMONE

Follicle-stimulating hormone is produced by pituitary and its secretion is controlled by gonadotropin-releasing hormone (GnRH) from the hypothalamus and by the negative feedback of estrogen (Fig. 6.4). It acts on granulosa cells to produce estrogen. In the initial phases of the menstrual cycle, the estrogen level is low, the FSH level is raised. When the follicle size is less than 6 mm, these follicles are FSH independent. By the sensitizing effect of androgen, these follicles become FSH sensitive at 6–9 mm and beyond 9–10 mm, these follicles become FSH dependent. AMH, produced by the granulosa cells of preantral and small antral follicles, inhibits factors affecting FSH sensitivity of the follicle. As AMH levels decrease with follicle growth, this inhibition would be removed.[16] This means that the follicular growth beyond 6 mm size suggests FSH action. Therefore, faster growth of the follicles indicates high FSH. Early follicular recruitment, fast growth of the follicle in early follicular phase, and follicle of larger than 10 mm on the baseline scan indicates high basal FSH levels. But it is important to remember that the follicle that is recruited early, may grow fast on stimulation, but is less likely to produce good quality follicle due to its shorter duration to maturity and this is seen in patients with aging ovaries.

Whereas a slow follicular growth rate indicates that the FSH level is lower than optimum. This is the situation in PCOS patients. Because of multiple follicular development and aromatization of excess androgen to estrogen, there is rise in estrogen level leading to negative feedback to FSH and, therefore, slow rise in FSH and, therefore, slow growth of follicles.

High basal FSH is, thus, suggested by early recruitment of follicle (Fig. 6.5).

LUTEINIZING HORMONE

Luteinizing hormone is also produced by pituitary. Its secretion is controlled by GnRH from hypothalamus and by positive feedback of estrogen and acts on theca cells to produce androgen and progesterone from cholesterol. LH is also responsible for proliferation of theca cells.

Elevated LH levels may be responsible for increased stromal vascularization due to neoangiogenesis, catecholaminergic stimulation, and leukocyte and cytokine activation. This means that LH is responsible for stromal vascularity.[17] This is the reason why PCOS patients who

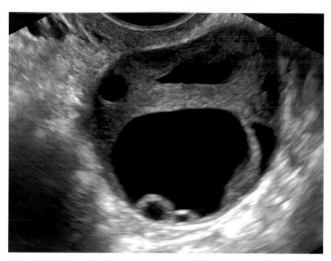

Fig. 6.5: B-mode ultrasound image of the ovary on 4 day of the cycle, demonstrating early recruitment of the follicle.

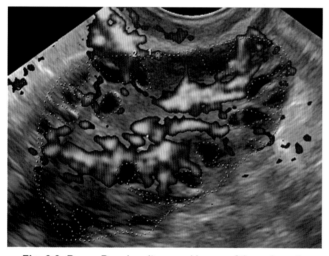

Fig. 6.6: Power Doppler ultrasound image of the polycystic ovary showing abundant ovarian stromal vascularity.

TABLE 6.1: Vascular parameters of the ovarian stromal vessels in PCOS and normal patients.		
Parameters	PCOS	Normal
RI	0.54 ± 0.04	0.78 ± 0.06
PI	0.89 ± 0.04	1.87 ± 0.38
PSV	11.9 ± 3.2	9.6 ± 2.1

(PCOS: polycystic ovary syndrome; PI: pulsatility index; PSV: peak systolic velocity; RI: resistance index)

What is the effect of high luteinizing hormone in polycystic ovarian syndrome?

It is known that PCOS is not a cause but a result of chronic anovulation. It is a process of evolution from adolescent aged multicystic ovaries to polycystic ovaries. As a result of marginally high androgen levels in early follicular phase in polycystic ovarian disease patients, there is recruitment of multiple antral follicles. But these follicles grow only up to 6–7 mm under the effect of androgen. These small follicles do secrete estrogen, and therefore, cumulative rise in estrogen causes a negative feedback for FSH. Low FSH is not enough for follicular maturation and leads to chronic anovulation. But all these follicles do not become dominant due to high LH and/or AMH levels. These follicles that were recruited but not matured, undergo atresia under the effect of raised LH and contribute to stroma as theca cells. This stroma tries to accommodate itself in the ovarian capsule and, therefore, starts becoming dense initially and then increases the ovarian volume. Polycystic ovarian morphology (PCOM) has been found to be a better discriminator than ovarian volume between PCOS and control women.[20] Patients having long-standing PCOS and long-standing anovulation have more dense stroma and this is a cardinal feature that has been shown as bright, highly echogenic stroma on transvaginal ultrasound (Fig. 6.7).[21] Ovarian stroma is considered to be hyperechoic when its echogenicity is more than that of normal myometrium. In a study by Franks et al., it is also shown that PCOM in normal women are not a morphological variant of normal ovaries but rather represent a functional entity of PCO.[21,22] Lam et al. have concluded in their study that the current criteria of 10-cc ovarian volume will fail to identify a group of ovulatory, normoandrogenic women still at risk of complications classically associated with PCOS such as ovarian hyperstimulation syndrome (OHSS), failed implantation, miscarriage, and hyperinsulinemia. To identify these women, further information, particularly about the ovarian stroma and the degree of vascularization, is required.[22,23]

have high LH levels, have increased stromal vascularity, as compared to the normal controls.

The vascular parameters of the ovarian stromal vessels in PCOS and normal patients are given in Figure 6.6 and Table 6.1.[18]

When assessed by 3D power Doppler, compared to the normal control women, PCOS women had higher AFC (median 16.3 per ovary vs 5.5 per ovary), ovarian volume (12.56 mL vs 5.6 mL), stromal volume (10.79 mL vs 4.69 mL), and stromal vascularization [vascularization index (VI) 3.85% vs 2.79%, vascularization flow index (VFI) 1.27 vs 0.85].[19]

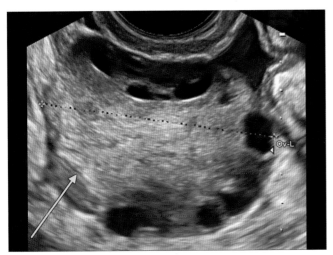

Fig. 6.7: B-mode ultrasound image of the ovary on days 3–4 of the cycle, showing antral follicles and hyperechoic stroma as shown by the arrow.

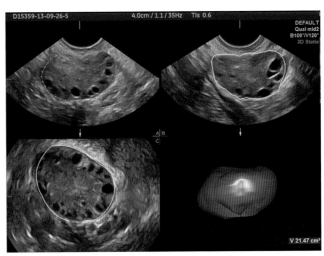

Fig. 6.9: 3D ultrasound acquired image of the ovary with VOCAL calculated volume of the ovary. (3D: three-dimensional; VOCAL: virtual organ computed-aided analysis).

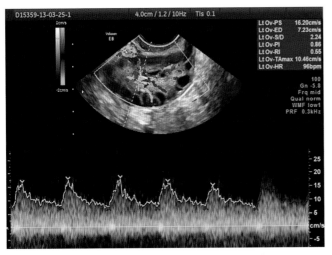

Fig. 6.8: Spectral Doppler image of the polycystic ovary, showing low resistance flow on the spectrum.

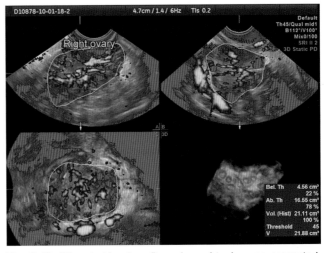

Fig. 6.10: "Threshold volume" used on virtual organ computed-aided analysis (VOCAL) acquired volume of the ovary to calculate the stromal volume. Above threshold value in the figure suggests stromal volume.

This means that high LH in PCOS patients can be identified by increased stromal vascularity, in the form of more blood vessels and low resistance flow[18] (Fig. 6.8) and stromal abundance, in the form of increased stromal echogenicity or increased stromal volume. Stromal volume can be assessed by 3D ultrasound. Ovarian volume is acquired by 3D ultrasound, a software called virtual organ computer-aided analysis (VOCAL) (Fig. 6.9) is used to calculate the volume of the ovary and further the "threshold volume" software is used to assess the threshold volume (Fig. 6.10).

Correlation of Antral Follicle Count with Hyperinsulinemia and Anti-Müllerian Hormone in Polycystic Ovarian Syndrome Patients

Hyperinsulinemic PCOS patients had an *increased vascularity* of the ovarian stroma.[16] Increased ovarian stromal blood flow in PCOS may be because of overexpression of vascular endothelial growth factor (VEGF), which modulates the permeability of theca cells and increase insulin-like growth factor-1 (IGF-1), apart from LH.[18,24,25] This, in turn, enhances gonadotropin-stimulated steroid production in granulosa cells and theca cells resulting in increased ovarian androgen production and subsequently increased AMH.[26]

It has been observed that the poor responders have poor ovarian stromal flow. Measurement of ovarian stromal flow in early follicular phase is related to subsequent ovarian response in in vitro fertilization (IVF) treatment. Those who had low stromal peak systolic velocity (PSV) in the early follicular phase were poor responders.[27] VI, flow index (FI), and VFI of the ovary were significantly related to ovarian response to stimulation.[28] Total ovarian VI and VFI were significantly lower in women aged more than or equal to 41 years.[29] And according to the Poseidon criteria, it is these groups of patients in whom LH needs to be added.[30] The explanation here may be that these patients have less flow and therefore, may have less bioactive LH or less LH receptors and the supplementation of LH, therefore, may be helpful for better response.

Less ovarian stromal flow indicates poor response to stimulation and need for LH supplementation.

ESTROGEN

It is known that the granulosa cells of follicle are responsible for estrogen secretion and therefore, increasing follicular size is associated with rising estrogen levels. Therefore, the simplest evidence that the estrogen level is high even on days 2–3 of the cycle, is either follicular growth to dominance or beyond or multiple follicles as in PCOS. It is worth while mentioning here that FSH is the cause and estrogen is the result of follicular growth.

The receptors of estrogen are in the endometrium and endometrial thickness can be used as a guide to estrogen levels on the baseline scan. Thin linear endometrium on baseline scan suggests adequate downregulation and low basal estrogen levels. For the patients on downregulation for IVF, if the baseline scan shows an endometrial thickness of more than 3 mm, it is an indicator of inadequate downregulation (Fig. 6.11).[31] This endometrial thickness usually correlates with 30–50 pg/mL of estrogen.

Thick multilayered endometrium on baseline scan indicates high estrogen.

Either an early recruited follicle (>10 mm in diameter) or multiple follicles of PCOS may be the cause of high estrogen and both these causes can be confirmed by ultrasound (see Figs. 6.1A and 6.5).

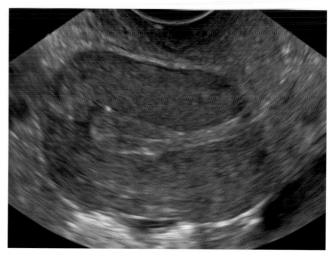

Fig. 6.11: B-mode image of the uterus on days 3–4 showing thick endometrium suggestive of high estrogen levels.

PROGESTERONE

In some cases, thick echogenic endometrium on baseline scan may be because of high progesterone (Fig. 6.12A). It can be confirmed on ultrasound showing corpus luteum with peri-corpus luteal low resistance flow in the ovary (Fig. 6.12B). In these cases, it is important to switch on the Doppler and confirm that the entire thickness of the endometrium visible on ultrasound, is actually endometrial tissue and not blood, normally seen in menstrual phase.

In both the earlier cases of thick endometrium, it is important to confirm that the endometrio-myometrial junctional zone is intact. This is so because, the common cause of thick endometrium on the baseline scan is acute endometritis and this shows irregular endometrio-myometrial junctional zone (Fig. 6.13).

PREOVULATORY PERIOD

This phase is defined by a mature follicle and endometrium. This can be confirmed biochemically by estrogen levels or by ultrasound. But it is in this phase that LH and progesterone levels may also be of concern, because early rise of progesterone or premature LH surge can be strong negative factors affecting embryo quality and implantation.

The hormonal assessments that may be indicated in this phase are:

- Estrogen
- Progesterone
- Luteinizing hormone.

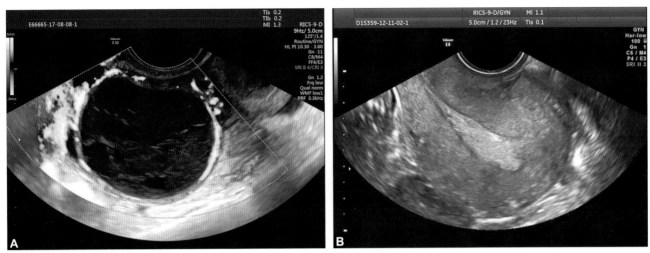

Figs. 6.12A and B: (A) HD flow ultrasound image of the ovary showing a residual corpus luteum with active flow suggesting progesterone secretion; and (B) B-mode ultrasound image of the uterus on the same day in the same patient showing hyperechoic thickened endometrium.

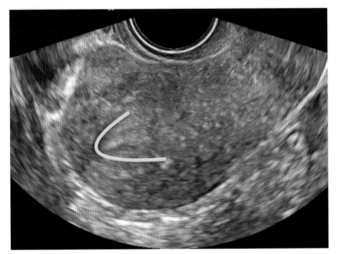

Fig. 6.13: B-mode ultrasound image of the uterus showing thick endometrium, the margins in the fundal region, shown by the yellow line. The endometrio-myometrial junction in the rest of the part is ill defined, the endometrium is almost isoechoic. All the findings put together may suggest acute endometritis.

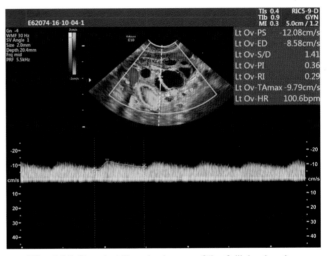

Fig. 6.14: Spectral Doppler image of the follicle showing low resistance perifollicular flow.

These are to assess follicular maturity, endometrial receptivity, and possibility of premature LH surge.

Follicular maturity biochemically is assessed by estrogen level and on ultrasound by B-mode and Doppler assessment of the follicle. It is known that the estrogen level gradually starts rising after 5th day of the menstrual cycle, when the dominant follicle is selected. Estrogen is responsible for perifollicular vascularity. Increase in perifollicular vascularity of dominant follicle in theca layer starts developing as early as 8th day of a normal length cycle. Fall in perifollicular RI starts 2 days before ovulation.[32] This is the time when the shoot up is seen in the estrogen level. At ovulation when estrogen level has just passed the peak, the RI is the lowest (Fig. 6.14). This means that the resistance index (RI) of the perifollicular vessels can be inversely correlated with the estrogen levels. Increase in PSV starts 29 hours before ovulation and continues for at least 72 hours after ovulation.[33,34] This can be explained by

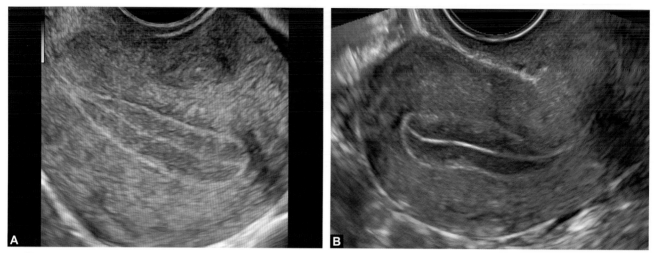

Figs. 6.15A and B: B-mode ultrasound image of the endometrium. (A) Grade A endometrium; and (B) Grade B endometrium.

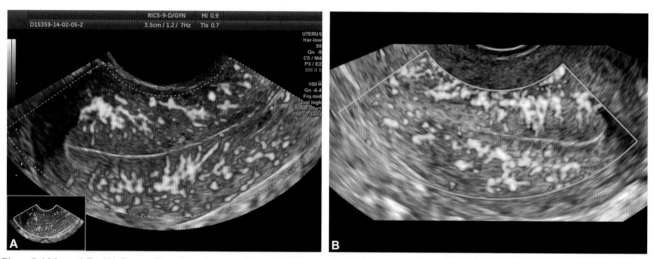

Figs. 6.16A and B: (A) Power Doppler ultrasound image of the endometrium, showing vascularity reaching the area intervening the three lines of the endometrium—zone 3 vascularity; and (B) HD flow image of the endometrium showing vessels reaching the dentral line of the endometrium—zone 4 vascularity.

the fact that LH is responsible for the influx of blood in the ovary and neoangiogenesis that is essential for the follicular and in turn ovum oxygenation. The increase in perifollicular PSV can be correlated with the increase in the LH levels at the time of surge. It is the combined action of estrogen and LH surge that leads to these final circulatory changes before ovulation. Vascular changes at the time of impending ovulation include increased vascularity of the inner wall of the follicle and a coincident surge in blood velocity just prior to eruption.[35] A marked increase in the PSV around the follicle, in the presence of a relatively constant pulsatility index (PI), could be a sign of follicle maturity and impending ovulation.[36] In stimulated cycles, the surge is surrogate and

that is by hCG or GnRH agonist. The influx of blood flow surrounding the follicle, therefore, follows trigger.

Thus, the increasing perifollicular blood flow and lowering resistance can be correlated with the rising estrogen levels whereas increasing LH level correlates with the rising perifollicular PSV.

At this stage, the endometrial vascularity also reaches the peak. When the endometrial receptors are well-developed, not only the endometrium appears multilayered with grade A or B morphology (Figs. 6.15A and B),[37] but also shows vascularity reaching zones 3–4 (Figs. 6.16A and B).[38] These blood vessels—spiral vessels also show low resistance with RI of less than 0.6. All these together with fluid seen in the

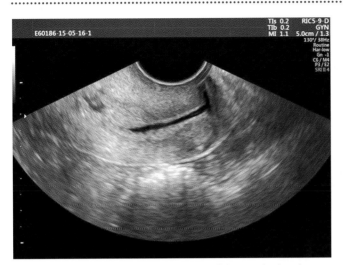

Fig. 6.17: B-mode ultrasound image of the cervix showing anechoic area in the cervical canal—cervical mucous.

cervical canal (Fig. 6.17) indicate sufficient estrogen levels and satisfactory development of estrogen receptors and, therefore, adequate estrogen priming of the endometrium.

But it is known that after the peak of LH surge, either natural or surrogate, there is a sudden downfall in the estrogen level, but the rise in the progesterone level is slow and reaches peak only in the mid-luteal phase. It is because of this that the uterine artery resistance increases after the LH surge[39,40] and the endometrial flow also decreases for 3–4 days, which then increases to reach the low resistance flow in the mid-luteal phase. This may be the need of physiology for implantation. Histological and embryological data suggests that relatively low partial pressure of oxygen (pO_2) environment may be necessary for successful implantation of human blastocyst.[41] Low endometrial VI and VFI is seen in pregnant group on the day of oocyte retrieval is considered a positive sign for endometrial receptivity.[42]

It is known according to two-cell two-hormone theory[43,44] that LH is responsible for conversion of granulosa cells to theca cells. In the preovulatory phase: this action of LH is seen whenever any follicle is exposed to LH. This means that if a mature follicle is exposed to LH, it leads to conversion of the granulosa cells of this follicle into theca cells and progresses it toward rupture leading corpus luteal formation. Instead if an immature follicle, that is dominant is exposed to LH, the granulosa cells of this follicle are converted into theca cells, and the follicle is converted into a luteinized unruptured follicle (LUF), which produces progesterone but not as much as corpus luteum, the medium-sized follicles share the receptors for FSH and LH and therefore, when exposed to LH/hCG

trigger, these further grow in size and if a follicle which is still not dominant, may be only an antral follicle, the follicle undergoes atresia and the theca cells of this follicle also contribute to stroma. Very interestingly, the response of the follicle to LH can be predicted by the pretrigger perifollicular vascular indices.

This means a correct time to use the surrogate LH surge (hCG or GnRH agonist) is of utmost importance. And the ultrasound features which would decide the follicular maturity on the pre-hCG scan are as follows (Figs. 6.18A to C):

- Follicular size of at least 18 mm.
  - Perifollicular RI 0.4–0.48[17] and PSV more than 10 cm/s.[45]
  - Perifollicular vascularity covering three-fourths of the follicular circumference.[46]

Follicular RI and PSV are more important in decision making than the size of the follicle.[46] Ovarian flow correlates well with oocyte recovery rates and hence, may be useful in determining the most appropriate time to administer hCG to optimize recovery rate. Oocytes from severely hypoxic follicles are associated with high frequency of abnormalities of organization of chromosomes on metaphase spindle and may lead to segregation disorders and catastrophic mosaics in embryo.[47]

According to certain studies, perifollicular PSV goes as high as 45 cm/s before an hour of ovulation[37] under the effect of rising LH. Rising PSV with steady low RI suggests that LH surge has already established and the follicle is close to rupture.[36]

Preovulatory Findings and Luteinizing Hormone

- Rise in perifollicular PSV suggests fast rising LH level and impending rupture.
- Fluffy outer margins of the endometrium is the another sign that indicates rising LH and also initial rise in preovulatory progesterone.

What is more interesting is that ultrasound not only gives information about the estrogen levels, follicular behavior, and LH response, it also gives information about development of estrogen receptors in the endometrium. This is not possible by any other biochemical tests.

ESTROGEN EFFECT ON ENDOMETRIUM

Estrogen is produced by the granulosa cells of the follicle, but endometrium is the receptor organ for estrogen.

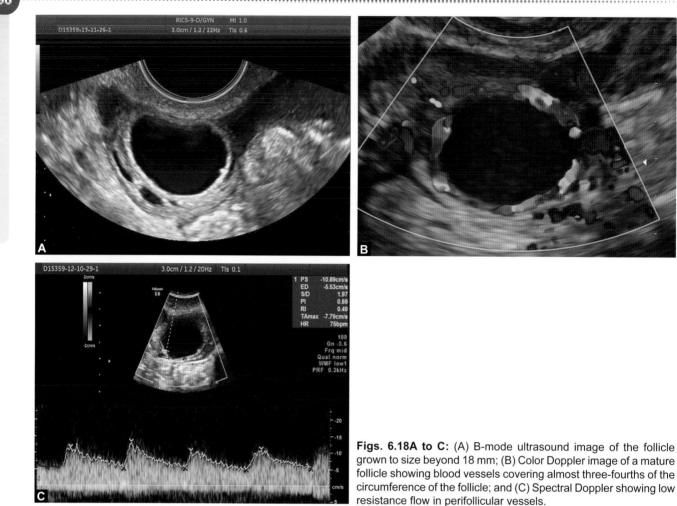

Figs. 6.18A to C: (A) B-mode ultrasound image of the follicle grown to size beyond 18 mm; (B) Color Doppler image of a mature follicle showing blood vessels covering almost three-fourths of the circumference of the follicle; and (C) Spectral Doppler showing low resistance flow in perifollicular vessels.

Increasing endometrial thickness and changing endometrial morphology to multilayered correlates with follicular growth and increasing estrogen levels.[37] Endometrium is the receptor organ for both estrogen and progesterone. Following the endometrium can also be a guide to predict estrogen and progesterone dominance. At the baseline scan, the endometrium is thin or the cavity contains blood (Fig. 6.19), but as the estrogen level starts rising with the growth of the follicle, the endometrium becomes multilayered and starts increasing in thickness. As the estrogen level rises and the multilayered endometrium grows, it changes in morphology. Initially, it is grade B[48] (Fig. 6.20A), when it is multilayered with sharp outer margin and hypoechoic intervening area, then it becomes multilayered with sharp outer margin and the intervening area grade A (Fig. 6.20B), isoechoic to the myometrium and when the estrogen level rises to supraphysiological levels, the endometrium becomes

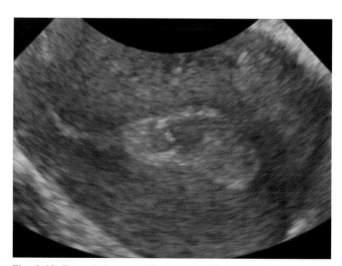

Fig. 6.19: B-mode image of the uterus with endometrium showing heterogeneous echogenicity, due to blood in the endometrial cavity.

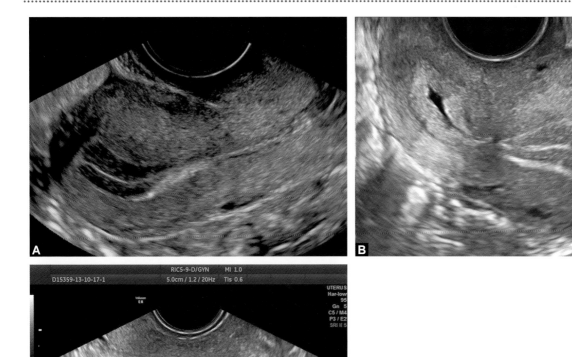

Figs. 6.20A to C: B-mode ultrasound image of the endometrium showing grade B (multilayered with hypoechoic intervening area), grade A (multilayered with isoechogenicity in the intervening area), and grade C (homogeneous isoechoic endometrium) endometrium, respectively.

homogeneous and isoechoic to the myometrium[37]—grade C (Fig. 6.20C). If the LH surge starts, there is a minimal rise in progesterone even before ovulation. LH rise leads to fluffiness of the outer margin of the endometrium (Fig. 6.21A) and when the progesterone exposure starts, the outer margin starts becoming hyperechoic (Fig. 6.21B). This hyperechogenicity progresses from periphery to the central line of the endometrium, to make it completely hyperechoic in the mid-luteal phase (Fig. 6.22). This means that the fluffy endometrium should normally be found only close to ovulation normally.

The vascularity of the endometrium also correlates with the estrogen levels also. Endometrial and subendometrial flow increases in the follicular phase and reaches its maximum approximately 3 days prior to ovulation (Fig. 6.23). This is the time when estrogen level starts rising fast for the final peak. The spiral vessels grow towards

the endometrium and penetrate the endometrium. Endometrial thickness and vascularity are indicators of estrogen receptors in endometrium.

It has been shown in several studies that when uterine artery PI is more than 3.2, implantation rates are extremely low and embryo transfer (ET) or intrauterine insemination (IUI) should be withheld.[49-51] If the upper limit of cut off for uterine artery PI is established at 3–3.3, prediction of nonreceptive uterus has specificity of 96–100%, positive predictive value (PPV) of 88–100%, sensitivity of 13–35%, and negative predictive value (NPV) of 44–56%.[52] As has been discussed earlier, with the start of the surge, there is increase in perifollicular PSV beyond 10 cm/s and this start of the surge also leads to increased resistance in uterine artery. Both together mean that the surge has started but when the follicular PSV is low and the uterine artery resistance is high, it means that the follicle is not yet mature.

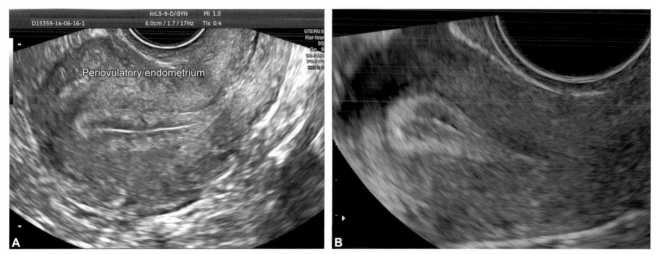

Figs. 6.21A and B: Ultrasound of the progressive secretory changes in the endometrium. (A) B-mode ultrasound showing multilayered endometrium with fluffy but nonhyperechoic outer margins of the endometrium; and (B) B-mode ultrasound showing multilayered endometrium with hyperechoic outer margins of the endometrium.

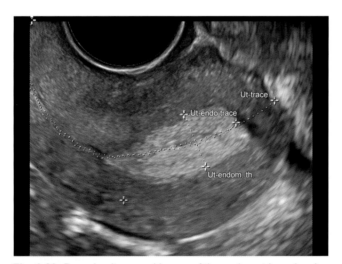

Fig. 6.22: B-mode ultrasound image of the endometrium showing hyperechoic secretory changes, normally seen in the mid-luteal phase of the menstrual cycle.

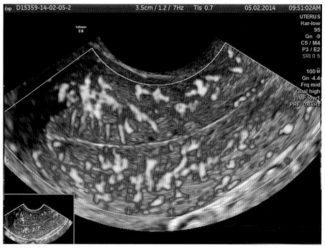

Fig. 6.23: Power Doppler image of the uterus showing vascularity in the preovulatory endometrium.

SECRETORY PHASE ASSESSMENT

Rupture of the follicle leads to formation of corpus luteum. Corpus luteum is responsible for progesterone production. The functional efficacy of the corpus luteum can be assessed by Doppler by assessing the peri-corpus luteal vascularity.

A clear correlation between RI of corpus luteum and plasma progesterone levels has been seen in natural cycle. RI of the corpus luteum can, therefore, be used as an adjunct to plasma progesterone assay as an index of luteal function.[53] A corpus luteum that is functionally normal and

produces adequate amount of progesterone shows corpus luteal flow with RI 0.35–0.50 and PSV 10–15 cm/s (Figs. 6.24A and B).

The receptor organ for progesterone also (like estrogen) is endometrium and its vascular studies can be a reliable clue to adequate progesterone production. Segmental uterine and ovarian artery perfusion demonstrates a significant correlation with histological and hormonal markers of uterine receptivity and may aid in assessment of luteal phase defect. Endometrium also becomes hyperechoic in the mid-luteal phase (Fig. 6.22) as a result of

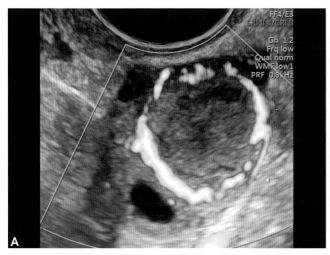 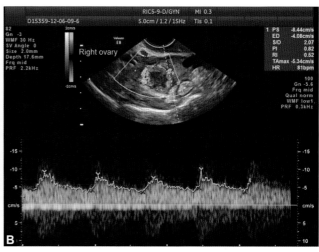

Figs. 6.24A and B: HD flow and spectral Doppler image of the corpus luteum showing normal flow pattern of the corpus luteum in the mid-luteal phase.

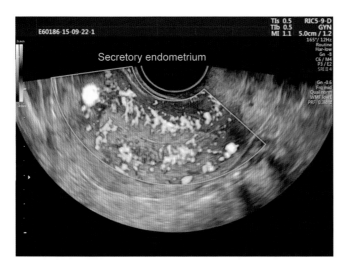

Fig. 6.25: HD flow image of the uterus showing vascularity in the secretory endometrium in the mid-luteal phase.

progesterone exposure. With adequate progesterone levels, that are achieved in the mid-luteal phase, the spiral arteries show RI of 0.48–0.52 (low resistance flow) (Fig. 6.25) and uterine artery shows PI of 2.0–2.5. This PI is lower than in the preovulatory phase because of smooth muscle relaxing effect of progesterone. Inadequate progesterone production and, therefore, corpus luteal inadequacy is suggested by high resistance flow in corpus luteal vessels. Whereas high spiral artery resistance would suggest inadequate response of endometrium to progesterone.

In luteal phase defect, because of low progesterone levels, the resistance in the peri-corpus luteal vessels is high. Because of low progesterone levels, there is inadequate

relaxation of the muscularis of the uterine artery and therefore, the uterine artery resistance is high along with higher resistance in its branches—the spiral vessels in luteal phase defect.

CORRELATION OF PROGESTERONE TO ULTRASOUND FINDINGS

- Blurring of outer margin of multilayered endometrium suggests initiation of progesterone secretion.
- Low resistance flow in corpus luteum, with echogenic endometrium and low resistance endometrial vascularity in mid-luteal phase suggests normal luteal phase.
- High resistance corpus luteal flow suggests corpus luteal inadequacy.
- High resistance endometrial flow in mid-luteal phase suggests either inadequate progesterone levels or inadequate progesterone receptors in endometrium.

The entire cycle monitoring can be summarized as:
On baseline scan:
- Early recruitment of the follicle—increased FSH
- Increased endometrial thickness—high estrogen/progesterone
- Increased stromal flow—high LH for a short period
- Increased stromal echogenicity—high LH and anovulation
- More antral follicles—high androgen
- High uterine artery resistance—high androgen

Pre-hCG scan:

- Good perifollicular flow—good estrogen production
- Good endometrium with good endometrial flow, cervical mucous—adequate estrogen receptors in endometrium
- Fluffy endometrial margins—early exposure to progesterone
- Increasing echogenicity of the follicle wall and increased RI—premature LH surge.

Luteal phase:

- Low corpus luteal RI—normal progesterone production
- High endometrial vascularity—adequate progesterone receptors
- Low corpus luteal vascularity—luteal phase defect
- Low endometrial vascularity—inadequate progesterone or inadequate progesterone receptors.

CONCLUSION

Ultrasound is an excellent tool for assessment of the menstrual cycle. Hormonal changes occurring day-to-day during the menstrual cycle reflects as morphological and vascular changes in the ovary and the uterus. Assessing these changes by transvaginal ultrasound and Doppler and correctly interpreting can explain the hormonal basis of these changes. Ultrasound with Doppler can, thus, be used as the only modality for cycle assessment in patients undergoing assisted reproduction technology and may be of help to reduce the cost of the cycle by avoiding certain hormonal assessments and still maintaining close and accurate watch on the hormonal changes occurring during treatment cycle.

REFERENCES

1. Jonard S, Robert Y, Cortet-Rudelli C, et al. Ultrasound examination of polycystic ovaries: is it worth counting the follicles? Hum Reprod. 2003;18:598-603.
2. Raju GA, Chavan R, Deenadayal M, et al. Luteinizing hormone and follicle stimulating hormone synergy: A review of role in controlled ovarian hyper-stimulation. J Hum Reprod Sci. 2013;6:227-34.
3. Battaglia C, Battaglia B, Morotti E, et al. Two- and three-dimensional sonographic and color Doppler techniques for diagnosis of polycystic ovary syndrome. The stromal/ovarian volume ratio as a new diagnostic criterion. J Ultrasound Med. 2012;31:1015-24.
4. Ozkan S, Vural B, Calişkan E, et al. Color Doppler sonographic analysis of uterine and ovarian artery blood flow in women with polycystic ovary syndrome. J Clin Ultrasound. 2007;35:305-13.
5. Haadsma ML, Bukman A, Groen H, et al. The number of small antral follicles (2-6 mm) determines the outcome of endocrine ovarian reserve tests in a subfertile population. Hum Reprod. 2007;22:1925-31.
6. Van Rooij IA, Broekmans FJ, te Velde ER, et al. Serum anti-Müllerian hormone levels: a novel measure of ovarian reserve. Hum Reprod. 2002;17:3065-71.
7. Hehenkamp WJ, Looman CW, Themmen AP, et al. Anti-Müllerian hormone levels in the spontaneous menstrual cycle do not show substantial fluctuation. J Clin Endocrinol Metab. 2006;91:4057-63.
8. La Marca A, Stabile G, Artenisio AC, et al. Serum anti-Müllerian hormone throughout the human menstrual cycle. Hum Reprod. 2006;21:3103-7.
9. van Rooij IA, Broekmans FJ, tr Velde ER, et al. Serum anti-Mullerian hormone levels: a novel measure of ovarian reserve. Hum Reprod. 2002;17:3065-71.
10. Gruijters MJ, Visser JA, Durlinger AL, et al. Anti-Müllerian hormone and its role in ovarian function. Mol Cell Endocrinol. 2003;211:85-90.
11. Panchal S, Nagori C. Comparison of anti-mullerian hormone and antral follicle count for assessment of ovarian reserve. J Hum Reprod Sci. 2012;5:274-8.
12. Aflatoonian A, Oskouian H, Ahmadi S, et al. Prediction of high ovarian response to controlled ovarian hyperstimulation: anti-Müllerian hormone versus small antral follicle count (2-6 mm). J Assist Reprod Genet. 2009;26:319-25.
13. Broer SL, Willem BJ, Hendriks D, et al. The role of antimullerian hormone in prediction of outcome after IVF: comparison with the antral follicle count. Fertil Steril. 2009;91:705-14.
14. Loverro G, Vicino M, Lorusso F, et al. Polycystic ovary syndrome: relationship between insulin sensitivity, sex hormone levels and ovarian stromal blood flow. Gynecol Endocrinol. 2001;15:142-9.
15. Hendriks DJ, Mol BW, Bancsi LF, et al. Antral follicle count in the prediction of poor ovarian response and pregnancy after in vitro fertilization: a meta-analysis and comparison with basal follicle-stimulating hormone level. Fertil Steril. 2005;83:291-301.
16. Battalgia C, Artini PG, Salvatori M, et al. Ultrasonographic patterns of polycystic ovaries: color Doppler and hormonal correlations. Ultrasound Obstet Gynecol. 1998;11:332-6.
17. Battalgia C, Artini PG, D'Ambrogio G, et al. The role of color Doppler imaging in the diagnosis of polycystic ovarian syndrome. Am J Obstet Gynecol. 1995;172:108-13.
18. Lam PM, Jhonson IR, Rainne-Fenning NJ. Three-dimensional ultrasound features of the polycystic ovary and the effect of different phenotypic expressions on these parameters. Hum Reprod. 2007;22:3116-23.
19. Legro RS, Chui P, Kunselman AR, et al. Polycystic ovaries are common in women with hyperandrogenic chronic anovulation but do not predict metabolic or reproductive phenotype. J Clin Endocrinol Metab. 2005;90:2571-9.
20. Buckett WM, Bouzayen R, Watkin KL, et al. Ovarian stromal echogenicity in women with normal and polycystic ovaries. Hum Reprod. 1999;14:618-21.
21. Franks S, Webber LJ, Goh M, et al. Ovarian morphology is a marker of heritable biochemical traits in sisters with polycystic ovaries. J Clin Endocrinol Metab. 2008;93:3396-402.

22. Lam PM, Raine-Fenning N. The role of three-dimensional ultrasonography in polycystic ovary syndrome. Hum Reprod. 2006;21:2209-15.

23. Zaidi J, Barber J, Kyei-Mensah A, et al. Relationship of ovarian stroma blood flow at baseline ultrasound to subsequent follicular response in an in vitro fertilization program. Obstet Gynecol. 1996;88:779-84.

24. Abd El Aal DE, Mohamed SA, Amine AF, et al. Vascular endothelial growth factor and insulin-like growth factor-1 in polycystic ovary syndrome and their relation to ovarian blood flow. Eur J Obstet Gynecol Reprod Biol. 2005;118:219-24.

25. Willis DS, Mason HD, Gilling-Smith C, et al. Modulation by insulin of follicle-stimulating hormone actions in human granulosa cells of normal and polycystic ovaries. J Clin Endocrinol Metab. 1996;81:302-9.

26. Pellatt L, Rice S, Dilaver N, et al. Anti-Müllerian hormone reduces follicle sensitivity to follicle-stimulating hormone in human granulosa cells. Fertil Steril. 2011;96:1246-51.

27. Merce LT, Barco MJ, Bau S, et al. Prediction of ovarian response and IVF/ICSI outcome by three-dimensional ultrasonography and power Doppler angiography. Eur J Obstet Gynecol Reprod Biol. 2007;132:93-100.

28. Ng EH, Chan CC, Yeung WS, et al. Effect of age on ovarian stromal flow measured by three-dimensional ultrasound with power Doppler in Chinese women with proven fertility. Hum Reprod. 2004;19:2132-7.

29. Humaidan P, Alviggi C, Fischer R, et al. The novel POSEIDON stratification of 'Low prognosis patients in Assisted Reproductive Technology' and its proposed marker of successful outcome. F1000Res. 2016;5:2911.

30. Dogan MM, Uygur D, Alkan RN, et al. Prediction of pituitary downregulation by evaluation of endometrial thickness in an IVF programme. Reprod Biomed Online. 2004;8:595-9.

31. Jokubkeine L, Sladkevicius P, Rovas L, et al. Assessment of changes in volume and vascularity of ovaries during the normal menstrual cycle using three-dimensional power Doppler ultrasound. Hum Reprod. 2006;21:2661-8.

32. Campbell S, Bourne T, Waterstone J, et al. Transvaginal color blood flow imaging of the preovulatory follicle. Fertil Steril. 1993;60:433-8.

33. Kupesic S, Kurjak A. Uterine and ovarian perfusion during the periovulatory period assessed by transvaginal color Doppler. Fertil Steril. 1993;60:439-43.

34. Bourne TH, Jurkovic D, Waterstone J, et al. Intrafollicular blood flow during human ovulation. Ultrasound Obstet Gynecol. 1991;1:53-9.

35. Tan SL, Zaidi J, Campbell S, et al. Blood flow changes in the ovarian and uterine arteries during the normal menstrual cycle. Am J Obstet Gynecol. 1996;175:625-31.

36. Bassil S, Magritte JP, Roth J, et al. Uterine vascularity during stimulation and its correlation with implantation in IVF. Hum Reprod. 1995;10:1497-501.

37. Smith B, Porter R, Ahuja K, et al. Ultrasonic assessment of endometrial changes in stimulated cycles in an in vitro fertilization and embryo transfer program. J In Vitro Fert Embryo Transf. 1984;1:233-8.

38. Applebaum M. The steel or teflon endometrium-ultrasound visualization of endometrial vascularity in IVF patients and outcome. Presented at the Third World Congress of Ultrasound in Obstetrics and Gynecology. Ultrasound Obstet Gynecol. 1993;3(Suppl 2):10.

39. Ng EH, Chan CC, Tang OS, et al. Relationship between uterine blood flow and endometrial and subendometrial blood flows during stimulated and natural cycles. Fertil Steril. 2006;85:721-7.

40. Graham CH, Postovit LM, Park H, et al. Adriana and Luisa Castellucci award lecture 1999: role of oxygen in the regulation of trophoblast gene expression and invasion. Placenta. 2000;21:443-50.

41. Ng EH, Chan CC, Tang OS, et al. The role of endometrial and subendometrial blood flows measured by three-dimensional power Doppler ultrasound in prediction of pregnancy during IVF treatment. Hum Reprod. 2006;21:164-70.

42. Fevold HL. Synergism of the follicle stimulating and luteinizing hormones in producing estrogen secretion. J Clin Endocrinol Metab. 1941;42:918.

43. Short RV. Steroids in the follicular fluid and the corpus luteum of the mare. A 'two-cell type' theory of ovarian steroid synthesis. J Endocrinol. 1962;24:59-63.

44. Chui D, Pugh N, Walker S, et al. Follicular vascularity—the predictive value of transvaginal power Doppler ultrasonography in an in vitro fertilization program: A preliminary study. Hum Reprod. 1997;12:191-6.

45. Nargund G, Bourne TH, Doyle PE, et al. Association between ultrasound indices of follicular blood flow, oocyte recovery and preimplantation embryo quality. Hum Reprod. 1996;11:109-13.

46. Van Blerkom J, Davis P, Alexander S. Inner mitochondrial membrane potential, cytoplasmic ATP content and free Ca2+ levels in metaphase II mouse oocytes. Hum Reprod. 2003;18(11):2429-40.

47. Bourne TH, Jurkovic D, Waterstone J, et al. Follicular blood flow during human ovulation. Ultrasound Obstet Gynecol. 1991;1:53.

48. Zaidi J, Campbell S, Pittrof FR, et al. Endometrial thickness, morphology, vascular penetration and velocimetry in predicting implantation in an in vitro fertilization program. Ultrasound Obstet Gynecol. 1995;6:191-8.

49. Tsai YC, Chang JC, Tai MJ, et al. Relationship of uterine perfusion to outcome of intrauterine insemination. J Ultrasound Med. 1996;15:633-6.

50. Cacciatore B, Simberg N, Fusaro P, et al. Transvaginal Doppler study of uterine artery blood flow in in vitro fertilization embryo transfer cycles. Fertil Steril. 1996;66:130-4.

51. Salle B, Bied-Damon V, Benchaib M, et al. Preliminary report of an ultrasonography and colour Doppler uterine score to predict uterine receptivity in an in-vitro fertilization programme. Hum Reprod. 1998;13:1669-73.

52. Glock JL, Brumsted JR. Colour flow pulsed Doppler ultrasound in diagnosing luteal phase defect. Fertil Steril. 1995;64:500-4.

53. Kupesić S, Kurjak A, Vujisić S, et al. Luteal phase defect: comparison between Doppler velocimetry, histological and hormonal markers. Ultrasound Obstet Gynecol. 1997;9:105-12.

Ultrasound and a Treatment Cycle

INTRODUCTION

Ultrasound is a patient friendly, easy to use repeatedly, and an affordable modality for monitoring of the patients on treatment for infertility, may it be intrauterine insemination (IUI) cycles or in vitro fertilization (IVF) cycles. Transvaginal route of ultrasound scan has markedly improved the information available on ultrasound scan due to the high frequency probe used that is placed close to the organs of interest and, therefore, gives high-resolution images. Moreover, when used with Doppler, it gives precise idea not only about the morphological changes but also about the vascular changes occurring during the entire cycle in the uterus and ovaries. It has been established beyond doubts that the vascular changes are instantaneous reflection of hormonal changes.

These hormonal changes are a continuous process during the menstrual cycle and, therefore, ultrasound monitoring also ideally should be done throughout the cycle. But for convenience, this discussion will be divided here into three parts:

1. Baseline scan
2. Preovulatory scan
3. Luteal phase scan.

BASELINE SCAN

This scan is done when ovarian hormonal (estrogen and progesterone) levels are at their baseline on days 2–3 of the menstrual cycle. The ovaries are silent, and have no active (dominant) follicle or corpus luteum at this stage. The scan is done using B-mode ultrasound with color Doppler, pulse Doppler, three-dimensional (3D) ultrasound, and 3D power Doppler. This scan assesses the ovarian reserve and response. It is also a key scan for ultrasound diagnosis of polycystic ovaries.

Assessment of ovarian reserve and response has been tried by several workers. Bologna criteria also defines poor responders as those with age more than 40 years, less than three follicles per ovary, and anti-Müllerian hormone (AMH) less than 0.5–1.1 ng/mL. One of the earliest studies, by Ravhon et al.[1] has used dynamic assessment of inhibin B and estradiol after buserelin acetate as predictors of ovarian response and have found these to be highly correlating with the ovarian response in IVF patients. The two major drawbacks of this study are that: (1) this required several blood tests at different times and (2) the study sample was pretty small (n = 37).

In 2002, Kupesic et al.[2] used 3D ultrasound for assessment of ovarian response in IVF cycles. The antral follicle count (AFC) and ovarian stromal flow parameters on the baseline scan were shown to be most predictive of the ovarian response after pituitary downregulation in this study, followed by total ovarian volume, ovarian stromal area, and age. This study could predict favorable IVF outcome in 50% (11/22) of patients and poor outcome in 85% (29/34) of patients. Using this, nomogram for dose calculation was evaluated by the same group in another study. The results of this study were in absolute favor of individualizing dose according to the dosage nomogram proving the reliability of ultrasound parameters and age and body mass index (BMI) for decision on stimulation doses. Whereas a study by Ng et al.[3] showed basal follicle-stimulating hormone (FSH) to be the most reliable parameter for assessment of ovarian response followed by AFC and BMI. Where AFC was predictive of number of follicles (serum estradiol level) on the day of human chorionic gonadotropin (hCG) and BMI was predictive of gonadotropins dosage. An ultrasound-based study on prediction of ovarian response in 2007 by Merce et al.[4] evaluated ovarian volume, AFC, and 3D power Doppler indices vascularization index (VI), flow index (FI), and vascularization flow index (VFI) for their reliability to calculate the number of follicles grown, oocyte retrieved embryos transferred. This study clearly showed the relevance of ovarian volume and AFC to the number of follicles matured and oocytes retrieved. It also mentioned that 3D power Doppler indices made the assessment of ovarian response to stimulation protocols easier.

But these studies do not have a precise dose calculation strategy.

Popovic-Todorovic et al.,[5] in 2003 combined age, BMI, cycle length and smoking status, and ultrasound features of the ovaries also to design a dosage nomogram of recombinant follicle-stimulating hormone (rFSH) for IVF/intracytoplasmic sperm injection (ICSI) patients. This was a prospective study and also had a larger sample volume than the previous two studies (n = 145). According to this study, total number of antral follicles and ovarian stromal blood flow were the two most significant predictors of ovarian response and ovarian volume was highly significant predictor of number of follicles and oocytes retrieved. La Marca et al. have shown that daily FSH dose may be calculated on the basis of age, AFC, and serum FSH levels in a patient.[6]

Another landmark study by Olivennes and Howles et al.,[7]—The CONSORT study used basal FSH, BMI, age, and AFC for individualizing FSH dose for ovarian stimulation. A dose calculator was developed using these factors as predictors and was evaluated in a prospective clinical trial.

The only study that worked on the dose calculations for IUI patients was by Freiesleben NL et al.[8] in 2008 with 159 patients. They evaluated age, spontaneous cycle length, body weight, BMI, smoking status, total ovarian volume, AFC, total Doppler score of ovarian stromal blood flow, baseline FSH, and estradiol as possible predictive factors of ovarian response. This study concluded that body weight and AFC may be used to achieve appropriate ovarian response for IUI in ovulatory patients. Study by the same investigators for IVF and ICSI patients concluded that AFC and age could predict the low response better whereas to predict hyperresponse AFC and cycle length were better parameters.

The parameters that we have used to calculate the dose for gonadotropins stimulation protocol for IUI cycles in our study are AFC, ovarian volume, stromal resistance index (RI)

and peak systolic velocity (PSV), and age and BMI. Before proceeding to the actual dose calculation protocol, a short justification for each parameter used would be considered relevant. As AMH has been already established as a reliable parameter for assessment of ovarian reserve, the AFC and ovarian volume that are considered for the assessment of the ovarian reserve would be compared with AMH.

Anti-Müllerian hormone and AFC both have reflections of primordial follicles and both are stable between cycles.[9] Serum AMH levels have been shown to strongly correlate with the number of antral follicles[10] and have appeared to be cycle independent.[9] In a meta-analysis by Broer et al., it has been shown that AMH has at least the same level of accuracy and clinical value for the prediction of poor response and nonpregnancy as AFC.[11] Both AMH and AFC are accurate predictors of excessive response to ovarian hyperstimulation.[12] Difference of correlation coefficient between AFC and AMH for ova retrieved on ovum pick-up (OPU) is minimally significant in nonpolycystic ovary (PCO) and is not significant in PCO group. Therefore, for both groups, AFC alone may suffice as a test for estimation of ovarian reserve.[13]

Doing AFC assessment alone would be more cost-effective for predicting the ovarian reserve in patients undergoing controlled ovarian stimulation with gonado-tropin-releasing hormone (GnRH) antagonist. AFC had the highest accuracy for predicting ovarian response in patients with abnormal ovarian reserve test and was statistically significant (number of oocyte aspirated, $p < 0.001$) than AMH ($p < 0.06$) and FSH ($p < 0.212$) in predicting ovarian response. For prediction of poor ovarian response, a model including AFC + AMH was found to be almost similar to that of ($p < 0.001$) using AFC alone.[14]

Precise calculation of AFC, therefore, can help in predicting the ovarian response. This can be done on two-dimensional (2D) ultrasound or by 3D with inversion mode rendering and Sono-AVC a specialized 3D ultrasound software for calculation of antral follicle number and volumes. Jayaprakasan et al. have shown that calculation of follicle number per ovary (FNPO) with 2D or 3D have given identical results.[15] Though 3D with Sono-AVC may be more precise in cases with AFC being more than 12–15. There is least chance of follicles being missed or being counted twice because of color coding when Sono AVC is used for calculating the AFC. But postprocessing is required for accurate calculations. It takes longer to perform, because of the need for postprocessing, and obtains values that are lower than those obtained by the 2D- and 3D-MPV techniques as it does not over count (Fig. 7.1).[16,17]

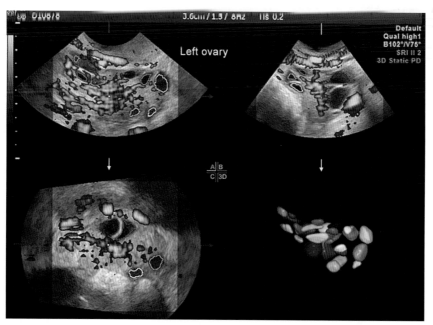

Fig. 7.1: Three-dimensional (3D) ultrasound image of the ovary with Sono-AVC for calculating antral follicle counts. (AVC: automated volume calculation)

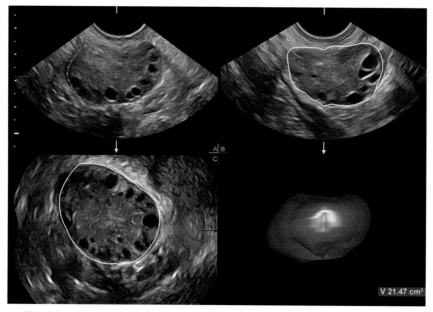

Fig. 7.2: 3D ultrasound calculated ovarian volume by a software called VOCAL. (3D: three-dimensional; VOCAL: virtual organ computer-aided analysis)

According to one study, ovarian volume less than 3 cc was significantly predictive of higher IVF cancelation rates more than 50%[18] (Fig. 7.2) and ovarian volume can be used in decision-making for stimulation protocol for ovarian induction. Moreover, it is also known that the patients who have larger ovaries and are PCOS have a higher risk of developing OHSS. AFC and ovarian volume provide direct measurements of ovarian reserve.[19] The mean ovarian diameter significantly correlated with age, day 3 FSH, day 3 LH, and day 3 estradiol.[20] But another study shows that ovarian volume is a poor predictor of number of oocytes obtained in an IVF cycle as compared to AFC.[21]

Inclusion of stromal blood flows (Fig. 7.3) as one of the decision-making parameters is also considered. It has been shown that measurement of ovarian stromal flow in early follicular phase is related to subsequent ovarian response

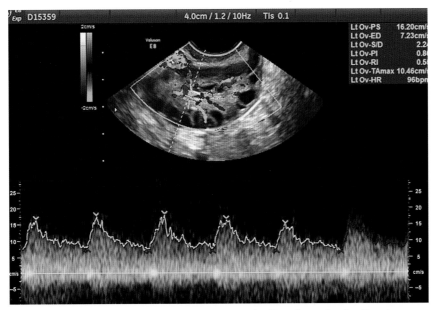

Fig. 7.3: Ovarian stromal flow as seen on color Doppler and pulse Doppler.

in IVF treatment.[22] Ovarian stromal blood flow velocity after 2–3 weeks of pituitary suppression is a true representative of baseline ovarian blood flow and predictive of ovarian responsiveness and outcome of IVF treatment.[23]

The ovarian stromal blood flow was found to be negatively correlated with age. Ovarian blood flow predicts ovarian responsiveness and hence provides a noninvasive and cost-effective prognostic factor of IVF outcome.[24]

Ovarian stromal PSV after pituitary suppression is predictive of ovarian responsiveness and outcome of IVF treatment.[23] Ovarian stromal PSV was the most important single independent predictor of ovarian response in patients with normal basal serum FSH level. Patients with PSV more than or equal to 10 cm/s had significantly higher median number of mature oocytes and higher clinical pregnancy rates. Ovarian stromal blood flow velocity after 2–3 weeks of pituitary suppression is a true representative of baseline ovarian blood flow and predictive of ovarian responsiveness and outcome of IVF treatment.[23]

Considering the 3D power Doppler indices that are representation of global vascularity of the organ of interest, it has been demonstrated that VI, FI, and VFI of the ovary were significantly related to ovarian response to stimulation.[4]

Kupesic has shown correlation between the ovarian stromal FI and number of mature oocytes retrieved in IVF cycles and pregnancy rates (Fig. 7.4).[2] This study has shown that stromal FI <11 indicates low responder, 11–14 indicates good, and > 15 has a high risk of ovarian hyperstimulation syndrome (OHSS). Women with polycystic ovary syndrome

(PCOS) had higher AFC (median 16.3 vs 5.5 per ovary), ovarian volume (12.56 mL vs 5.6 mL), stromal volume (10.79 mL vs 4.69 mL), and stromal vascularization (VI 3.85% vs 2.79%, VFI 1.27 vs 0.85). Though 2D power Doppler indices were not higher in PCOS than in controls.[25,26]

Total ovarian VI and VFI were significantly lower in women aged more than or equal to 41 years.[27] Quantification of ovarian stromal blood flow by 3D power Doppler US in women with endometriosis may provide an important prognostic indicator in those undergoing IVF.[28] Undetectable basal ovarian stromal blood flow in at least one ovary is related to low ovarian response in infertile women undergoing IVF-embryo transfer (ET).[29]

The role of the ovarian stromal flow in variable ovarian response can be explained by a simple understanding. If the blood flow to the ovary is abundant, more percentage of the gonadotropins loaded into the patient's system will reach the ovary and, therefore, total amount of gonadotropins to be used for the patient may be less and vice versa. Therefore, if blood flow to the ovary is more (low RI and high PSV), the patient is a good responder, but if the flows to the ovaries are less, she is a poor responder.

Total number of antral follicles achieved the best predictive value for favorable IVF outcome, followed by ovarian stromal FI, total ovarian stromal area, and total ovarian volume.[2] AFC, ovarian volume, and ovarian 3D power Doppler flow indices did not significantly change after a short-term treatment of GnRH agonist for pituitary downregulation.[30]

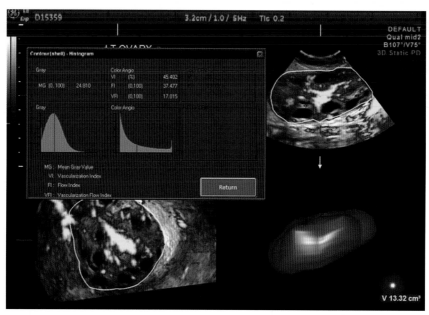

Fig. 7.4: 3D power Doppler ultrasound image with VOCAL calculated volume with volume histogram (blue box) showing VI, FI, and VFI parameters. (3D: three-dimensional; FI: flow index; VI: vascularization index; VFI: vascularization flow index; VOCAL: virtual organ computer-aided analysis)

And, therefore, these parameters can be used as reliable parameters for assessment of the ovarian reserve and response to decide the stimulation protocol in non-down regulated IUI cycles, as well as in agonist and antagonist down regulated IVF cycles also. The ovarian stromal flow is less in obese patients as compared to controls.[26] This means that the obese patients require higher doses for stimulation. Elevated luteinizing hormone (LH) levels may be responsible for increased stromal vascularization due to neoangiogenesis, catecholaminergic stimulation, and leukocyte and cytokine activation.[31] Does this mean that when the LH is low, ovary may show less flow and it is in these patients, that there is a need to add LH to their stimulation.

PREOVULATORY SCAN

A follicle that is of more than 10 mm in diameter, grows at a rate of 2–3 mm/day, has no internal echogenicity and has thin (pencil line-like) walls, is not only more likely to become the leading follicle but will also give mature healthy ovum. The dominance of the follicle is selected by day 5 of the cycle and the dominance becomes apparent by day 7 of the cycle. Increase in perifollicular vascularity of dominant follicle in theca layer starts developing as early as 8th day of the cycle. That means a dominant follicle can be identified by the initiation of blood flow surrounding it. This sign can be used

to differentiate between early recruitment of the follicle and old follicle of the previous cycle on the baseline scan. If it is a follicle of more than 9 mm and shows few blood vessels around, it means it is a freshly recruited follicle and it is known that the follicle growth beyond 9–10 mm is dependent on FSH, so it is an indicator of rising FSH and aging ovary.

A Mature Follicle

Follicular maturity is conventionally assessed by its size, measured as inner-to-inner diameter of a follicle (Fig. 7.5). The follicle size, when assessed by follicle diameter, three orthogonal diameters are measured and the mean is considered as the mean follicular diameter. Follicular diameter of 17–18 mm is considered as adequate generally for gonadotropin-stimulated cycle and for clomiphene-stimulated cycles, 18–20 mm diameter may be optimum.[29] A follicle that has thin regular walls and anechoic contents are considered good in quality. But this is only evaluation of the anatomy of the follicle. It is essential to evaluate that at that follicular size, ovum inside is functionally mature or not. This can be assessed by the assessment of the blood flow.

Increase in perifollicular vascularity of dominant follicle in theca layer starts developing as early as 8th day of the cycle. Fall in perifollicular RI starts 2 days before ovulation, reaches nadir at ovulation, remains low for 4 days, and then with gradual rise reaches 0.5 in mid-luteal phase (Fig. 7.6).[32]

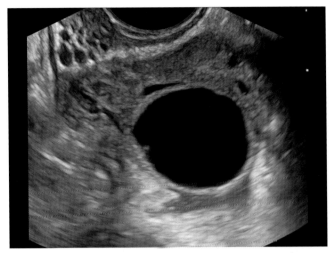

Fig. 7.5: B-mode ultrasound image of a mature follicle.

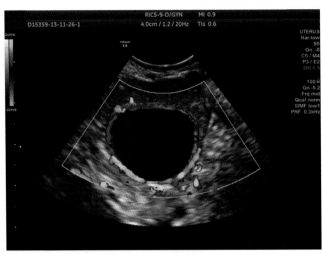

Fig. 7.7: Perifollicular vascularity seen on color Doppler.

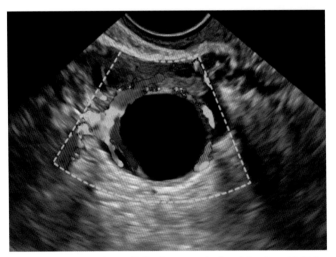

Fig. 7.6: Increase in perifollicular vascularity of dominant follicle seen on color Doppler.

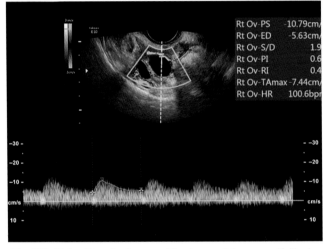

Fig. 7.8: Pulse Doppler image of the low resistance perifollicular flow.

When functionally mature, the follicle shows blood vessels covering at least three-fourths of the follicular circumference (Fig. 7.7). Chui et al. graded the follicular flow on the day of oocyte collection as grades 1–4 when in a single cross area slice the flow covered less than 25%, 25–50%, 50–75%, and more than 75% of follicular circumference. The conception was related to grades 3–4 vascularity.[33]

On pulse Doppler, these blood vessels show RI of 0.4–0.48[33] and PSV of more than 10 cm/s (Fig. 7.8).

The pulse repetition frequency (PRF) settings for color Doppler are set at 0.3 and wall filter at the lowest for infertility scans. The perifollicular vessels are only those that obliterate the follicular wall with color. If the follicular wall is seen and the vessel is seen just besides it, it is not a perifollicular vessel. Ovarian flow correlates well with oocyte recovery rates and hence may be useful in determining the most appropriate time to administer trigger to optimize recovery rate. It has been quoted in a study by Nargund et al.[25,33] that embryos produced by fertilization of the ova obtained from the follicles which had a perifollicular PSV of less than 10 cm/s, are less likely to be grade 1 embryos and also have higher chance of chromosomal malformations. In the same study, it has been shown that the probability of developing a grade 1 or 2 embryo is 75% if PSV was more than 10 cm/s, 40% if PSV was less than 10 cm/s, and 24% if there was no perifollicular flow. There is yet another study that supports this finding. Oocytes from severely hypoxic follicles are associated

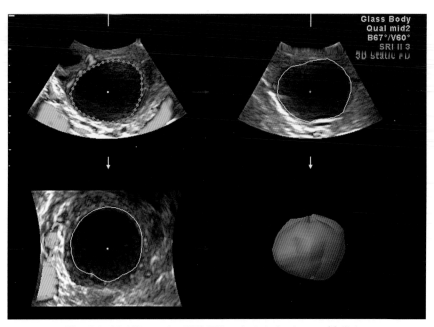

Fig. 7.9: 3D US acquired VOCAL calculated volume of follicle.
(3D: three-dimensional; US: ultrasound; VOCAL: virtual organ computer-aided analysis)

with high frequency of abnormalities of organization of chromosomes on metaphase spindle and may lead to segregation disorders and catastrophic mosaics in embryo.[34] Our data of more than 1,000 IUI cycles has shown that when the perifollicular RI more than 0.53 and PSV less than 9 cm/s, 12 hours before hCG injection, the conception rates were only 8.3% and 10%, respectively as compared to 32.8% and 28.2%, respectively and individually when perifollicular RI was less than 0.50 and PSV was more than 11 cm/s. We have, therefore, always preferred to wait with no extra medication when patient is on clomiphene citrate stimulation or continue with the same dose of gonadotropin till we get desired perifollicular RI and PSV.[35] Sometimes one may have to wait till follicular size of 24–25 mm before optimum flows are achieved (Fig. 7.9).

It has been shown that follicular fluid concentration of leptin, a follicular angiogenesis-related factor is inversely related to the stromal blood FI.[28]

It has also been suggested that the follicles containing oocytes capable to produce a pregnancy have a perifollicular vascular network more uniform and distinctive.[36] Although it is possible to assess the follicular flow as expressed by the PSV and perifollicular color map,[37] 3D power Doppler provides a more detailed quantitative information about the ovarian vascularization and perifollicular blood flow.[38,39]

In our study,[40] we have found perifollicular VI of between 6 and 20 and perifollicular FI more than 35 as most optimum values to achieve pregnancy. 68.4% of patients conceived when the VI was between 6 and 18 and 50% when it was between 18 and 20. However, the pregnancy rates were less than 25% when VI was less than 6 and only 7.4% when VI was more than 20. It was only 7.4% of patients with FI less than 27 who conceived whereas beyond 27, the conception rates rose consistently. It was 50% with FI between 27 and 35, 70% when FI was between 35 and 43, and almost all patients had conceived when FI was more than 43. Although it is possible to assess the follicular flow as expressed by the PSV and perifollicular color map,[38] it is the 3D power Doppler that gives the most precise information about the vascularization and follicular blood flow.[39]

Human chorionic gonadotropin plays a major role in inducing influx of blood within follicles. At the LH surge, the perifollicular PSV is 10 cm/s. This means that if the follicle is said to be functionally mature when PSV is 10 cm/s, that is the time when the LH surge starts and under the effect of that LH, the perifollicular PSV keeps on rising constantly.[40,41] The follicular PSV starts shooting up about 29 hours before ovulation.

This derives that a rising PSV with steady low RI suggests that the follicle is close to rupture.

Implantation has been the weakest link in the success of infertility treatment. Endometrium is a receptor organ for majority of the hormones involved in fertility and, therefore, study of its morphology and vascularity is thought to explain

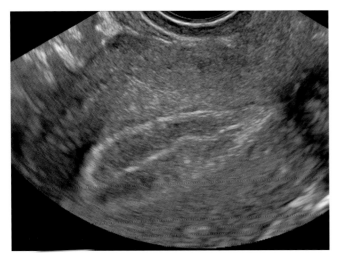

Fig. 7.10: B-mode ultrasound image of grade A endometrium.

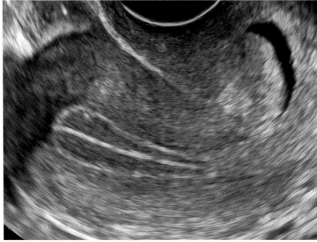

Fig. 7.11: B-mode ultrasound image of grade B endometrium.

the mysteries of implantation failure. Therefore, like follicle, endometrium is also assessed by transvaginal 2D US and color Doppler before planning for hCG during any assisted reproductive technologies.

B-mode Features of Endometrium with Good Receptivity

An endometrial thickness of 8–10 mm is considered optimum for implantation.[42,43]

Morphology of the endometrium is as important as thickness of the endometrium. An intact endometrio-myometrial junction is an important marker for a healthy endometrium and breach or irregularity of endometrio-myometrial junction is an indication of unhealthy endometrium and, therefore, poor receptivity.

Popularly multilayered endometrium is considered as a desired endometrial pattern. Morphologically, the endometrium is graded as the best grade A, when it is a triple line endometrium and the intervening area is as hypoechoic as the anterior normal myometrium (Fig. 7.10). The echogenicity is attributed to the development of multiple vessels penetrating in the endometrium producing multiple tissue interfaces and, therefore, causing the echogenicity and due to glycogen storage in the endometrial columnar epithelium and due to stromal edema (Fig. 7.11).[44] The endometrium is graded as intermediate or grade B (Fig. 7.12) when it is multilayered or triple line with hypoechoic intervening area. In grade C which was once thought to be most unfavorable endometrium would be a homogeneous isoechoic endometrium.[45] Though some studies have shown no significant difference in pregnancy rates among different morphological patterns.

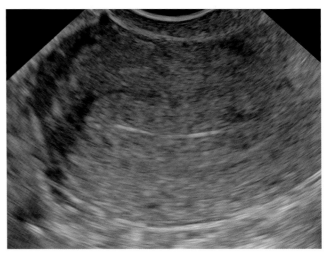

Fig. 7.12: B-mode ultrasound image of grade C endometrium.

Doppler Features of Endometrium with Good Receptivity

There are several reports by different groups[46] that agree on the fact that implantation rates can be more correlated to the vascularity of the endometrium rather than the thickness and morphology of the endometrium. Segmental uterine artery perfusion demonstrates significant correlation with hormonal and histological markers of uterine receptivity, reaching the highest sensitivity for subendometrial blood flow.[2]

Nearly the same time as follicular vascularity, the spiral arteries start extending toward the endometrium. This is the effect of estrogen. Endometrial and subendometrial flow increases in the follicular phase and reaches its maximum 3 days prior to ovulation and this correlates with the estrogen peak. But the endometrial neoangiogenesis differ in natural and stimulated cycles. In stimulated cycles, there may be 35% less in endometrial and subendometrial vascularity as compared to non-stimulated cycles.[47]

On color Doppler, endometrium with good receptivity shows vascularity in zones 3 and 4 or may be called subendometrial and endometrial layers (Fig. 7.13).

The zones of vascularity are defined according to Applebaum[46] as: zone 1 when the vascularity on power Doppler is seen only at endometrio-myometrium junction, zone 2 when vessels penetrate through the hyperechogenic endometrial edge, zone 3 when it reaches intervening hypoechogenic zone, and zone 4 when the vessels reach the endometrial cavity. The pregnancy rates related to the zones of vascular penetration was documented as 26.7% for zone 1, 36.4% for zone 2, and 37.9% for zone 3.

One more comparison of two studies have also shown similar results, as shown below:[48]

- *Zone 1*: 3.5–7.5% (5.2%)
- *Zone 2*: 15.8–29.7% (28.7%)
- *Zone 3*: 24.2–47.8% (52%)
- *Zone 4*: 67.3% (74%).

Endometrial Vascularity: Its Relation to Implantation Rates (Table 7.1)[49]

Zaidi et al. found that absence of flow in the endometrial and subendometrial zones on day of hCG indicate total failure of implantation.[50] In our data of more than 1,000 IUI cycles, when color Doppler studies were done 12 hours before the trigger we have found only 7.3% pregnancy rates for zone 1 and 13.4% for zone 2 vascularity. The conception rates with zones 3 and 4 vascularity, were comparable and were 35.8% and 38.3%, respectively. When pregnancy is achieved in absence of endometrial and subendometrial flow more than half of these pregnancies will finish as spontaneous miscarriage.[48]

This vascularity should cover at least 5-mm^2 area of the endometrium. Below this cutoff, the pregnancy rates are extremely low.[51] Those women with an intra-endometrial

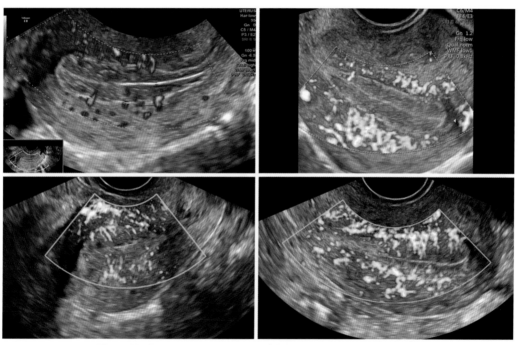

Fig. 7.13: Power Doppler images of the grades 1–4 endometrium.

TABLE 7.1: Endometrial vascularity: its relation to implantation rates.

Vascularity in	Zone 1	Zone 2	Zone 3	Zone 4
Percentage of patients	6.69%	20.73%	58%	14.47%
Beta human chorionic gonadotropin (βhCG)	19%	21.87%	39.77%	70.14%
Gestational sac	9.6%	14.58%	36.8%	68.65%
Abortions	50%	23.8%	5.6%	1.5%

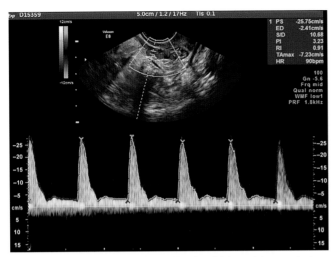

Fig. 7.14: Pulse Doppler image showing high resistance uterine artery flow waveform.

TABLE 7.2: Ultrasound features of mature follicle and endometrium.

	Follicle	Endometrium
Size/thickness	16–18 mm	8–10 mm
Morphology	Thin wall, no internal echoes, and halo	Grade A/B
Vascularity	Three-fourths circumference	Zones 3–4
RI	0.4–0.48	<0.5
PSV	>10 cm/s	–
Uterine artery PI	–	<3.2
Volume	3–7 cc	3–7 cc
3D morphology	Cumulus	Intact endometrial-myometrial junction
3D PD	More symmetrical the better	Higher the better

(3D: three-dimensional; PI: pulsatility index; PSV: peak systolic velocity; RI: resistance index; PD: power Doppler)

power Doppler area (EPDA) less than 5 mm^2, achieved a significantly lower pregnancy rate (23.5% vs 47.5%, p = 0.021) and implantation rate (8.1% vs 20.2%, p = 0.003) than those with an EPDA more than 5 mm^2.[51]

While the reported correlation between vascularity in the endometrium and subendometrium and pregnancy rates is controversial, it has been concluded in two studies that no difference was found in patients with good prognosis for cycle outcome, but in patients with poor embryo quality, better endometrial vascularity seemed to improve the cycle outcome.[4,52]

The vessels that reach the endometrium are the spiral arteries. The pulse Doppler of these arteries should have an RI of < 0.6 for the endometrium to be called mature for implantation. Moreover, the pulse Doppler analysis of the uterine artery waveform is done and its RI should not be more than 0.9 and PI should be less than 3.2 (Fig. 7.14).

Several authors have shown that the optimum uterine receptivity was obtained when average PI of the uterine artery was between 2 and 3 on the day of transfer or on the day of hCG.[53,54] Coulam et al. have also shown that no pregnancy was achieved after ET when uterine artery PI was above 3.3 in an IVF program on the day of trigger.[55] Cacciatore et al. suggest that implantation is unlikely when PI is more than 3.3 and RI is more than 0.95 or when no velocities are seen at the end of the diastole.[37] Tsai and colleagues evaluated the prognostic value of uterine perfusion on day of trigger for IUI cycles and showed that no pregnancy occurred when the PI of ascending branch of uterine artery was more than 3. Fecundity rate was 18% when PI was less than 2 and 19.8% when PI was between 2 and 3.[56]

Endometrial volume by 3D ultrasound volume calculation of the endometrium may help to correlate the cycle outcome with more reliable quantitative parameter rather than endometrial thickness.

A study by Raga et al.[57] shows pregnancy and implantation rates were significantly lower when endometrial volume less than 2 mL, while no pregnancy was achieved when endometrial volume was less than 1 mL. Study by Kupesic et al. also shows no pregnancy when endometrial volume was less than 2 mL, or when exceeded 8 mL.[58]

Kupesic et al. also reported a subendometrial FI of less than 11 on the day of ET as a cutoff level for predicting poor implantation.[58] Ng et al. concluded that number of embryos replaced and endometrial VFI were the only two predictive factors for pregnancy.[59] According to another study, VFI on the day of trigger is more sensitive than volume, VI and FI for prediction of pregnancy. VFI more than 0.24 has:

- Sensitivity of 83.3%
- Specificity of 88.9%
- Positive predictive value (PPV) 93.8%
- Negative predictive value (NPV) 72.3%
- For prediction of pregnancy with 33% pregnancy rate.[60]

Table 7.2 summarizes the features of pre-trigger mature follicle and receptive endometrium.

Secretory Phase Assessment

It is very important to mention here that the Doppler study for assessment of endometrial receptivity must be done

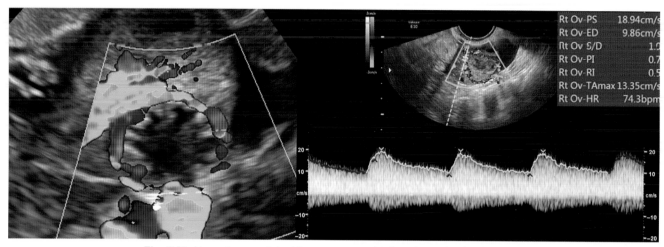

Fig. 7.15: Normal corpus luteal flow seen on color Doppler and pulse Doppler.

before the trigger. This can be explained by physiology. It is known that with the LH surge, there is fall in the estrogen level and progesterone takes about 4–5 days to reach a plateau. These are the two steroids responsible for endometrial vascularity and in absence of both, evidently the endometrial vascularity decreases. This is a need for implantation. Histological and embryological data suggests that relatively low partial pressure of oxygen (pO_2) environment may be necessary for successful implantation of human blastocyst.[61]

Ng et al. have also reported a low endometrial VI and VFI in pregnant group on the day of oocyte retrieval and also a nonsignificant trend of higher implantation and pregnancy rates in patients with absent subendometrial and endometrial flow. This probably can be explained on the basis that hCG administration/LH peak causes increased uterine artery resistance and hence decrease in endometrial perfusion also on the day of oocyte retrieval.[62]

It is with the rise of the progesterone that the endometrial vascularity starts increasing. Endometrial vascularity in luteal phase is due to progesterone. Adequate development of progesterone receptors with adequate progesterone secretion is represented as low resistance flow in the endometrium in the luteal phase.

MID-LUTEAL PHASE

Rupture of the follicle leads to formation of corpus luteum. Corpus luteum is responsible for progesterone production. The functional efficacy of the corpus luteum can be assessed by Doppler by assessing the pericorpus luteal

vascularity. Segmental uterine and ovarian artery perfusion demonstrates a significant correlation with histological and hormonal markers of uterine receptivity and may aid assessment of luteal phase defect.[63] A clear correlation between RI of corpus luteum and plasma progesterone levels has been seen in natural cycle. RI of the corpus luteum can, therefore, be used as an adjunct to plasma progesterone assay as an index of luteal function.[64]

A corpus luteum that is functionally normal and produces adequate amount of progesterone shows corpus luteal flow with RI 0.35–0.50 and PSV 10–15 cm/s (Fig. 7.15).

Soon after rupture of the follicle, the outer margin of the endometrium starts becoming fluffy and blurred. The endometrium also becomes hyperechoic as a result of progesterone exposure. But with adequate progesterone levels in the mid-luteal phase, the spiral arteries show RI of 0.48–0.52 (low resistance flow) and uterine artery shows PI of 2.0–2.5. This PI is lower than in the preovulatory phase because of smooth muscle relaxing effect of progesterone.

Inadequate progesterone production and, therefore, corpus luteal inadequacy is suggested by high resistance flow in corpus luteal vessels.[64] In luteal phase defect because of low progesterone levels, the resistance in the pericorpus luteal vessels is high. Because of low progesterone levels, there is inadequate relaxation of the muscularis of the uterine artery and, therefore, the uterine artery resistance is high along with higher resistance in its branches—the spiral vessels (Figs. 7.16A and B).

Corpus luteal flow and spiral artery flow in normal cycle and luteal phase defect are described in Tables 7.3 and 7.4.[63]

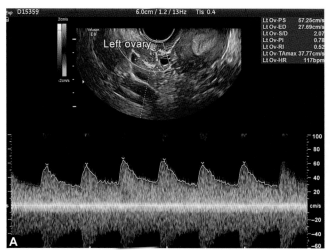
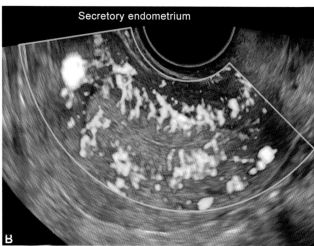

Figs. 7.16A and B: (A) Low resistance blood flow of the corpus luteum demonstrated on pulse Doppler; and (B) HD power Doppler showing blood flow in the secretory endometrium.

TABLE 7.3: Corpus luteal flow in normal cycle and in luteal phase defect.

	Normal	LPD
Perifollicular phase	0.56 ± 0.06	0.58 ± 0.04
LH peak day	0.44 ± 0.04	0.58 ± 0.04
Mid-luteal phase	0.42 ± 0.06	0.58 ± 0.04
Late luteal phase	0.50 ± 0.04	0.58 ± 0.04

(LH: luteinizing hormone; LPD: luteal phase defect)

TABLE 7.4: Spiral artery flow in normal cycle and in luteal phase defect.

Phase	Control RI	LPD RI
Periovulatory	0.53 ± 0.04	0.70 ± 0.06
Mid-luteal	0.50 ± 0.02	0.72 ± 0.06
Late luteal	0.51 ± 0.04	0.72 ± 0.04

(LPD: luteal phase defect; RI: resistance index)

CONCLUSION

Ultrasound is an excellent tool for assessment of the menstrual cycle. Hormonal changes occurring day-to-day during the menstrual cycle reflects as morphological and vascular changes in the ovary and the uterus. Assessing these changes by transvaginal ultrasound and Doppler and correctly interpreting can explain the hormonal basis of these changes. Ultrasound with Doppler can, thus, be used as the only modality for cycle assessment in patients undergoing assisted reproduction technology and may be of help to reduce the cost of the cycle by avoiding certain hormonal assessments and still maintaining close and accurate watch on the hormonal changes occurring during treatment cycle.

But it is very important to understand here that Doppler used for cycle monitoring is not to cancel the cycle when optimum parameters are not achieved. It is to optimize the time of trigger, and IUI. One should safely wait till the optimum Doppler parameters are achieved for both follicle and endometrium. If in the process the follicle ruptures, the chances of conception are low and, therefore, in such cases, it is best to advise natural intercourse rather than do an IUI. Though a proper counseling with the patient for the same is important. For IVF, one can wait till optimum parameters are achieved as the patients are already down-regulated. To our experience of more than 9,000 documented pregnancies with IUI, using Doppler for follicular monitoring increases the pregnancy rates by 20–25%.

REFERENCES

1. Ravhon A, Lavery S, Michael S, et al. Dynamic assays of inhibin B and oestradiol following buserelin acetate administration as predictors of ovarian response in IVF. Hum Reprod. 2000;15:2297-301.
2. Kupesic S, Kurjak A. Predictors of IVF outcome by three-dimensional ultrasound. Hum Reprod. 2002;17:950-5.
3. Ng EH, Tang OS, Chan CC, et al. Ovarian stromal blood flow in the prediction of ovarian response during in vitro fertilization treatment. Hum Reprod. 2005;20:3147-51.
4. Merce LT, Barco MJ, Bau S, et al. Prediction of ovarian response and IVF/ICSI outcome by three dimensional ultrasonography and power Doppler angiography. Eur J Obstet Gynecol Reprod Biol. 2007;132:93-100.

5. Popovic-Todorovic B, Loft A, Lindhard A, et al. A prospective study of predictive factors of ovarian response in 'standard' IVF/ICSI patients treated with recombinant FSH. A suggestion for recombinant FSH dosage normogram. Hum Reprod. 2003;18:781-7.

6. La Marca A, Grisendi V, Giulini S, et al. Individualization of the FSH starting dose in IVF/ICSI cycles using the antral follicle count. J Ovarian Res. 2013;6:11.

7. Olivennes F, Howles CM, Borini A, et al. Individualizing FSH dose for assisted reproduction using a novel algorithm: the CONSORT study. Reprod Biomed Online. 2009;18:195-204.

8. Freiesleben NL, Lossl K, Bogstad J, et al. Predictors of ovarian response in intrauterine insemination patients and development of a dosage nomogram. Reprod Biomed Online. 2008;17:632-41.

9. La Marca A, Stabile G, Artenisio AC, et al. Serum anti-Müllerian hormone throughout the human menstrual cycle. Hum Reprod. 2006;21:3103-7.

10. van Rooij IA, Broekmans FJ, te Velde ER, et al. Serum anti-Müllerian hormone levels: a novel measure of ovarian reserve. Hum Reprod. 2002;17:3065-71.

11. Broer SL, Mol BW, Hendriks D, et al. The role of antimullerian hormone in prediction of outcome after IVF: comparison with the antral follicle count. Fertil Steril. 2009;91:705-14.

12. van Disseldorp J, Lambalk CB, Kwee J, et al. Comparison of inter- and intra-cycle variability of anti-Mullerian hormone and antral follicle counts. Hum Reprod. 2010;25:221-7.

13. Panchal S, Nagori C. Comparison of anti-mullerian hormone and antral follicle count for assessment of ovarian reserve. J Hum Reprod Sci. 2012;5:274-8.

14. Krishnakumar J, Agarwal A, Nambiar D, et al. Comparison of antral follicle count, antimullerian hormone and day 2 follicle stimulating hormone as predictor of ovarian response and clinical pregnancy rate in patient with an abnormal ovarian reserve test. Int J Reprod Contracept Obstet Gynecol. 2016;5:2762-7.

15. Jayaprakasan K, Hilwah N, Kendall NR, et al. Does 3D ultrasound offer any advantage in the pretreatment assessment of ovarian reserve and prediction of outcome after assisted reproduction treatment? Hum Reprod. 2007;22:1932-41.

16. Rainne-Fenning NJ. What is in a number? The polycystic ovary revisited. Hum Reprod. 2011;26:3118-22.

17. Deb S, Jayaprakasan K, Campbell BK, et al. Intraobserver and interobserver reliability of automated antral follicle counts made using three-dimensional ultrasound and SonoAVC. Ultrasound Obstet Gynecol. 2009;33:477-83.

18. Lass A, Skull J, McVeigh E, et al. Measurement of ovarian volume by transvaginal sonography before ovulation induction with human menopausal gonadotrophin for in-vitro fertilization can predict poor response. Hum Reprod. 1997;12:294-7.

19. van Rooji IA, Broekmans FJ, tr Velde ER, et al. Serum anti-Mullerian hormone levels: a novel measure of ovarian reserve. Hum Reprod. 2002;17:3065-71.

20. Fratelli JL, Levi AJ, Miller BT. A prospective novel method of determining ovarian size during in vitro fertilization cycles. J Assist Reprod Genet. 2002;19:39-41.

21. Kwee J, Elting ME. Schats R, et al. Ovarian volume and antral follicle count for the prediction of low and hyper responders with in vitro fertilization. Reprod Biol Endocrinol. 2007;5:9.

22. Zaidi J, Barber J, Kyei-Mensah A, et al. Relationship of ovarian stromal blood flow at baseline ultrasound to subsequent follicular response in an in vitro fertilization program. Obstet Gynecol. 1996;88:779-84.

23. Engmann L, Sladkevicius P, Agrawal R, et al. Value of ovarian stromal blood flow velocity measurement after pituitary suppression in the prediction of ovarian responsiveness and outcome of in vitro fertilization treatment. Fertil Steril. 1999;71:22-9.

24. Arora A, Gainder S, Dhaliwal L, et al. Clinical significance of ovarian stromal blood flow in assessment of ovarian response in stimulated cycle for in vitro fertilization. Int J Reprod Contracept Obstet Gynecol. 2015;4:1380-3.

25. Nargund G, Bourne TH, Doyle PE, et al. Association between ultrasound indices of follicular blood flow, oocyte recovery and preimplantation embryo quality. Hum Reprod. 1996;11:109-13.

26. Lam PM, Johnson IR, Rainne-Fenning NJ. Three dimensional ultrasound features of the polycystic ovary and the effect of different phenotypic expressions on these parameters. Hum Reprod. 2007;22:3116-23.

27. Ng EH, Chan CC, Yeung WS, et al. Effect of age on ovarian stromal flow measured by three-dimensional ultrasound with power Doppler in Chinese women with proven fertility. Hum Reprod. 2004;19:2132-7.

28. Wu MH, Tsai SJ, Pan HA, et al. Three dimensional power Doppler imaging of ovarian stromal blood flow in women with endometriosis undergoing in vitro fertilization. Ultrasound Obstet Gynecol. 2003;21:480-5.

29. Luciano GN, Tarek AG. Ultrasonography and IVF. In: Botros RM, Rizk B (Eds). Ultrasonography in Reproductive Medicine and Infertility. Cambridge: Cambridge University Press; 2010.

30. Ng EH, Chan CC, Shan Tang O, et al. Effect of pituitary downregulation on antral follicle count, ovarian volume and stromal blood flow measured by three-dimensional ultrasound with power Doppler prior to ovarian stimulation. Hum Reprod. 2004;19:2811-5.

31. Aleem FA, Predanic M. Transvaginal colour Doppler determination of the ovarian and uterine blood flow characteristics in polycystic ovary disease. Fertil Steril. 1996;65:510-6.

32. Jokubkeine L, Sladkevicius P, Rovas L, et al. Assessment of changes in volume and vascularity of ovaries during the normal menstrual cycle using three-dimensional power Doppler ultrasound. Hum Reprod. 2006;21:2661-8.

33. Nargund G, Doyle PE, Bourne TH, et al. Ultrasound derived indices of follicular blood flow before hCG administration and the prediction of oocyte recovery and preimplantation embryo quality. Hum Reprod. 1996;11:2512-7.

34. Van Blerkom J, Antezak M, Schrader R. The developmental potential of human oocyte is related to the dissolved oxygen content of follicular fluid: association with vascular endothelial growth factor levels and perifollicular blood flow characteristics. Hum Reprod. 1997;12:1047-55.

35. Panchal S, Nagori C. Follicular monitoring. J Ultrasound Obstet Gynecol. 2012;6:300-12.

36. Vlaisavljević V, Reljic M, Gavrić Lovrec V, et al. Measurement of perifollicular blood flow of the dominant preovulatory follicle using three-dimensional power Doppler. Ultrasound Obstet Gynecol. 2003;22:520-6.

37. Cacciatore B, Simberg N, Fusaro P, et al. Transvaginal Doppler study of uterine artery blood flow in in vitro fertilization embryo transfer cycles. Fertil Steril. 1996;66:130-4.

38. Merce LT. Ultrasound markers of implantation. Ultrasound Rev Obstet Gynecol. 2002;2:110-23.

39. Merce LT, Barco MJ, Kupesic S, et al. 2D and 3D power Doppler ultrasound from ovulation to implantation. In: Kurjak A, Chervenak F (Eds). Textbook of Perinatal Medicine. London: Parthenon Publishing; 2005.

40. Panchal SY, Nagori CB. Can 3D PD be a better tool for assessing the pre-HCG follicle and endometrium? A randomized study of 500 cases. Presented at 16th World Congress on Ultrasound in Obstetrics and Gynecology, 2006, London. J Ultrasound Obstet Gynecol. 2006;28:504.

41. Lunenfeld E, Schwartz I, Meizner I, et al. Intra-ovarian blood flow during spontaneous and stimulated cycles. Hum Reprod. 1996;11:2481-3.

42. Dickey RP, Olar TT, Taylor SN, et al. Relationship of biochemical pregnancy to preovulatory endometrial thickness and pattern in patients undergoing ovulation induction. Hum Reprod. 1993;8:327-30.

43. Boué J, Boue A, Lazar P. Retrospective and prospective epidemiological studies of 1500 karyotyped spontaneous human abortions. Teratology. 1975;12:11-26.

44. Fleischer AC, Kepple DM, Aenoco AL, et al. Transvaginal Ultrasound. St Louis: Mosby; 1992. pp. 21-43.

45. Smith B, Porter R, Ahuja K, et al. Ultrasonic assessment of endometrial changes in stimulated cycles in an in vitro fertilization and embryo transfer program. J In Vitro Fert Embryo Transf. 1984;1:233-8.

46. Applebaum M. The 'steel' or 'teflon' endometrium—ultrasound visualization of endometrial vascularity in IVF patients and outcome. Presented at the Third World Congress of Ultrasound in Obstetrics and Gynecology. Ultrasound Obstet Gynecol. 1993;3:10.

47. Ng EH, Chan CC, Tang OS, et al. Comparison of endometrial and subendometrial blood flow measured by three-dimensional power Doppler ultrasound between stimulated and natural cycles in the same patients. Hum Reprod. 2004;19:2385-90.

48. Chien LW, Au HK, Chen PL, et al. Assessment of uterine receptivity by the endometrial-subendometrial blood flow distribution pattern in women undergoing in vitro fertilization-embryo transfer. Fertil Steril. 2002;78:245-51.

49. Nagori CB, Panchal S. Endometrial vascularity: Its relation to implantation rates. Int J Infertil Fetal Med. 2012;3:48-50.

50. Zaidi J, Campbell S, Pittrof R, et al. Endometrial thickness, morphology, vascular penetration and velocimetry in predicting implantation in an in vitro fertilization program. Ultrasound Obstet Gynecol. 1995;6:191-8.

51. Yang JH, Wu MY, Chen CD, et al. Association of endometrial blood flow as determined by a modified colour Doppler technique with subsequent outcome of in-vitro fertilization. Hum Reprod. 1999;14:1606-10.

52. Mercé LT, Barco MJ, Bau S, et al. Are endometrial parameters by three-dimensional ultrasound and power Doppler angiography related to in vitro fertilization/embryo transfer outcome? Fertil Steril. 2008;89:111-7.

53. Steer CV, Campbell S, Tan SL, et al. The use of transvaginal colour flow imaging after in vitro fertilization to identify optimum uterine conditions before embryo transfer. Fertil Steril. 1992;57:372-6.

54. Zaidi J, Pittrof R, Shaker A, et al. Assessment of uterine artery blood flow on the day of human chorionic gonadotrophin administration by transvaginal colour Doppler ultrasound in an in vitro fertilization program. Fertil Steril. 1996;65:377-81.

55. Coulam CB, Stern JJ, Soenksen DM, et al. Comparison of pulsatility indexes on the day of oocyte retrieval and embryo transfer. Hum Reprod. 1995;10:82-4.

56. Tsai YC, Chang JC, Tai MJ, et al. Relationship of uterine perfusion to outcome of intrauterine insemination. J Ultrasound Med. 1996;15:633-6.

57. Raga F, Bonilla-Musoles F, Casan EM, et al. Assessment of endometrial volume by three-dimensional ultrasound prior to embryo transfer: clues to endometrial receptivity. Hum Reprod. 1999;14:2851-4.

58. Kupesic S, Bekavac I, Bjelos D, et al. Assessment of endometrial receptivity by transvaginal colour Doppler and three-dimensional power Doppler ultrasonography in patients undergoing in vitro fertilization procedures. J Ultrasound Med. 2001;20:125-34.

59. Ng EH, Chan CC, Tang OS, et al. Relationship between uterine blood flow and endometrial and subendometrial blood flows during stimulated and natural cycles. Fertil Steril. 2006;85:721-7.

60. Wu HM, Chiang CH, Huang HY, et al. Detection of subendometrial vascularization flow index by three-dimensional ultrasound may be useful for predicting the pregnancy rate for patients undergoing in vitro fertilization-embryo transfer. Fertil Steril. 2003;79:507-11.

61. Graham C, Postovit IM, Park H, et al. Adrina and Luisa Castellucci award lecture 1999: role of oxygen in regulation of trophoblast gene expression and invasion. Placenta. 2000;21:443-50.

62. Ng EH, Chan CC, Tang OS, et al. The role of endometrial and subendometrial blood flows measured by three-dimensional power Doppler ultrasound in prediction of pregnancy during IVF treatment. Hum Reprod. 2006;21:164-70.

63. Kupesić S, Kurjak A, Vujisić S, et al. Luteal phase defect: comparison between Doppler velocimetry, histological and hormonal markers. Ultrasound Obstet Gynecol. 1997;9:105-12.

64. Glock JL, Brumsted JR. Colour flow pulsed Doppler ultrasound in diagnosing luteal phase defect. Fertil Steril. 1995;64:500-4.

Doppler in Normal and Abnormal Early Pregnancy

INTRODUCTION

Pregnancy starts from the time when oocyte is fertilized by sperm in the fallopian tube. It is known that the fertilized ovum takes about 4–5 days to travel from the tube to the endometrial cavity and to implant. During this period, it keeps on growing. The first 12 weeks of life in the womb is the most dynamic period as far as fetal growth is concerned. Beyond 12 weeks, it is no more called an early pregnancy. The growth and development of this early pregnancy can be assessed by B-mode ultrasound, but the prognosis of the pregnancy can be predicted by B-mode as well as Doppler.

The earliest prediction of the presence of pregnancy can be done in the mid-luteal phase of the cycle. The corpus luteum is formed after the rupture of the follicle and ovulation. The corpus luteal function reaches its maximum in the mid-luteal phase. The function of the corpus luteum, chiefly is progesterone production. A clear correlation between resistance index (RI) of corpus luteum and plasma progesterone levels has been seen in natural cycle. The RI of the corpus luteum can, therefore, be used as an adjunct to plasma progesterone assay as an index of luteal function.[1] The RI of the corpus luteum in the mid-luteal phase is less than 0.5 (Fig. 8.1), when the progesterone production is normal. In the patients who conceive, this RI remains low or may further decrease beyond the mid-luteal phase. Whereas in nonconception cycles, the RI of the corpus luteum increases beyond the mid-luteal phase toward the end of the cycle.

In the mid-luteal phase, the endometrium is about 14–16 mm, sometimes more, and it is homogeneous and hyperechoic and also shows posterior enhancement. The

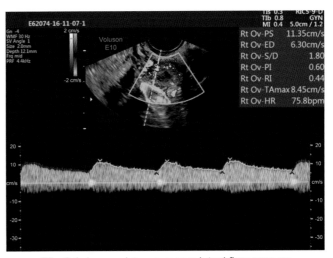

Fig. 8.1: Low resistance corpus luteal flow seen on color and pulsed Doppler.

spiral arteries (endometrial vessels) show low resistance flow in normal mid-luteal phase with RI of less than 0.52 (Fig. 8.2).[1] If the embryo has already implanted, this resistance will keep on decreasing until the end of the cycle, but in nonconception cycles, the resistance will gradually increase toward the end of the cycle. Spiral artery peak systolic velocity (PSV) of more than 5 cm/s can be a positive predictor of pregnancy in mid-luteal phase.[1] Along with the low resistance in the spiral vessels, the uterine artery also shows a comparatively low resistance flow, with maximum pulsatility index (PI) of 2.5 (Fig. 8.3). This remains low throughout the rest of the cycle in conception cycle and increases toward the end of the cycle in nonconception cycles. Low corpus luteal RI indicates normal progesterone

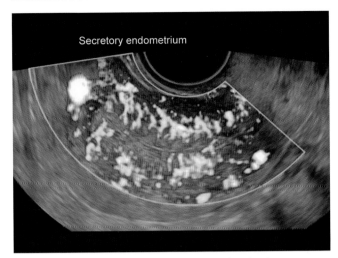

Fig. 8.2: Secretory endometrium showing low resistance flow with vascularity.

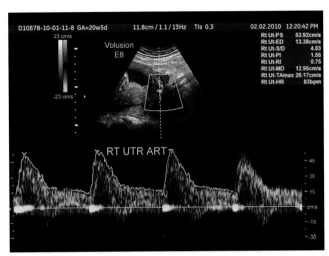

Fig. 8.4: Increased diastolic flow and leading to low resistance flow in the uterine artery.

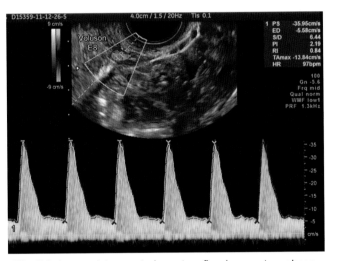

Fig. 8.3: Low resistance uterine artery flow in secretory phase.

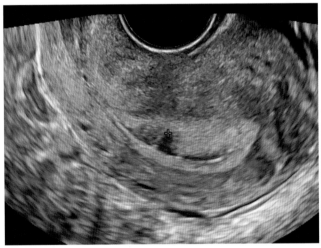

Fig. 8.5: B-mode ultrasound image of the endometrium showing asymmetrical thickening of the endometrium.

production, whereas low spiral artery and uterine artery RI indicate adequate development of progesterone receptors in the endometrium. Progesterone is a smooth muscle relaxant and is responsible, therefore, for decreased tone in the muscularis of the uterine artery and, thus, leading to low resistance flow. This means that these low resistance vessels in the luteal phase are indicators of adequate progesterone production and also of development of adequate progesterone receptors. During the entire 1st trimester, the uterine artery resistance decreases. With adequate placentation, the diastolic notch of the uterine artery waveform also smoothens out and the diastolic flows in uterine artery increase as a result of conversion of spiral arteries into low resistance villous vessels, a primary change required for normal placentation (Fig. 8.4).[2]

Apart from this, Honemeyer et al. have also described a "color comet sign".[2] As discussed earlier, implantation occurs in 4–5 days after ovulation. Therefore, when ultrasound scan is done in the mid-luteal phase, the implantation has already occurred. This leads to asymmetrical thickening of the endometrium (Fig. 8.5), with localized area of increased echogenicity also. The "color comet sign" is two or more vessels heading and converging toward this one point/small area on the endometrium (Fig. 8.6). This may be used as a sign of early conception, even before the gestational sac appears.

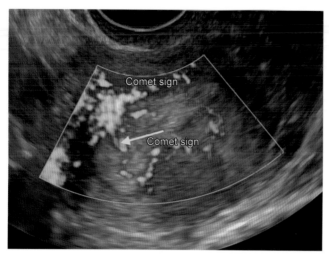

Fig. 8.6: HD flow showing color comet sign of early pregnancy.

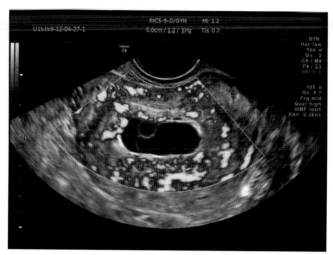

Fig. 8.8: Vascularity surrounding the true gestational sac with yolk sac as seen on three-dimensional (3D) power Doppler.

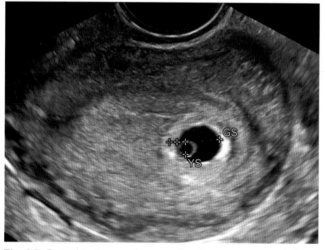

Fig. 8.7: B-mode ultrasound image of early pregnancy, gestational sac with yolk sac showing eccentric location of the gestational sac, and abutting of the endometrial cavity.

Though it must be remembered that these are only predictors of a conception cycles, not confirmation of pregnancy. Pregnancy can be confirmed clinically by missed periods and by positive urine pregnancy test or high serum beta-human chorionic gonadotropin (beta-hCG) levels in serum. Beta-hCG levels in serum [serum human chorionic gonadotropin (ShCG)] of more than 10 IU are considered as a very sensitive diagnostic test for pregnancy, though it does not indicate a normal/abnormal early pregnancy. Serum beta-hCG levels rise until 8–9 weeks in normal early pregnancy and then decrease and remain low during the 2nd and 3rd trimesters. Confirmation of intrauterine pregnancy can only be done by ultrasound. For

the assessment of very early pregnancy, transvaginal route is to be preferred. ShCG level of more than 1,500 mIU/mL is reached 10–14 days after conception and at this level, intrauterine gestational sac is always seen by transvaginal scan.

Intrauterine gestational sac is seen as an anechoic round structure in the fundal half of the endometrial cavity, with hyperechoic thick margins (Fig. 8.7), due to decidual reaction in the thick hyperechoic endometrium. The central anechoic area, which the gestational sac, may contain the yolk sac and the embryonic pole, depending on the age of gestation. Normal gestational sac shows not only a well-vascularized endometrium, but also a ring of vascularity around the gestational sac, with low resistance flow (RI < 0.5) (Fig. 8.8). Though it is important to mention here that if a good ring of vascularity is seen around the gestational sac, it is not mandatory to assess the RI in these vessels.

The purpose of this early scan is to confirm the intra-uterine location of the pregnancy and also to prognosticate it. It is, therefore, essential to assess the corpus luteal flow. This is because along with the rising serum beta-hCG levels, in the early pregnancy, till at least 10 weeks, the estrogen and progesterone levels also rise (Fig. 8.9).[3]

All these hormones are essential to support the early pregnancy till the placenta takes over. Progesterone is secreted by corpus luteum and, therefore, it is essential to assess the corpus luteal flow in early pregnancy along with the assessment of the intrauterine gestational sac. It has been documented that low progesterone levels (<12 ng/mL) prior to 7 weeks of gestation may be indicative of bad prognosis of pregnancy.[4] And if progesterone production

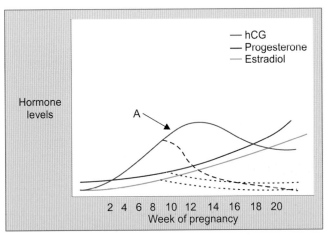

Fig. 8.9: Status of different hormones in pregnancy.
Source: Adapted from Kumar P, Magon N. Hormones in pregnancy. Niger Med J. 2012;53:179-83.

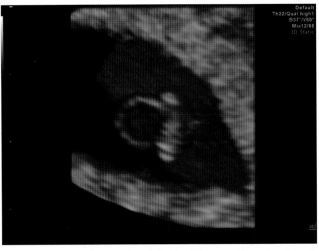

Fig. 8.11: Three-dimensional (3D) ultrasound image of early pregnancy showing elongated embryonic pole with cephalic and caudal poles and yolk sac.

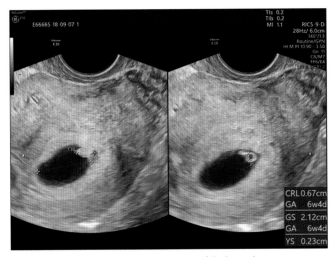

Fig. 8.10: B-mode ultrasound image of 5–6 weeks pregnancy, showing yolk sac and embryonic pole.

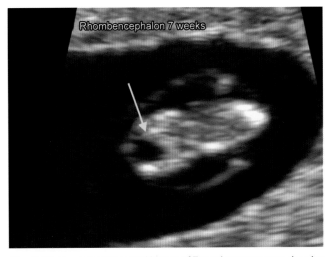

Fig. 8.12: B-mode ultrasound image of 7 weeks pregnancy showing anechoic structure in the cephalic pole—rhombencephalon (arrow).

from corpus luteum can be correlated with the corpus luteal RI,[1] rise in the corpus luteal flow resistance at anytime, therefore, before 7–8 weeks of pregnancy, can be an indication of a pregnancy at risk. Beyond 9 weeks, corpus luteal RI starts increasing as the placenta starts taking over the function and by the end of 12 weeks, corpus luteum completely regresses.

Ultrasound scan in the 1st trimester is done to confirm the intrauterine location of the pregnancy, viability of the pregnancy, to confirm normal growth and development, and to diagnose abnormalities. As for the last indication, diagnosis of abnormalities in the 1st trimester, we shall discuss only those, in this chapter, for the diagnosis of which Doppler has a role to play. To diagnose abnormalities, clear

idea about the role of ultrasound in the study of normal development is essential.

At 4 weeks of gestation, the tiny gestational sac appears with hyperechoic margin of decidual reaction, abutting the endometrial cavity (*see* Fig. 8.7). Doppler will show a low resistance flow in the blood vessels encircling the gestational sac (*see* Fig. 8.8). In the 5th week, the yolk sac develops and by the end of 5th week, embryonic pole can be identified (Fig. 8.10). The embryonic pole elongates and then curves during the 6th week (Fig. 8.11), the cephalic and caudal poles are identified, and the neural tube also starts developing. In the 7th week, rhombencephalon develops (Fig. 8.12) and it is this early during the pregnancy that the circulation is seen in the cephalic pole of the embryo.

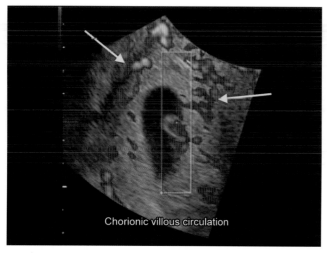

Fig. 8.13: Power Doppler image of the early pregnancy showing chorionic circulation.

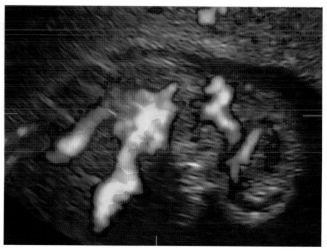

Fig. 8.15: Doppler image of 9 weeks fetus showing circulation in the entire body.

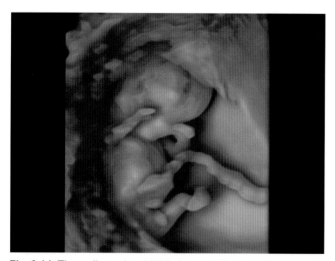

Fig. 8.14: Three-dimensional (3D) ultrasound image of 9–10 weeks gestation showing fetus with limb buds and physiological umbilical hernia.

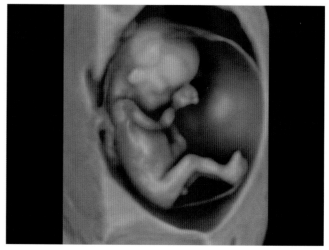

Fig. 8.16: Three-dimensional (3D) ultrasound image of 11 weeks fetus.

At this stage, even the arterial and venous circulation can be identified in the chorionic villi (Fig. 8.13). During the following 2 weeks, the limb buds develop, physiological umbilical hernia starts developing, cord insertion can be identified (Fig. 8.14), and the circulation in the entire embryonic body can be seen on power Doppler (Fig. 8.15). At 9 weeks, the entire circle of Willis is seen. From 8–10 weeks of development, the fetal limbs show development of all the three segments. Cord insertion becomes absolutely clear when the umbilical hernia disappears at 11 weeks (Fig. 8.16). At 12 weeks, absent end-diastolic flow in umbilical artery is at this stage is a normal finding (Fig. 8.17).[5]

ABNORMAL EARLY PREGNANCY

- Pregnancies with abnormal prognosis
- Pregnancies of abnormal location
- Pregnancies with vesicular moles and chorioangiomas
- Pregnancies with uterine abnormalities
- Pregnancy associated with other pelvic abnormalities.

Doppler does not have significantly different findings in early pregnancy in presence of uterine abnormalities and in presence of other pelvic pathologies, than a normal intrauterine pregnancy. So, we shall discuss the role of Doppler in the first three situations in this chapter.

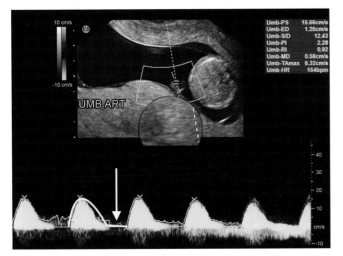

Fig. 8.17: Spectral Doppler of the umbilical artery at 11 weeks pregnancy showing absent diastolic flow.

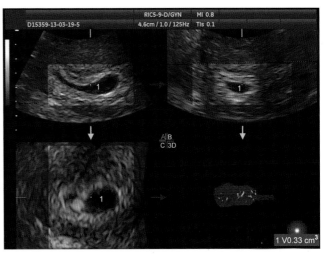

Fig. 8.18: Three-dimensional (3D) ultrasound volume of the gestational sac with sono-AVC software used to calculate the volume of the gestational sac.

Pregnancies with Abnormal Prognosis

Pregnancy prognosis can be predicted by normal or abnormal growth pattern of the pregnancy. Gestational sac, yolk sac, amniotic sac, and embryonic pole all have their normal defined appearances and growth rate. Variations in these beyond physiological limits predict abnormal prognosis of pregnancy.

Gestational Sac

At 4.3–4.5 weeks from the last date of menstruation, gestation sac appears and is 2–3 mm in diameter at this time.[6] It normally is well-defined round structure with regular, thick, hyperechoic walls (more echogenic than normal myometrium) (*see* Fig. 8.7). The hyperechoic walls are due to development of decidual reaction. It is normally situated in the fundus/upper body of the uterus and is abutting the endometrial cavity (*see* Fig. 8.7). It abuts the endometrial cavity because it is implanted in one of the two lips of endometrium. Normal growth rate of the gestational sac is 1–2 mm/day. The size of the gestational sac is measured as inner margin of the hyperechoic decidual margin to the inner margin of hyperechoic wall across the gestational sac. It is most reliable to measure three orthogonal diameters and take the mean of three as the actual gestational sac diameter. Volume assessment of the gestational sac by the three-dimensional (3D) ultrasound supported virtual organ computer-aided analysis (VOCAL) or Sono-AVC software (Fig. 8.18) may be considered the most reliable parameter for assessment of gestational sac size.[7] Gestational sac may be considered abnormal and may also be considered to indicate bad prognosis when it is too large (Fig. 8.19), showing a difference of more than 6 days compared to the gestational age calculated by embryonic pole crown-rump length (CRL). It is also considered abnormal when it is too small, difference of more than 6 days as compared to CRL. Abnormal gestational sac size is associated with trisomy and triploidy.[8]

At a particular point of time, the gestational sac size is not abnormal, but on serial assessments, the growth rate is slow or too fast, in those cases, also it is an indication of bad prognosis (<0.7 mm a day). It is important to mention here that normally when the gestational sac is 6–7 mm, yolk sac should be seen and when it is 10 mm and above, the embryonic pole should be seen. But gestational sac of larger than 10 mm with no yolk sac and gestational sac larger than 16 mm in diameter with no embryonic pole are definitely considered as poor prognostic indicators[9] for pregnancy. Though according to most guidelines, the pregnancy is not announced to have a bad prognosis till the gestational sac of 20 mm does not show the yolk sac and the gestational sac of 25 mm does not show the fetal pole.[10] Decidual layer thickness of less than 3 mm is also a sign of defective decidualization and, therefore, may indicate a bad pregnancy prognosis (Fig. 8.20). At any time in the 1st trimester, the thickness of the decidual ring (trophoblastic layer) in mm should be equal to the number of gestational weeks. Discrepancy of more than 3 mm in this thickness is considered a sign of bad prognosis. A normally growing gestational sac shows an almost complete ring of color on

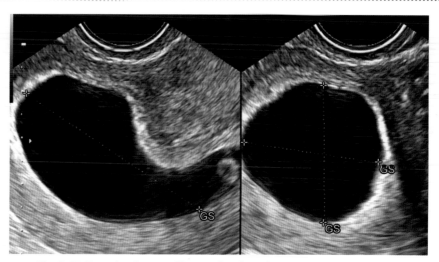

Fig. 8.19: B-mode ultrasound image showing a large gestational sac with a comparatively very small yolk sac and no embryonic pole.

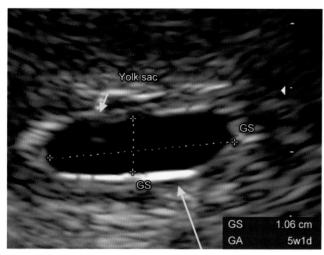

Fig. 8.20: B-mode image of the gestational sac with yolk sac and thin chorionic plate, suggesting a bad prognosis.

Doppler, with a low resistance flow, where the RI is always less than 0.5. The velocity of these blood flows increase as the pregnancy advances. As the pregnancy advances, in the later half of the 1st trimester, the trophoblast differentiates into chorion frondosum (decidua basalis) and chorion leave (decidua capsularis). The chorion frondosum develops into placenta later. Normally, the low resistance vascularity develops in the chorion frondosum. The vascularity in the chorion leave is markedly less compared to the chorion frondosum as appreciated on Doppler.

A bad prognosis of pregnancy can be predicted by decreasing blood flow in the form of increasing resistance or decrease in the blood flow abundance. This may occur in

perisac bleeding. This may also lead to irregular sac margins. Though abnormal margins of the sac can also be seen due to uterine contraction, overfull bladder (rare), or myomas.

Perisac hematoma in early pregnancy may or may not be associated with per vaginal bleeding. When vaginal bleeding is present, it is called threatened abortion. Sonography can identify perigestational hemorrhage in 5–22% as a cause of vaginal bleeding in women with threatened abortion. Whether vaginal bleeding is present or not, the prognosis of pregnancy with hematoma is dependent on the size and location of perisac hematoma. Location of hematoma is more predictive of pregnancy outcome than the size of the hematoma.[11] Hematomas in the supracervical area may have much better prognosis than those in the retrochorionic (deep to chorion frondosum) area. Those in the vicinity of chorion frondosum have a worse prognosis than those related to chorion leave (Fig. 8.21).

On B-mode ultrasound, perisac hematoma is seen as an anechoic cystic area, sometimes with low-level echogenicities. This needs to be differentiated from the residual endometrial cavity (Fig. 8.22), that may still be seen till 8 weeks of pregnancy, when the endometrial cavity completely abuts. Even a nongrowing twin sac (vanishing twin) or a blighted ovum in a twin pregnancy may give similar appearance but the thick decidual reaction and the roundish shape may help to differentiate these from hematoma.[11]

Subchorionic hematoma may lead to compression of spiral arteries and, therefore, increased resistance in the spiral arteries. These hematomas have a tendency to get absorbed and then the circulation normalizes.

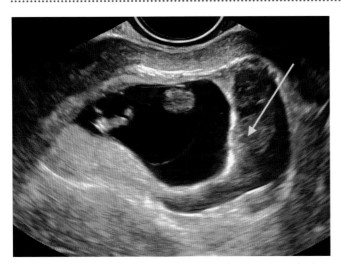

Fig. 8.21: B-mode ultrasound image showing gestational sac with perisac hematoma as shown by the arrow.

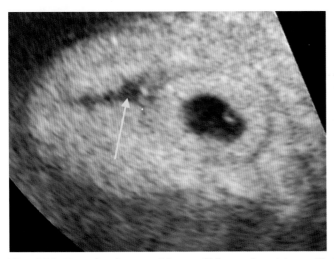

Fig. 8.22: B-mode ultrasound image if the endometrium with eccentrically situated gestational sac and residual endometrial cavity as shown by the arrow.

Improvements of blood flow indices are, therefore, predictive of normal pregnancy outcome.[12] But, in severely incomplete transformation of uteroplacental arteries and abnormal villous, development associated with the premature entry of a large amount of maternal blood inside the placenta, which progressively dislocates the entire gestational sac[13] ends in complete abortion. Therefore, low impedance perisac blood flow and pooling of blood are signs of failing pregnancy. Risk of miscarriage increases to 4–33% if subchorionic hematoma is seen.[14]

Yolk Sac

The yolk sac that can be seen on ultrasound, is the secondary yolk sac.

It is the first visible embryonic structure and is a confirmatory sign of a true gestational sac. As mentioned earlier, it is normally seen when gestational sac is 6–9 mm or serum beta-hCG levels of 7,000–1,000 mIU/mL. This usually happens in the 5th week of gestation, since last menstrual period (LMP). It is located outside the amniotic cavity in the extraembryonic coelom. It grows at a rate of 0.1 mm a day, and maximum up to 6 mm. It usually disappears at 12–13 weeks of gestation.

Yolk sac has nutritive, lymphatic, etc. several functions for the embryo. Therefore, an abnormal yolk sac is an indicator of bad prognosis of pregnancy. Though it is important to mention here that pregnancies with abnormal yolk sacs may also progress normally and so whenever the yolk sac is abnormal, a closer observation is required, not a termination of pregnancy. A yolk sac less than 2 mm or more than 6 mm in diameter, thick-walled, irregular, or solid looking yolk sac is considered to indicate a bad prognosis (Figs. 8.23A to D).[2,15] Whereas degenerative changes in the yolk sac with lack of translucency and abundant calcification in a yolk sac with a fetal pole showing no cardiac activity, indicate long-standing fetal demise.[16,17]

Routinely Doppler study for yolk sac is not done. But it usually shows a low velocity (4.1–7.5 cm/s), high resistance blood flow with absent diastolic blood flow (PI: 3.24 ± 0.94). But it has been documented by Kurjak et al. that irregular blood flow, permanent diastolic flow, or venous blood flow signals in the yolk sac are indicators of bad prognosis of pregnancy.[18]

Absent yolk sac in a gestational sac of larger than 10 mm mean diameter often results in a blighted ovum. But when the gestational sac of 15 mm is seen without yolk sac, it is almost always a blighted ovum (Fig. 8.24). In some cases, the gestational sac will not grow to this size and will not have a yolk sac. In these cases, if volume of the sac is less than 2.5 mL and is not increasing in size by at least 75% over a period of 1 week, it is diagnosed as a blighted ovum. It may be thought that since this is a failed pregnancy, the perisac blood supply may be of high resistance. But it is interesting to note here that the perisac blood flow around the blighted ovum shows low resistance flow.[19] The explanation given is that in these pregnancies, there is normal development of the intervillous spaces, the low resistance circulation pattern. As contrary to the normal pregnancies, the circulation through the high resistance fetal system is absent in a pregnancy with blighted ovum (anembryonic pregnancy) and, therefore, the resistance in the perisac vessels is even lower than in the normal gestational sac.

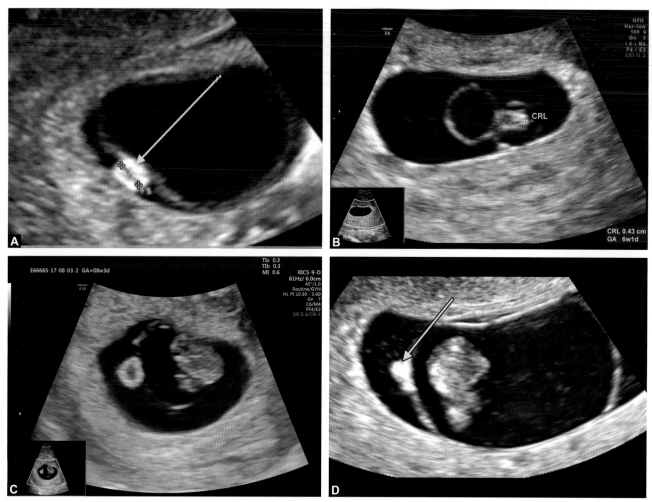

Figs. 8.23A to D: (A) Tiny yolk sac; (B) Large yolk sac; (C) Thick-walled yolk sac; and (D) Solid yolk sac.

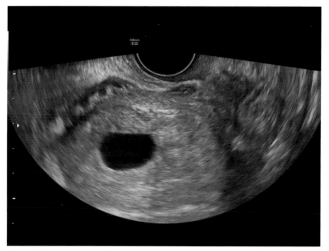

Fig. 8.24: B-mode ultrasound image showing a gestational sac of 13 mm mean diameter with no yolk sac or embryonic pole—blighted ovum.

Embryonic Pole

Embryonic pole usually appears at the gestational sac diameter of 10–15 mm or serum beta-hCG levels are 10,800 mIU/mL,[20] about 5 weeks and 5 days from LMP, and normally grows at a rate of 1 mm/day. Embryonic pole can be earliest seen by transvaginal probe, when it is hardly 1–1.5 mm in length and is often recognized only by the presence of cardiac activity. The cardiac activity can be observed on real-time B-mode ultrasound or can be documented by M-mode ultrasound (more preferred) or pulsed Doppler. Presence of an embryonic pole without a cardiac activity is a sign of failed pregnancy-missed miscarriage. But if a transabdominal scan is done and the embryonic pole is less than 7 mm, a second scan after 7 days is to be done, before confirming the missed miscarriage.[21] The follow-up to confirm absence of cardiac activity may be differed to

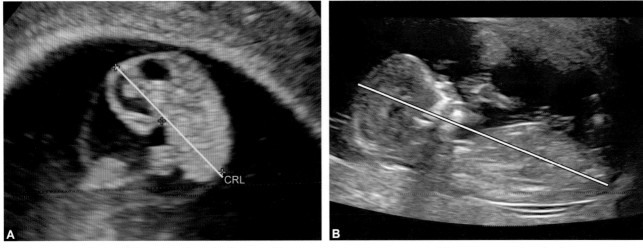

Figs. 8.25A and B: B-mode ultrasound images showing measurement of the crown-rump length at (A) 8 weeks 4 days; and (B) 11 weeks of gestation

10 days when the sac size is more than 12 mm and to 14 days when the sac size is less than 12 mm.[21]

Its growth is measured as CRL and is a reliable parameter of normal pregnancy growth till 11–12 weeks. CRL is measured in the mid-sagittal plane from top of the head to the end of the rump of the embryo on transvaginal scan (Figs. 8.25A and B).[22]

It is used as a most reliable pregnancy dating parameter from 8 weeks to 11 weeks. CRL is considered to be more reliable after it reaches 18–22 mm in length.[3] Embryos with a difference of, CRL calculated gestational age and gestational age calculated by dates, of more than 1 week have a high risk of abortion.[23] The vascular endothelial growth factor (VEGF) family of proteins, together with their receptors and the tyrosine kinase with immunoglobulin and epidermal growth factor homology domains (TIE) receptors, are crucial for embryonic development.[24] Comparing the controls with the missed miscarriage or the blighted ovum patients, later two groups show diminished placental trophoblastic VEGF immunoreactivity; weaker VEGFR-1 and -2 immunoreactivity in decidual vascular endothelium; reduced placental trophoblastic Tie-1 receptor immunoreactivity; and reduced decidual vascular endothelial TIE-1 and -2 receptor immunoreactivity.[24]

Heart Rate

The heart rate changes from the time of appearance at about 6 weeks to 9–10 weeks. In 5th week, it is slow-like peristalsis, may be 60–80 beats/min, and reaches 100 beats/min at the end of 5th week, it reaches 105–130 beats/min at the end

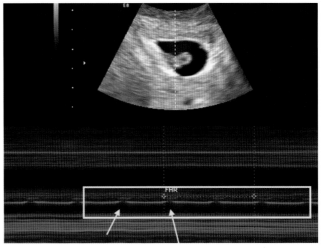

Fig. 8.26: M-mode image of 6 weeks gestation showing cardiac activity—beats indicated by arrows.

of 6th week and at 9 weeks reaches 160–170 beats/min to finally settle between 120 beats/min and 160 beats/min.[25]

Though cardiac activity can be documented on B-mode ultrasound, heart rate can be counted on M-mode (Fig. 8.26), but still in difficult cases, when it is not possible to document by these modalities, color Doppler is the method of choice for its documentation and pulse Doppler can be used for the calculation of the heart rate. Late appearance of cardiac activity or marked persistent bradycardia (<100 beats/min), or persistent tachycardia (>200 beats/min), may be considered as markers of either chromosomal abnormalities or bad pregnancy prognosis.[26] As mentioned earlier, absent cardiac activity with a fetal pole indicates intrauterine fetal demise and is a missed miscarriage.

Fetal demise in a pregnancy with absent cardiac activity may be declared when no cardiac activity is documented in the embryo/fetus in the gestational sac with yolk sac and fetal pole on two subsequent scans done at an interval of 7 days.[21]

No change is seen in intervillous blood flow in these cases than normal pregnancy, though in long-standing missed miscarriage progressive accumulation of fluid, results in low impedance in intervillous flow and spiral arteries.[19]

Amniotic Sac

Though amniotic sac is not specifically documented by many because it is thin and normal amniotic sac diameter is approximately equal to CRL in very early pregnancy.[2]

It is important to know that a thick, echogenic amniotic sac[27] or a large amniotic sac are indicators of poor prognosis of pregnancy.[28] In normal pregnancy, the embryo is usually documented before the amniotic sac, because in the early pregnancy, the amniotic sac is small and well-apposed to the embryo (Fig. 8.27). But if the amniotic sac is seen without an embryo, it is abnormal. This gestational sac may show two ring-like structures adjacent to each other—often described as "two bubble sign" (Fig. 8.28) or empty amnion sign and raises a suspicion of missed miscarriage especially beyond the gestational sac size of 16 mm.[29,30]

Pregnancies of Abnormal Location

Pregnancies that do not implant in the endometrial cavity, but implant elsewhere are pregnancies of abnormal location and are called ectopic pregnancies. Ectopic pregnancies may occur in the fallopian tubes, interstitium of the tubes, angle of the endometrial cavity, cornu of congenitally abnormal uterus, cervix, ovary, or in the peritoneal cavity. Clinically, these are diagnosed by a history of missed period, with abdominal pain or fainting attacks and biochemically by low beta-hCG levels (not corresponding with the duration of amenorrhea) and by slow rising rate of beta-hCG.[21] This might be correlated with the fact that in ectopic gestations, the actual pregnancy is younger than the period of amenorrhea. Though normal levels of serum beta-hCG may be found, if the ectopic pregnancy is live. Combination of clinical examination, serum beta-hCG assay, and TVS has a sensitivity of 100% for diagnosis of ectopic pregnancy.[31] In one large prospective study of 6,621 patients, ectopic pregnancy was correctly diagnosed by TVS with a sensitivity of 90.9% and specificity of 99.9%.[32] In one another study, TVS was found to have a sensitivity of 96%, specificity of

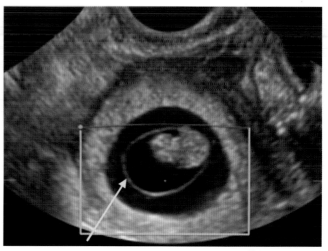

Fig. 8.27: B-mode ultrasound image of 7 weeks pregnancy showing embryo in short axis and amniotic sac as marked by arrow.

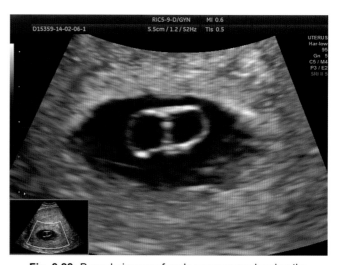

Fig. 8.28: B-mode image of early pregnancy showing the double bubble sign due to empty amniotic sac.

88%, positive predictive value (PPV) of 89%, and negative predictive value (NPV) of 95%.[33]

Tubal Pregnancy

This entity constitutes 95% of all ectopic pregnancies.

On ultrasound, empty endometrial cavity may or may not show increased endometrial thickness due to decidual-like reaction but the symmetrical thickening of endometrial cavity is an indication of extrauterine pregnancy (Fig. 8.29). This may be well-appreciated on 3D ultrasound image. In medial longitudinal plane, it was found asymmetrical in 84% of intrauterine pregnancies and symmetrical in 90% of ectopic pregnancies.[34] Though the sac may also be absent in spontaneous abortion with early pregnancy.[35] In all

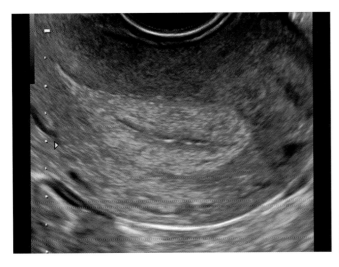

Fig. 8.29: B-mode ultrasound image of the uterus showing hyperechoic endometrium with both leaves of endometrium equal in thickness—symmetrical endometrium.

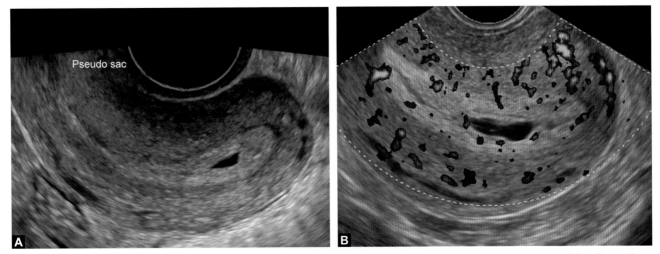

Figs. 8.30A and B: (A) B-mode ultrasound image of the uterus showing central anechoic area in the endometrial cavity; and (B) The anechoic lesion changes shape shows no flow on power Doppler suggestive of a pseudosac.

those cases in which the gestational sac is not seen in the endometrial cavity or not even located outside the uterus, follow-up after 1 week or if patient develops symptoms is recommended.[36] With an empty uterus in a patient with serum beta-hCG levels of more than 3,000 mIU/mL, the chance of ectopic pregnancy is very high, but there is still a 0.5% likelihood ratio of intrauterine pregnancy.[21]

Pseudogestational sac is seen in 10–20% of patients with ectopic pregnancy.[35] Pseudogestational sac can be identified as an anechoic, gestational sac-like structure in the endometrial cavity, but absence of the double decidual sign, change in shape with uterine contractions, its location in the center of the endometrial cavity, and no peripheral flow differentiate it from the true gestational sac (Figs. 8.30A

and B).[2] Therefore, Doppler may be a useful to differentiate a true sac from the pseudosac.

If the pregnancy is in the fallopian tube, adnexa shows a mass lesion. In a patient with missed period and positive pregnancy test, with serum beta-hCG more than 1,500 IU, and an empty endometrial cavity, an adnexal mass unless proved otherwise is suspected to be an ectopic pregnancy. It may appear only as an extraovarian roundish isoechoic mass in its early stages, this mass may show a hyperechoic center, or may actually show a typical gestational sac, with or without yolk sac and embryonic pole as it grows (Figs. 8.31A to C). Fetal pole with cardiac activity is seen in only about 15–28% of ectopic gestations (live ectopic).[37] But an ectopic gestational sac with fetal pole but no cardiac activity may be seen in about 46–71% of ectopic pregnancies.[38] There may also be free fluid around the mass or in the pouch of Douglas (Fig. 8.32).

On Doppler, the endometrium shows no evidence of increased velocity or low resistance vascularity. There is no significant change in the uterine artery Doppler parameters also.[39] If the pseudogestational sac is seen, it usually shows no peripheral blood flow, but if it does, it is a high resistance flow with RI more than 0.55. It has been shown in one study that a PSV less than 21 cm/s excludes the possibility of a true sac.[40]

Adnexa shows randomly dispersed multiple small vessels in adnexa with RI less than 0.42 on Doppler. More grown the pregnancy is, more is the vascularity. Extent of the vascularity tells about the invasion of the trophoblastic tissue in the surrounding tissues. The mass typically shows a low resistance, high velocity flow and ring of color (Fig.

8.33).[41] This Doppler parameters can be used as a guide for growth or otherwise of ectopic pregnancy on follow-up also. In small adnexal lesions, or those difficult to confirm as ectopic pregnancy with B-mode and Doppler, use of intravascular contrast agents, especially when used with contrast mode activation on the scanner is very useful. It picks up smaller and very low velocity vessels to facilitate the visualization of these lesions.[42]

Tubal ectopic pregnancies may abort into the abdominal cavity or may rupture the tube due to trophoblast invasion. In both the cases, patient may present with acute abdominal pain with or without a fainting attack. In growing tubal ectopics, the blastocyst grows mainly between the lumen of the tube and the peritoneal covering, both longitudinally and circumferentially.[43] The bleeding occurs also when the growing trophoblast invades the vessels. In tubal abortion, it may be difficult to find a well-defined mass in the adnexa,

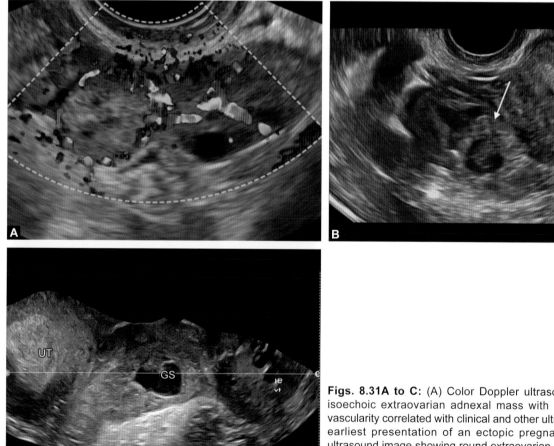

Figs. 8.31A to C: (A) Color Doppler ultrasound image of an isoechoic extraovarian adnexal mass with peripheral ring of vascularity correlated with clinical and other ultrasound findings—earliest presentation of an ectopic pregnancy; (B) B-mode ultrasound image showing round extraovarian adnexal mass with central anechoic gestational sac and possibly embryonic pole; and (C) Ectopic pregnancy on B-mode ultrasound seen as extraovarian adnexal mass with gestational sac and fetal pole.

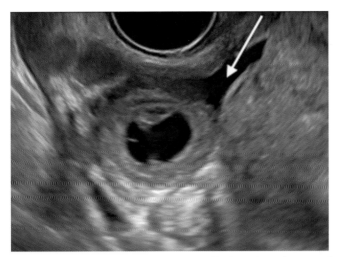

Fig. 8.32: Free fluid marked by arrow with the adnexal mass of ectopic pregnancy confirmed by central anechoic gestational sac and yolk sac in it.

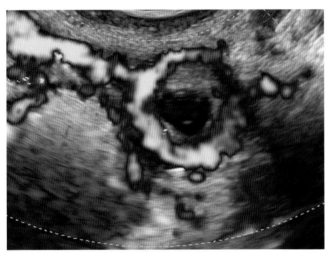

Fig. 8.33: Power Doppler image showing ectopic gestational sac with vascular ring.

usually with free fluid in pelvis. If the mass is found, it shows high resistance (RI > 0.6), low velocity vessels, and does not show a typical complete ring of color.

At least two-thirds of the ectopic pregnancies have a tendency to resolve on their own. The rest may require a medical or surgical line of treatment depending on the location and growth of the pregnancy and also depending on the patient's presentation. Usually patients without any acute symptoms and with declining serum beta-hCG level and decreasing vascularity can be treated conservatively.[44] Whether it is a conservative management or it is medical or surgical treatment, decreasing vascularity, increasing resistance, or decreasing abundance of vascularity can be

assuring signs for regression of the ectopic pregnancy. For the assessment of the decreasing abundance of the flow, 3D power Doppler can be used as more informative modality. Assessing the vascularization index (VI), flow index (FI), and vascularization flow index (VFI) gives objective information about the abundance, average intensity of flow, and perfusion of the area of interest, respectively. The assessment of these parameters along with RI and PSV of the perilesional vessels are done every alternate days in the 1st week after the diagnosis of the tubal pregnancy and then as the parameters start decreasing, the interval can be increased till complete resolution of the lesion. Using this follow-up method, serum beta-hCG assessment can be done only once a week. If the parameters show increase in vascularity, or there is increase in the size of the mass lesion, it indicates growing pregnancy and, therefore, requires active intervention. This strategy can be used for the patients who are clinically stable and on ultrasound do not show embryonic pole and cardiac activity in the ectopic gestational sac.

Involution of anembryonic ectopic pregnancy can result into arteriovenous malformation (AVM) of mesosalpinx.[45] A suitable candidate for expectant management must have an ectopic pregnancy with no evidence of rupture, be clinically stable and asymptomatic, and have consistently declining serum beta-hCG concentrations.[46] A low serum progesterone is also a possible marker of suitability for the expectant approach. Follow-up should be between one time and three times weekly with beta-hCG measurement and ultrasonography as required. Expectant management is reported to be most useful when the initial beta-hCG is less than 1,000 IU/L.[46] Success rates between 47% and 82% are reported, depending on the patient's initial status.[47]

Chorionic villi of tubal implantation invade into the tubal wall and mesosalpinx and cytotrophoblast invades into the arteries and veins, destroys vessel walls and causes AVM.[48] These may be well-appreciated on 3D Power Doppler angiography.[45]

The ectopic pregnancies apart from tubes may also be located in the interstitial part of the tube, in the cervix, in the ovary, in the abdominal cavity anywhere, or in the scar of the uterus. Wherever it is, the common findings are symmetrical lips of the endometrium with no increase in endometrial vascularity and no change in uterine artery Doppler flow parameters. The diagnostic sign for a live ectopic pregnancy is Doppler showing a ring of color, with low resistance flow.

Interstitial pregnancy constitutes 1.1–6.3% of all ecto-pics.[49] It is very essential to diagnose this precisely because it

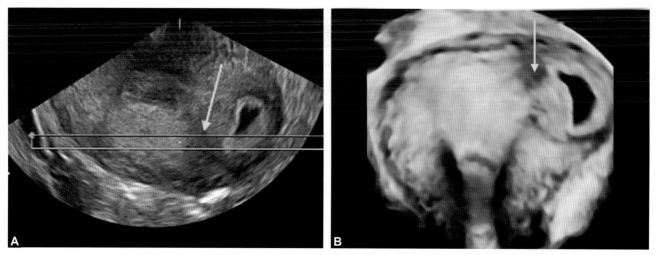

Figs. 8.34A and B: (A) B-mode image; and (B) Three-dimensional (3D) image of interstitial ectopic pregnancy, confirmed by presence of myometrium (as marked by arrow) between the lateral margin of endometrium and gestational sac.

has highest risk of rupture and massive hemorrhage, finally requiring only hysterectomy as treatment. Interstitial and angular pregnancy on B-mode can be differentiated on transverse section of the uterus at the level of uterine cornu. The gestational sac on this section, if is seen in continuity with the endometrium (medial margin of the gestational sac covered by endometrium), is suggestive of angular pregnancy, whereas if there is myometrial tissue seen (>1 cm) in between the endometrium and the gestational sac on this section is indicative of interstitial pregnancy (Figs. 8.34A and B).[50] If one can locate a plane where an echogenic band is seen as continuation of the endometrial cavity, the interstitium of the tube, and a trophoblastic reaction on it, this may be the most convincing sign of interstitial pregnancy.[51] 3D ultrasound and 3D power Doppler can be of help for correct diagnosis.[52,53]

In interstitial pregnancies, local injection of methotrexate in low doses is considered the most preferred treatment. Color Doppler helps in approaching the gestational sac from the medial aspect and traversing thicker layer of myometrium, thus, decreasing the risk of rupture and bleeding.[54] Expectant management has also been reported in interstitial pregnancy.[51]

Cervical pregnancy is a rare condition occurs in one in 50,000 pregnancies.[55] Cervical pregnancy is implanted in the cervical lip and, therefore, appears eccentric in cervical canal. It is this eccentric location and the peripheral vascularity that differentiates it from the gestational sac in process of abortion (Fig. 8.35).[56] The developing pregnancy in the cervix that leads to bulging of the cervix gives an hourglass appearance to the uterus. Doppler aids in the

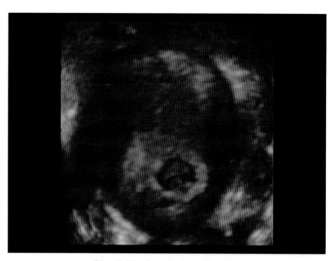

Fig. 8.35: Cervical pregnancy.

diagnosis by demonstrating the uterine vessels entering the uterus at the level of the internal os, the vascular ring surrounding the gestational sac, and the cardiac activity also (if this pregnancy is sufficiently grown and live).[13,54]

Ovarian pregnancy is very rare (<3% of all ectopic pregnancies).[57,58] It is difficult to differentiate from the corpus luteum, that has a similar B-mode appearance, thick walls, and anechoic center. Both have a ring of low resistance vascularity. Hyperechoic trophoblastic ring in the ovarian tissue is the only differentiating sign between the two.

Abdominal pregnancies constitute only 1% of all ectopic gestations. These are the most difficult to diagnose. It is to be suspected when the gestational sac is not seen in relation with the uterus, ovary, or adnexal soft tissue. Free fluid may or may not be seen around. But very typically, this gestational sac is not surrounded by myometrium. It may be a result of tubal abortion or may have primarily implanted in the abdomen. When live, shows a ring of vascularity with low resistance flow on color Doppler. These pregnancies may progress but have high chances of malformations, severe oligohydramnios, and disseminated intravascular coagulation (DIC) leading to abdominal hemorrhage.

Trophoblastic Diseases

Trophoblastic diseases can be classified as hydatidiform (vesicular) mole—complete, partial, or invasive mole, choriocarcinoma, placental site trophoblastic tumor (PSTT), and epithelioid trophoblastic tumor (ETT).

Complete Hydatidiform Mole

This comprises of 80% of gestational trophoblastic diseases (GTDs). The chorionic villi are converted into molar vesicles or hydropic villi, with no embryo or umbilical cord, but amnion may be present. It may also be one of the twin or triplet pregnancies.[59] This typically presents with missed period and positive urine or serum pregnancy tests, with very high beta-hCG levels. Patients may present with vaginal bleeding, pelvic discomfort, and hyperemesis gravidarum. Patients with vesicular mole typically show markedly high beta-hCG levels, not corresponding to the gestational age.

On ultrasound, in early stages, shows a gestational sac with no embryo but with thick walls showing small cystic areas. In very early stages, it may be confused for a blighted ovum on ultrasound due to a cystic area with absence of yolk sac and fetal pole. But as it grows, the chorionic plate thickens with multiple cystic areas (Fig. 8.36). Cystic areas are hydropic villi and may vary from 1 mm to 30 mm in size. Hydatidiform mole appears as a hyperechoic lesion filling up the entire uterus, when the cysts are very small and then when the cysts grow it shows multiple small anechoic areas giving a snowstorm appearance or a honeycomb appearance on B-mode ultrasound.[60] At this stage, the gestational sac is not seen if it is a complete vesicular mole. This may also be known as molar pregnancy. Typically, active corpus luteum is seen in the ovaries. But high serum beta-hCG levels may also lead to multiple theca lutein cysts. These are seen as multilocular cystic lesions with thin septae and vascularity (Fig. 8.37). As long as the vesicular mole is benign and/or not invasive, the endometrio-myometrial junction appears intact.

On Doppler, the endometrium with vesicular mole shows abundant color signals, but do not resemble the normal spiral vessels (Fig. 8.38). Among the color signals,

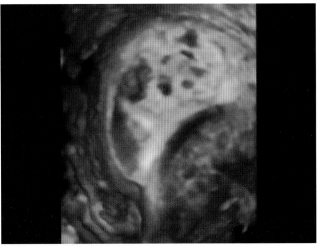

Fig. 8.36: Three-dimensional (3D) ultrasound image of the hyperechoic endometrium with multiple cystic areas and well-defined endometrio-myometrial junction—vesicular mole.

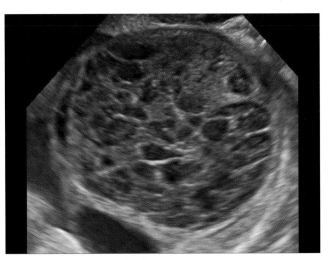

Fig. 8.37: Theca lutein cyst on B-mode ultrasound.

multiple anechoic cystic structures are seen. On power Doppler, it is a low resistance flow, but the velocity is also low (RI < 0.42).[61] The uterine, arcuate, radial, and spiral arteries also show low resistance flow.[62] Increase in resistance after chemotherapy indicates its responsiveness to treatment even before the tumor size decreases.[63] The corpus luteum also shows low resistance flow and a typical ring of color, like in normal pregnancy.

In patients with complete mole, the possibility of development of choriocarcinoma or invasive mole increases and this can be diagnosed by persistently high serum beta-hCG levels after evacuation of the mole.

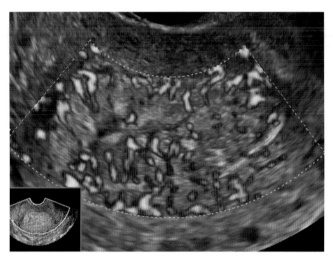

Fig. 8.38: Power Doppler image of vesicular mole with microcysts giving hyperechoic appearance and shows abundant vascularity.

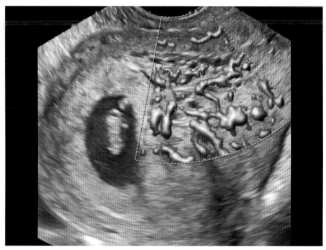

Fig. 8.39: HD flow Doppler image of the uterus showing small gestational sac with embryonic pole, but markedly thick endometrium with multiple small anechoic cystic areas, well-defined endometrio-myometrial junction, and abundant vascularity—partial mole.

Partial Hydatidiform Mole

It is partial conversion of chorionic villi into molar vesicles. The serum beta-hCG levels are unduly high in partial mole also. In cases of partial mole, the gestational sac is seen, embryo/fetus is also seen, but the trophoblastic layer appears very thick and edematous in some parts of the trophoblast. This can be differentiated from a complete mole of a twin or a triplet pregnancy on B-mode. In a complete mole of multiple pregnancy, a sac margin appears as a septum between the fetus and the hyperechoic mole. This septum-like structure is not seen in partial mole (Fig. 8.39). The molar part of the placenta shows the same B-mode and Doppler features like a complete mole. This can be better appreciated by 3D ultrasound than by B-mode. This is actually a situation, more difficult to diagnose than the complete mole. And detailed scans are required to exclude fetal anomalies also as these are fairly common in pregnancies with partial mole. Theca lutein cysts are typically not seen in these patients.

Invasive Hydatidiform Mole

It refers to invasion of the molar vesicles into the myometrium after the evacuation of complete or partial mole or during pregnancy. This leads to persistence of raised serum beta-hCG level. Patients may present with vaginal bleeding and on per vaginal examination, uterus may appear bulky. On ultrasound, the enlarged uterus is filled with a solid looking hyperechoic mass with multiple anechoic areas (molar cysts). The endometrio-myometrial junction is not identifiable (Fig. 8.39). It is a highly vascular tumor with low resistance flow in the blood vessels. Due to these findings, on ultrasound, it is not possible to differentiate it from choriocarcinoma, though the corpus luteal flow is high resistance in these cases.

Placental Site Trophoblastic Tumor

It is a rare uterine tumor of proliferated intermediate trophoblasts.[64] It follows an abortion, delivery, or a hydatidiform mole. These patients have serum low beta-hCG but high human placental lactogen (HPL) levels.[65] Though not typically malignant, recurrence and metastasis may occur in these cases. But as long as it is confined to the uterus, the prognosis is excellent after hysterectomy. Patients present with vaginal bleeding with bulky uterus. On ultrasound, it is not possible to confirm the diagnosis. Doppler shows low resistance flow. But it is a very rare tumor. On B-mode, it appears a solid uterine mass with anechoic areas (lacunae). Doppler is seen filling the lacunae and also the blood flow is seen around the mass, with low resistance flow (Figs. 8.40A and B). Myometrial invasion is not seen.

Epithelioid Trophoblastic Tumor

It has a similar clinical presentation and ultrasound and Doppler image as PSTT.

CONCLUSION

Ultrasound with Doppler is a modality of choice for assessment and prognostication of the early pregnancy. It has an

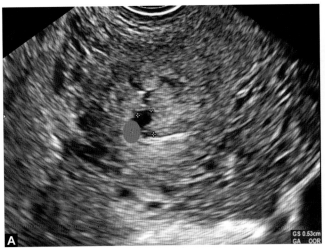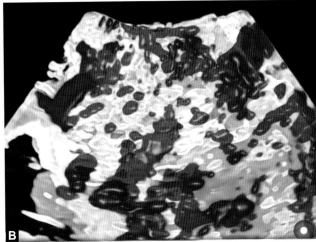

Figs. 8.40A and B: Placental site trophoblastic tumor. (A) B-mode it appears a solid uterine mass with anechoic areas (lacunae) and ill-defined endometrio-myometrial junction; and (B) Doppler is seen filling the lacunae.

important role for assessment of the normal growth of the embryo to fetus, for detection of abnormalities, ectopic pregnancies, and trophoblastic tumors.

REFERENCES

1. Glock JL, Brumsted JR. Color flow pulsed Doppler ultrasound in diagnosing luteal phase defect. Fertil Steril. 1995;64:500-4.
2. Honemeyer U, Kurjak A, Monni G. Normal and abnormal early pregnancy. DSJUOG. 2011;5:356-84.
3. Kumar P, Magon N. Hormones in pregnancy. Niger Med J. 2012;53:179-83.
4. Arck PC, Rucke M, Rose M, et al. Early risk factors for miscarriage: a prospective cohort study in pregnant women. Reprod Biomed Online. 2008;17:101-13.
5. Azumendi G, Kurjak A. Three-dimensional sonoembryology. DSJUOG. 2008;2:62-86.
6. Timor-Tritsch IE, Farine D, Rosen MG. A close look at early embryonic development with the high frequency transvaginal transducer. Am J Obstet Gynecol. 1988;159:676-81.
7. Rolo LC, Nardozza LM, Araujo Júnior E, et al. Gestational sac volume by 3D-sonography at 7-10 weeks of pregnancy using the VOCAL method. Arch Gynecol Obstet. 2009;279:821-7.
8. Nyberg DA, Mack LA, Laing FC, et al. Distinguishing normal from abnormal gestational sac growth in early pregnancy. J Ultrasound Med. 1987;6:23-7.
9. Levi CS, Lyons EA, Zheng XH, et al. Endovaginal ultrasound: demonstration of cardiac activity in embryos of less than 5.0 mm in crown rump length. Radiology. 1988;167:383-5.
10. Jeve Y, Rana R, Bhide A, et al. Accuracy of first-trimester ultrasound in the diagnosis of early embryonic demise: a systematic review. Ultrasound Obstet Gynecol. 2011;38: 489-96.
11. Kurjak A, Schulman H, Zudenigo D, et al. Subchorionic hematomas in early pregnancy: clinical outcome and flow patterns. J Matern Fetal Med. 1996;5:41-4.
12. Kurjak A, Zudenigo D, Predanic M, et al. Assessment of the fetomaternal circulation in threatened abortion by transvaginal color Doppler. Fetal Diagn Ther. 1994;9:341-7.
13. Jauniaux E, Taidi J, Jurkovic D, et al. Comparison of color Doppler features and pathological findings in complicated early pregnancy. Hum Reprod. 1994;9:2432-7.
14. Pearlston M, Baxi L. Subchorionic hematoma: a review. Obstet Gynecol Surv. 1993;48:65-8.
15. Varelas FK, Prapas NM, Liang RI, et al. Yolk sac size and embryonic heart rate as prognostic factors of first trimester pregnancy outcome. Eur J Obstet Gynecol Reprod Biol. 2008;138:10-3.
16. Lindsay DJ, Lovett IS, Lyons EA, et al. Yolk sac diameter and shape at endovaginal US: predictors of pregnancy outcome in first trimester. Radiology. 1992;183:115-8.
17. Harris RD, Vincent LM, Askin FB. Yolk sac calcification: a sonographic finding associated with intrauterine embryonic demise in the first trimester. Radiology. 1988;166:109-10.
18. Kurjak A, Kupesic S. Parallel Doppler assessment of yolk sac and intervillous circulation in normal pregnancy and missed abortion. Placenta. 1998;19:619-23.
19. Kurjak A, Kupesic S. Doppler assessment of the intervillous blood flow in normal and abnormal early pregnancy. Obstet Gynecol. 1997;89:252-6.
20. Illescas MT, Martinez TP, Bajo Arenas JM. Miscarriage and Threatened Miscarriage. Madrid: SEGO; 2011.
21. Rodgers SK, Chang C, DeBardeleben JT, et al. Normal and Abnormal US Findings in Early First-Trimester Pregnancy: Review of the Society of Radiologists in Ultrasound 2012 Consensus Panel Recommendations. Radiographics. 2015;35:2135-48.
22. Illescas T. 11-14 weeks' scan. In: Abuhamad A (Ed). Advanced Ultrasound in Obstetrics and Gynecology, 1st edition. New Delhi: Jaypee Brothers Medical Publishers (P) Ltd; 2015.
23. Koornstra G, Exalto N. Echography in the first pregnancy trimester has prognostic value. Ned Tijdschr Geneeskd. 1991;135:2231-5.

24. Vuorela P, Carpén O, Tulppala M, et al. VEGF, its receptors and the Tie receptors in recurrent miscarriage. Basic Science Reprod Med. 2000;6:276-82.

25. Doublet PM, Benson CB. Outcome of first trimester pregnancies with slow embryonic heart rate at 6-7 weeks gestation and normal heart rate by 8 weeks at US. Radiology. 2005;236:643-6.

26. Doubilet PM, Benson CB, Chow JS. Long-term prognosis of pregnancies complicated by slow embryonic heart rates in the early first trimester. J Ultrasound Med. 1999;18:537-41.

27. Laing FC, Frales MC. Ultrasound evaluation during the first trimester of pregnancy. In: Callen PW (Ed). Ultrasound in Obstetrics and Gynecology, 4th edition. Philadelphia: Saunders; 2000. pp. 105-45.

28. Harrow MM. Enlarged amniotic cavity: a new sonographic sign of early embryonic death. AJR Am J Roentgenol. 1992;158:359-62.

29. McKenna KM, Feldstein VA, Goldstein RB, et al. The empty amnion: a sign of early pregnancy failure. J Ultrasound Med. 1995;14:117-21.

30. Yegul NT, Filly RA. Further observation on 'empty amnion sign'. J Clin Ultrasound. 2010;38:113-7.

31. Bernhart K, Mennuti MT, Benjamin D, et al. Prompt diagnosis of ectopic pregnancy in an emergency department setting. Obstet Gynecol. 1994;84:1010-5.

32. Jehle D, Krause R, Braen GR. Ectopic pregnancy. Emerg Med Clin North Am. 1994;12:55-71.

33. Hopp H, Schaar P, Entezami M, et al. Diagnostic reliability of transvaginal ultrasound in ectopic pregnancy. Geburtshilfe Frauenheilkd. 1995;55:666-70.

34. Rempen A. The shape of the endometrium evaluated with three-dimensional ultrasound: an additional predictor of extrauterine pregnancy. Hum Reprod. 1998;13:450-4.

35. Kurjak A, Kupesic S. Ectopic pregnancy. In: Kurjak A (Ed). Ultrasound in Obstetrics and Gynecology. Boston: CRC Press; 1990. pp. 225-35.

36. Preisler J, Kopeika J, Ismail L, et al. Defining safe criteria to diagnose miscarriage: prospective observational multicentre study. BMJ. 2015;351:h4579.

37. Thoma ME. Early detection of ectopic pregnancy visualizing the presence of a tubal ring with ultrasonography performed by emergency physicians. Am J Emerg Med. 2000;18:444-8.

38. Nyberg D. Ectopic pregnancy. In: Nyberg DA, Hill LM, Bohm Velez M (Eds). Transvaginal Sonography. St Louis: Mosby Year Book; 1992. pp. 105-35.

39. Jurkovic D, Bourne TH, Jauniaux E, et al. Transvaginal color Doppler study of blood flow in ectopic pregnancies. Fertil Steril. 1992;57:68-73.

40. Dillon EH, Feyock AL, Taylor KJ. Pseudogestational sacs: Doppler US differentiation from normal or abnormal intrauterine pregnancies. Radiology. 1990;176:359-64.

41. Kemp B, Funk A, Hauptmann S, et al. Doppler sonographic criteria for viability in symptomless ectopic pregnancies. Lancet. 1997;349:1220-1.

42. Ordón MR, Gudmundsson S, Helin HL, et al. Intravascular contrast agent in the ultrasonography of ectopic pregnancy. Ultrasound Obstet Gynecol. 1999;14:348-52.

43. Budowich M, Johnson TR, Genadry R. The histopathology of developing tubal ectopic pregnancy. Fertil Steril. 1980;34:169-73.

44. Stovall TG, Link WF. Expectant management of ectopic pregnancy. Obstet Gyencol Clin North Am. 1991;18:135-44.

45. Shih JC, Shyu MK, Cheng WF, et al. Arteriovenous malformation of mesosalpinx associated with a vanishing ectopic pregnancy: diagnosis of three-dimensional color power angiography. Ultrasound Obstet Gynecol. 1999;13: 63-6.

46. Horne AW, Shaw JL, Murdoch A, et al. Placental growth factor: a promising diagnostic biomarker for tubal ectopic pregnancy. J Clin Endocrinol Metab. 2011;96:E104-8.

47. Shalev E, Peleg D, Tsabari A, et al. Spontaneous resolution of ectopic tubal pregnancy: natural history. Fertil Steril. 1995;63:15-9.

48. Mazur MT, Kurman RJ. Disease of the fallopian tube. In: Kerman RJ (Ed). Blaustein's Pathology of the Female Genital Tract, 4th edition. New York: Springer-Verlag; 1994. pp. 541-3.

49. Agarwal SK, Wisot AL, Garzo G, et al. Cornual pregnancies in patients with prior salpingectomy undergoing in vitro fertilization and embryo transfer. Fertil Steril. 1996;65:659-60.

50. Timor-Tritsch IE, Monteagudo A, Matera C, et al. Sonographic evaluation of cornual pregnancies treated without surgery. Obset Gynecol. 1992;79:1044-9.

51. Hafner T, Aslam N, Ros JA, et al. The effectiveness of non-surgical management of early interstitial pregnancy: a report of ten cases and review of the literature. Ultrasound Obstet Gynecol. 1999;13:131-6.

52. Jurkovic D, Geipel A, Gruboeck K, et al. Three-dimensional ultrasound for the assessment of uterine anatomy and detection of congenital anomalies: a comparison with hysterosalpingography and two-dimensional sonography. Ultrasound Obstet Gynecol. 1995;5:233-7.

53. Lawrence A, Jurkovic D. Three-dimensional ultrasound diagnosis of interstitial pregnancy. Ultrasound Obstet Gynecol. 1999;14:292-3.

54. Timor-Tritsch IE, Monteagudo A, Mandeville EO, et al. Successful management of viable cervical pregnancy by local injection of methotrexate guided by transvaginal ultrasonography. Am J Obstet Gynecol. 1994;170:737-9.

55. Kupesic S, Kurjak A. Color Doppler assessment of ectopic pregnancy. In: Kurjak A, Kupesic S (Eds). An Atlas of Transvaginal Color Doppler. London: Parthenon Publishing; 2000. pp. 137-47.

56. Jurkovic D, Hacket E, Campbell S. Diagnosis and treatment of early cervical pregnancy: a review and a report of two cases treated conservatively. Ultrasound Obstet Gynecol. 1996;8:373-80.

57. Kase NG. Ectopic pregnancy: In: Speroff L, Glass RH, Kase NG (Eds). Clinical Gynecologic Endocrinology and Infertility. London: Williams and Wilkins; 1999. pp. 1149-67.

58. Timor-Tritsch IE, Monteagudo A. Ectopic pregnancy. In: Kupesic S, de Zeigler D (Eds). Ultrasound and Infertility. UK: Parthenon Publishing; 2000. pp. 215-39.

59. Weaver DT, Fisher RA, Newlands ES, et al. Amniotic tissue in complete hydatidiform moles can be angiogenetic. J Pathol. 2000;191:67-70.

60. Stevens FT, Katzorke N, Tempfer C, et al. Gestational Trophoblastic Disorders: An Update in 2015. Geburtshilfe Frauenheilkd. 2015;75:1043-50.

61. Kurjak A, Zalud I, Salhagic A, et al. Transvaginal color Doppler in the assessment of abnormal early pregnancy. J Perinat Med. 1991;19:155-65.

62. Kurjak A, Zalud I, Predanic M, et al. Transvaginal color and pulsed Doppler study of uterine blood flow in the first and early second trimesters of pregnancy: normal versus abnormal. J Ultrasound Med. 1994;131:43-7.

63. Kundo S. Personal communication. In: Maeda K (Ed). Gestational Trophoblastic Disease. Dubrovnik: Donald Inter-University School of Medical Ultrasound; 1995.

64. Feltmate CM, Genset DR, Goldstein DP, et al. Advances in the understanding of placental site trophoblastic tumor. J Reprod Med. 2002;47:337-41.

65. Santoso JT, Coleman RI. Handbook of Gynecology Oncology. New York: Tata McGraw Hill; 2001.

Doppler in Fetal Echocardiography

INTRODUCTION

Fetal echocardiography is a wide subject and the entire discussion from its basics is out of the scope of this book. Assuming that the reader is acquainted with the basics of the fetal echocardiography, the B-mode, we shall here concentrate on the Doppler applications in fetal echocardiography.

The study of the heart for its normalcy requires study of its anatomy on the B-mode but it is known that heart has a very important function—receive blood from the entire body to circulate it through lungs and to pump it all to circulate to the entire body. Therefore, echocardiography is incomplete without a Doppler study.

It is also important to understand the normal fetal circulation before discussing the applications of Doppler in fetal echocardiography.

EQUIPMENT SETTINGS

High-resolution linear array, curved array, or sector scanners can be used for this examination. 4–8 MHz is the preferred frequency range for this examination.

The settings for two-dimensional *(2D) imaging/gray scale* are set at high contrast. The angle of the scanning field should be wide enough to include the transverse section of the thorax. The focal depth is kept sufficient so the area of interest is seen in the center of the screen, and the focal point is adjusted at the level of the heart. Orient region of interest (ROI) collinear to beam. Select smallest possible angle of insonation. Zoom the image so that the heart is seen large enough to identify all the structures but not too large

that the sharpness of the image is lost. Maternal abdominal fat or scars, anterior fetal spine or limbs may make the visualization of fetal heart difficult. Using harmonics, speckle reduction imaging (SRI) and compound resolution imaging (CRI) increases the sharpness of the image.

As heart has an anatomy to study and also the blood flows to be understood, cardiac examination cannot be complete without *color Doppler*. For color Doppler, high wall filter, high pulse repetition frequency (PRF), low persistence, and low color sensitivity settings are done. The color box should be big enough only to include the heart. The gains and PRF are so set that chambers of the heart are adequately filled with color but there is no aliasing. The color balance is adjusted so that both the gray scale and color can be defined adequately at a time. Using B-mode and color dual display can be helpful to correlate the anatomy and the blood flows better. Using *zoom and cine loop* examination can be very helpful with both gray scale and color Doppler.

For pulse Doppler, select small spectral sample volume to include the area of interest only [usually 3 mm for atrioventricular (AV) valves and smaller 1 mm for pulmonary veins] with angle not more than 60°. PRF and wall filters should be high as for color Doppler. Sweep speed is set high. Remember angle corrections are required only for absolute values and not for study of waveform pattern or ratios. Spectral sample volume is placed just downstream of valve to study the flow through the valve. It is placed upstream to demonstrate regurgitation in outflow tracts. For tricuspid regurgitation, the sample volume is placed across the valve. It may be placed by the help of color Doppler.

M-MODE STUDY

Fetal echocardiography cannot be considered complete without M-mode evaluation. The M-mode cursor is aligned perpendicular to the interventricular (IV) septum at the level of AV valves (Fig. 9.1). Interpreting M-mode correctly is based on identifying and correlating each line of M-mode with the anatomical structure on gray scale (Fig. 9.2).

MEASUREMENTS

Outer biventricular diameter is measured and right and left ventricular inner diameter is measured on B-mode.

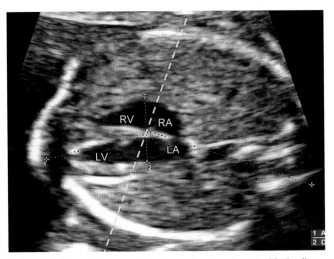

Fig. 9.1: B-mode image of the four chamber heart with the line showing the placement of the M-mode cursor.

Ventricular chamber size is measured at end-diastole when ventricular size is the largest on M-mode. Ventricular wall thickness and thickness of the IV septum are measured. Ventricular contractility is measured by measuring the systolic and diastolic outer dimensions and then subtracting systolic from diastolic measurement and then dividing it with diastolic measurement. Rhythm disturbances are assessed by correlating ventricular and atrial cycles when cursor passes through one atrium and one ventricle at 30° to the IV septum on four-chamber view. M-mode can also be used with color Doppler to understand the regurge better (Fig. 9.3).

B-mode scanning is the most important and color Doppler should be used only after B-mode diagnosis for demonstration and confirmation of a particular pathology. Color may be required sometimes for identification of anatomy only when evaluation of the heart is done at 11–14 weeks scan (Figs. 9.4A and B) Though with high-resolution probes and improving technology, early fetal echocardiography can be done at 11–14 weeks with the nuchal scan with transvaginal probe with 5–9 MHz frequency range.

Before discussing the role of color Doppler for diagnosis of cardiac abnormalities, it is essential to understand the normal anatomy and circulation of blood in the heart and its inflow and outflow tracts.

Systematic study requires several views of the heart on ultrasound that would show anatomy of the heart and circulation through it.

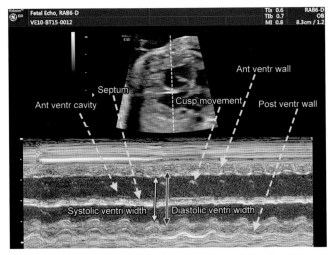

Fig. 9.2: M-mode ultrasound of the heart correlating the B-mode image with the layers seen on the M-mode. (Ant: anterior, Post: posterior, Ventr: ventricular).

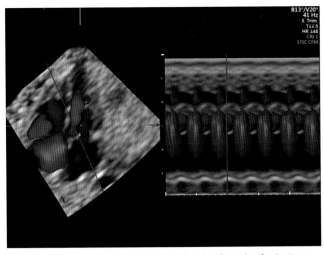

Fig. 9.3: M-mode of the heart with color Doppler for better understanding of valvular abnormalities.

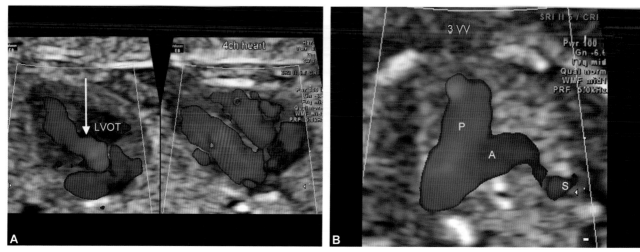

Figs. 9.4A and B: (A) Early echocardiography with color Doppler showing left ventricular outflow tract (LVOT) in the image on the left and four-chamber heart view in the image on the right; and (B) Early echocardiography with color Doppler showing three vessel view.

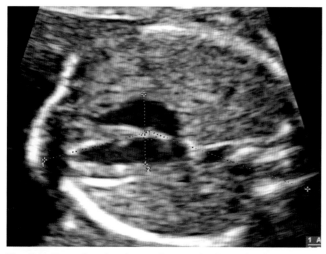

Fig. 9.5: Four-chamber heart view on the B-mode ultrasound in the transverse section of the thorax, showing only one rib on both the sides.

These are:
- Four-chamber view
- Left ventricular outflow tract (LVOT)
- Right ventricular outflow tract (RVOT)
- Three vessel view
- Short-axis view
- Arch views.

A correct four-chamber view will have only one rib in the transverse section of the heart (Fig. 9.5). If one can see multiple rib ends, it means it is an oblique section and will give erroneous calculation of cardiac size and axis and also erroneous impression about the symmetry of the cardiac

chambers. Apart from that, it should show symmetrical transverse section of thorax with all the four chambers of the heart and two pulmonary veins entering the left ventricle. Normally on this view, the chamber closest to the spine is the left atrium and the chamber closest to the sternum is the right ventricle.

What to see on four chamber heart?
- Cardiac area approximately one-third of thoracic area.
- Cardiac axis 25–65°.
- Both ventricles approximately same in size, ratio 1:1.1 to 1:1.2. Morphological right ventricle is identified by thicker walls due to chordae tendineae/moderator band and is close to the anterior thoracic wall. On color Doppler, both the ventricles show equal filling with color during systole.
- Both atria are approximately same in size. Morphological left atrium is the one in which the flap of foramen ovale opens and it is the chamber closest to the spine.
- Interatrial septum shows foramen ovale in its mid-part, the flap of that opens into morphological left atrium. The upper and lower third of the atrial septum is always seen as a thin line from posterior atrial wall and from the crux of the heart, respectively. Normal diameter of foramen ovale is 75–100% of the aortic root diameter. The blood flow direction is from right to left atrium across the foramen ovale. On pulse Doppler, it shows a peak systolic velocity (PSV) of approximately 45 cm/s.
- *Interventricular septum*: It has muscular part, membranous part, inlet part, and outlet part. But on this view, the muscular part and the inlet part are only seen.

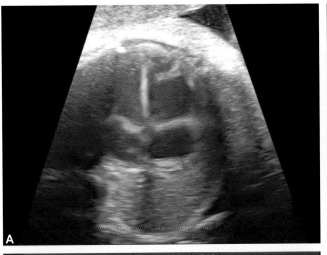

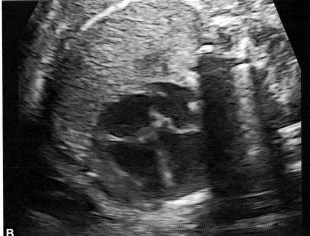

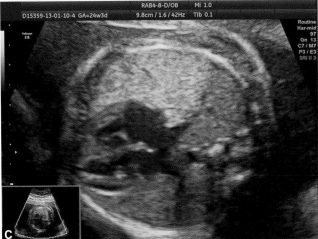

Figs. 9.6A to C: Four-chamber heart view on B-mode ultrasound. (A) Apical four-chamber view; (B) Basal four-chamber view; and (C) Oblique four-chamber view.

The septum must be seen in its full width from side-to-side by sweeping the beam to stamp it as normal. Whenever a breach is seen in the continuity of the ventricular septum, it is necessary to confirm the flow across by color Doppler, to confirm or exclude the diagnosis of ventricular septal defect (VSD). This can be best established on lateral or oblique four-chamber heart view rather than apical or basal four-chamber heart view (Figs. 9.6A to C).

- *Atrioventricular valves:*
  - *Mitral valve:* Tricuspid valve = 1:1.1 to 1:1.2. Septal cusp of the tricuspid valve is attached slightly more toward the apex than the septal cusp of the mitral valve at the IV septum and the attachment of the septal cusps of both the valves with the septum make a cross that is known as crux of the heart (Fig. 9.7). On color Doppler, flow is always seen across both these valves from atrial to ventricles during ventricular

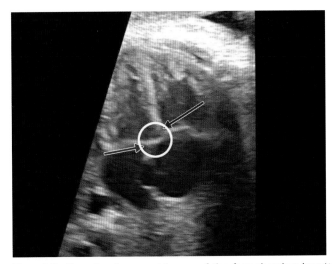

Figs. 9.7: B-mode ultrasound image of the four-chamber heart view, showing the attachment of the septal cusp of mitral valve (red arrow), septal cusp of tricuspid valve (blue arrow), and the crux in the circle.

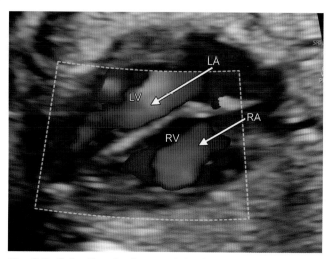

Fig. 9.8: Color Doppler image of the four chamber heart with blue color showing flow from the atria to the ventricles through the atrioventricular (AV) valves, with the arrows showing the flow direction.

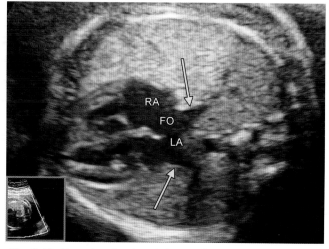

Fig. 9.10: Four-chamber heart view on B-mode ultrasound, with arrows showing pulmonary veins entering the left atrium.

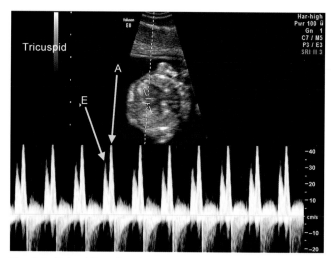

Fig. 9.9: Pulsed Doppler ultrasound image of the flow across the tricuspid valve. The arrows mark the E and the A waves on the spectrum.

diastole (Fig. 9.8). No flow is seen across these valves during ventricular systole normally. Normal waveform through the AV valve is double-peaked (Fig. 9.9) forward flow where the first one—"e" wave represents early diastolic filling of the ventricle and "a" wave represents filling of the ventricle by atrial contraction with no reverse flow throughout the cardiac cycle.

• *Pulmonary venous drainage:* Normally two (lower) pulmonary veins are seen entering the left atrium one

from either side of the descending aorta in this view (Fig. 9.10). Partial anomalous pulmonary venous drainage cannot be excluded on antenatal scan as it is difficult to see all the four pulmonary veins entering into the left atrium antenatally. On color Doppler, the flow will be seen in the veins, draining the blood toward the left atrium. The velocity in these vessels is markedly lower than that in the outflow tracts and, therefore, requires a lower PRF setting to demonstrate these flows.

• *Atrioventricular concordance:* Morphological right ventricle is connected to the morphological right atrium (RA) with the tricuspid AV valve and vice versa for left side.

Left Ventricular Outflow Tract

A vessel arising out of the left ventricle running anteriorly to right from the ventricle (Fig. 9.11) at a level cranial to the four chamber heart. Further, it curves cranially and gives off three neck branches. The posterior wall of the aorta shows continuity with the anterior leaflet of mitral valve and anterior wall is contiguous with IV septum. This is the membranous part of the IV septum (Fig. 9.11). The velocity of the blood flow through the arteries is 30 cm/s at 12 weeks. It increases throughout the gestation. The flow in aorta is always a little higher than in the pulmonary trunk.

Right Ventricular Outflow Tract

Vessel arising out of right ventricle, perpendicular to the aorta and runs posteriorly to right and divides into two

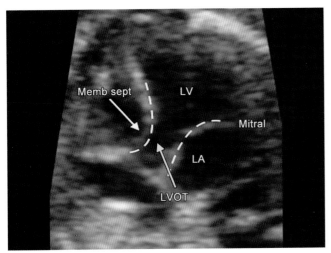

Fig. 9.11: B-mode ultrasound image of left ventricular outflow tract (LVOT)—its medial wall continuous with the interventricular septum and the lateral wall with the mitral valve cusp as shown by dotted lines. (Memb sept: membranous septum, LV: left ventricle, LA: left atrium).

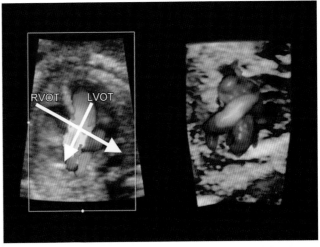

Fig. 9.13: Color Doppler and the three-dimensional (3D) color Doppler image of the crossover of the outflow tracts. (RVOT: right ventricular outflow tract; LVOT: left ventricular outflow tract)

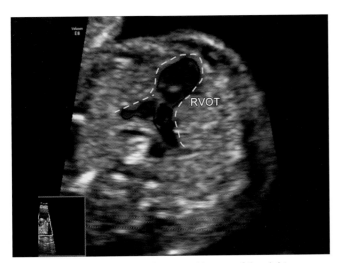

Fig. 9.12: B-mode ultrasound image of the right ventricular outflow tract (RVOT), with bifurcation.

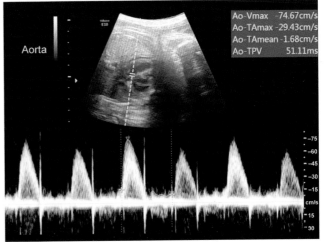

Fig. 9.14: Pulsed Doppler ultrasound image of the flow across the outflow tract.

soon after its origin (Fig. 9.12). RVOT divides into the duct and the pulmonary artery, this divides into right and left pulmonary artery. The second branch seen on bifurcation continues as right pulmonary artery and the left branch is directed cranially.

It is also necessary to confirm that morphological right ventricle gives out the pulmonary trunk and morphological left ventricle gives out the aorta. Confirming crossing over of two outflow tracts is very important (Fig. 9.13). The pulmonary valve is separated from the tricuspid valve by a complete muscular ring called infundibulum.

Outflow tracts show systolic single peaked forward flow due to ventricular systole (Fig. 9.14). *Normal velocities in the outflow tracts are* 60–70 cm/s, though that in the ductus arteriosus is 90–135 cm/s in systole and 15–25 cm/s in diastole.

Three-vessel View

At a level cephalic to the right ventricular and left ventricular outflow tracts, on the axial section of the thorax, three vessels are seen from forward left to rear right pulmonary trunk and aorta are seen in long axis and superior vena cava

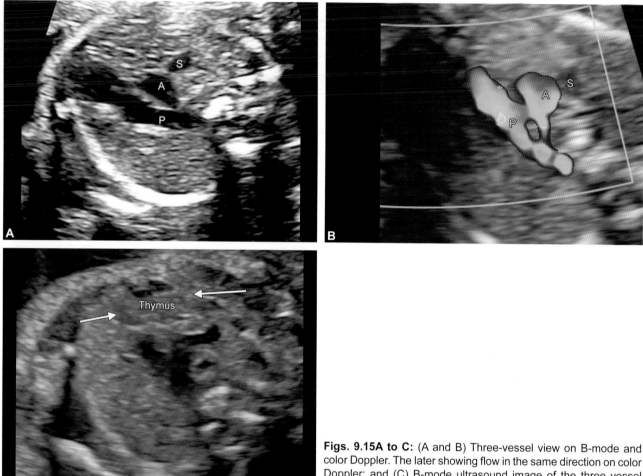

Figs. 9.15A to C: (A and B) Three-vessel view on B-mode and color Doppler. The later showing flow in the same direction on color Doppler; and (C) B-mode ultrasound image of the three vessel trachea view also showing thymus anteriorly.

(SVC) is seen in transverse/oblique section (Fig. 9.15A). The vessels show reducing caliber from pulmonary trunk to SVC. To be more specific at 12 weeks—both great arteries are almost same in size, at 16 weeks—pulmonary trunk is a little bigger than the aorta and this relationship then persists forever. At 20 weeks, pulmonary trunk is about 3.5 mm and aorta is 3 mm.

On color Doppler, the direction of flow is same in aorta and pulmonary trunk in this view normally (Fig. 9.15B). The aortic arch crosses the midline in front of the trachea from right to left and hooks over the left bronchus.

- *Three vessel trachea section* shows aorta and pulmonary trunk getting close to join by ductus arteriosus, forming a "V". Ductus arteriosus is seen as a vessel running posteriorly to the left of the spine from the bifurcation of the pulmonary trunk.

- Slightly higher level also shows trachea, just anterior to the spine. Slight sweep of the transducer shows the right and the left pulmonary artery.

- Sliding the probe transverse further upward shows aortic arch in transverse section with trachea in the concavity of "c". Slight caudal and left tilt from this shows aortic arch and duct together, with thymus anterior to the great vessels (Fig. 9.15C).

Short-axis View

As described in Yagel's technique,[1] it shows aorta in the center in transverse section and pulmonary trunk with bifurcation surrounding it that is also known as circle and sausage view (Figs. 9.16A and B). A section taken little inferior to this will show aortic root in the center protected

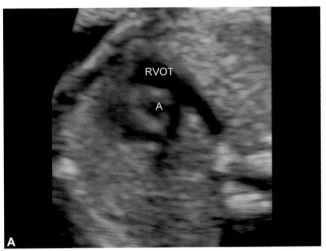 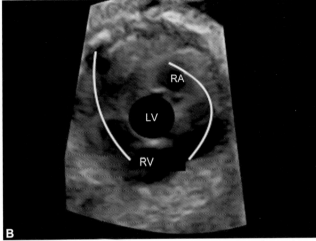

Figs. 9.16A and B: (A) B-mode ultrasound image showing aorta in the center with the right ventricular outflow tract (RVOT) with bifurcation, encircling it on the short-axis view of the heart; (B) Short-axis view of the heart on B-mode ultrasound, at a level, lower than the previous, showing left ventricular outflow tract (LVOT) in the center surrounded by the right ventricle (RV) and right atrium (RA).

by a complete circle formed by the right side of the heart. This view may be used for detection of subpulmonary VSD.

Arch/Longitudinal Views

- Aortic arch view can be achieved by rotating the probe 90° from the transverse aortic arch view (Fig. 9.17A).
- Ductal arch can be seen by rotating the probe 90° from ductus arteriosus in transverse view (Fig. 9.17B). On sagittal section of the fetus, heart is seen as a three-chambered structure and aorta is seen arising from the middle chamber, the left ventricle and is cane/"U" shaped. It gives off three neck vessels from the transverse part of the arch. Ductus arch is seen arising from the anterior most chamber, the right ventricle of the heart and is "hockey shaped" or has a flat curve. Both the arches can be seen connecting to each other, forming a "Y" anterior to the spine.
- *Right atrium inflow tracts:* Angulating the probe a little toward fetal right side from this view shows SVC and inferior vena cava (IVC) entering the RA (Fig. 9.17C). But let us first quickly go through the normal flows through the heart as these are observed on fetal echocardiography.

FETAL CIRCULATION (FIG. 9.18)[2]

Inferior and SVC bring unsaturated blood from lower and upper part of the body to RA. Saturated blood from umbilical vein enters ductus venosus (DV). This is a trumpet-shaped branchless structure with the narrowest part only 2 mm in diameter and opens into the RA. The shape helps to create a high speed jet of blood, which is directed from the RA, through foramen ovale to left atrium, unmixed with the unsaturated blood. Left atrium also receives blood from pulmonary veins. Right ventricle receives blood from RA and left ventricle from left atrium. Right ventricle gives out pulmonary trunk which apart from right and left pulmonary artery also gives out a third branch—ductus arteriosus. Left ventricle gives out aorta, which gives out coronaries and neck vessels in turn and then through ductus arteriosus, it is connected to pulmonary trunk. This causes mixture of blood from pulmonary trunk and aorta which is ultimately supplied to the unprivileged lower half of the body. Because of any abnormalities in the heart, the atrial changes precede the ventricular changes.

Keeping basics of this circulation in mind, Doppler can be used to confirm the abnormalities suspected on B-mode echocardiography based on deviations from this normal circulatory pattern.

Let us start from the most easy to achieve sectional plane of fetal echocardiography and also a single plane that gives maximum information—four-chamber heart view.

The most striking change from normal is chamber asymmetry. A chamber asymmetry is a result of abnormality in inflow or outflow to that particular chamber.

COMMON ABNORMALITIES INVOLVING THE RIGHT HEART

- Tricuspid anomalies including Ebstein's anomaly.
- Dysplastic tricuspid valve.

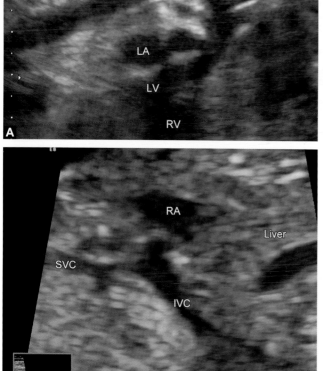

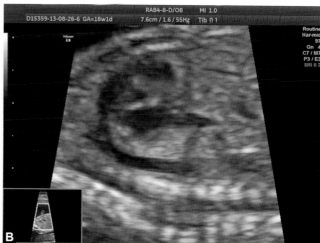

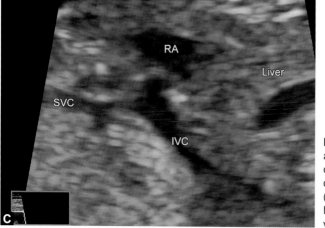

Figs. 9.17A to C: (A) Sagittal plane of the fetus showing the aortic arch with deep curve and neck branches and arising from the central chamber (LV) on this view; (B) Ductus arch showing flat curve, no neck branches, and arising from the anterior chamber (RV) on this view; and (C) Venous arch—right atrial inflow tracts—IVC and SVC. (IVC: inferior vena cava; LV: left ventricle; RV: right ventricle; SVC: superior vena cava; LA: left atrium)

- Unguarded tricuspid valve with almost no valvular tissue.[3]
- Tricuspid atresia.
- Pulmonary valve atresia with intact ventricular septum—hypoplastic right heart.
- Pulmonary stenosis.

Ebstein's Anomaly

It is characterized by low placed septal cusp of tricuspid valve leading to malalignment of the three cusps of tricuspid valve (Fig. 9.19A). Color Doppler shows regurgitation into RA (Fig. 9.19B). This is flow from ventricle to atrium on systole. Due to this, RA appears enlarged but it is actually atrialization of right ventricle. It is progressive in antenatal life. Pulmonary trunk may be small/normal depending on the functional size of the right ventricle. Severe right ventricular dysfunction may lead to severe pulmonary

stenosis/atresia which is ductus-dependent. This will represent on three vessel view as reversal of pulmonary trunk to aortic ratio. On the three vessel view on color Doppler, reversal of the flow is seen in the pulmonary trunk through the ductus arteriosus. The increased preload in the RA also leads to reversal of flow in DV leading to A-wave reversal on pulsed Doppler (Fig. 9.19C). It may often be associated with severe cardiac enlargement and lung hypoplasia. Atrial septal defect (ASD) may be associated with Ebstein's anomaly.

Dysplastic Tricuspid Valve

On B-mode, the tricuspid valve appears thickened. On ventricular diastole, the valve cusps movements are not comparable to that of the mitral valve cusps. This leads to stenotic effect on the flow from the RA to right ventricle. On color Doppler, this is seen as turbulent flow from atrium to

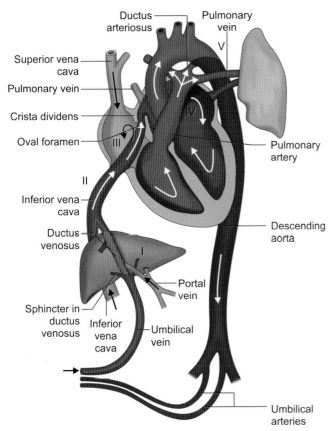

Fig. 9.18: Fetal circulation.
Source: Adapted from Navadia C. Fundamentals of Cardiology: Concise Review for USMLE and General Medical Boards, 2nd edition. India: MedRx Education; 2016.

ventricle during diastole or flow with aliasing effect due to high velocity jet (Fig. 9.19D).

Unguarded Tricuspid Valve with Almost no Valvular Tissue

This leads to an open way across the tricuspid valve, leading to severe regurgitation that can be appreciated on color Doppler.

Tricuspid Atresia

On ultrasound, tricuspid valve is seen but it is not functional, it does not open and close with the systole and diastole of the heart. So, naturally on color Doppler, no flow is seen across this valve during systole or diastole. Right ventricle is hypoplastic (Fig. 9.20). The ventricle is sometimes so hypoplastic that it may be barely identified. RA is normal/ large with restrictive ASD. Septal defects are common.

Pulmonary Valve Atresia with Intact Ventricular Septum: Hypoplastic Right Heart

Right ventricle is small and hypoplastic with decreased contractility even in early gestation but may be progressive and may appear normal till 20 weeks. IV septum is intact (Fig. 9.21). On color Doppler, no forward flow is seen through tricuspid and pulmonary valve as both are atretic. On three vessel view, aorta and pulmonary trunk show flow in opposite directions (Fig. 9.18) with turbulence at ductus as pulmonary trunk is filled through ductus arteriosus.[4]

Pulmonary Stenosis

There is thickening and doming of pulmonary valve. Pulmonary artery is small as seen on RVOT and on three vessels view plane, with increased Doppler velocities than in aorta showing turbulence on color Doppler (Figs. 9.22A and B). Reversed flow in ductus arteriosus is seen in severe cases (Fig. 9.18) and then it is a ductus-dependent disease that is when pulmonary stenosis is critical.[5] PSV may exceed 200 cm/s. Forward ductus flow may be noted. Pulmonary stenosis also is a progressive condition and as it progresses may lead to reversed flow in ductus and tricuspid regurgitation.[6] Dysplasia of the pulmonary valve may also lead to pulmonary regurgitation.

Septal defects are common.

In cases of atretic pulmonary valve, but patent pulmonary artery (a ductus-dependent condition), aortopulmonary collaterals may be seen filling the pulmonary artery on Doppler on transverse or coronal planes.

LEFT HEART ABNORMALITIES

- Aortic stenosis
- Coarctation
- Interrupted aortic arch
- Hypoplastic left heart
- Mitral valve disease.

Aortic Stenosis

It refers to narrowing at or around the level of the valve. Aortic valve is thickened and shows doming. Left ventricle may be hypertrophied and there may be asymmetric septal hypertrophy (Fig. 9.23). This is due to the fact that left ventricle continuously is pushing against a tightly stenotic valve. Thickening of the ventricular septum may obstruct

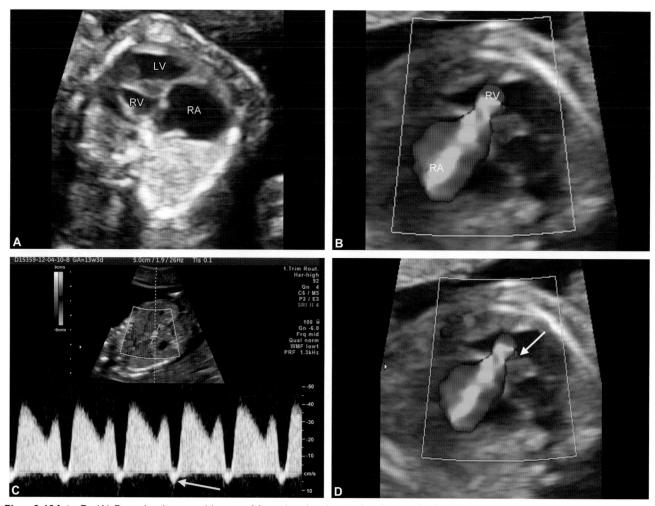

Figs. 9.19A to D: (A) B-mode ultrasound image of four chamber heart showing marked evident enlargement of the right atrium; (B) Color Doppler image showing backflow of the blood from the RV to RA during systole-tricuspid regurge; (C) Pulsed Doppler image of the ductus venosus flow showing reversed "A" wave; and (D) Color Doppler image showing tricuspid regurgitation with the arrow showing mixing of colors due to high velocity jet. (RA: right atrium; RV: right ventricle).

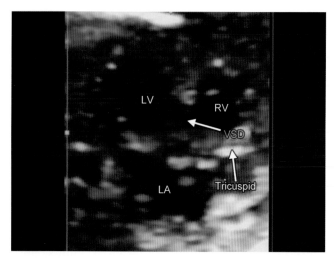

Fig. 9.20: Four-chamber heart view showing very small right atrium with hyperechoic closed tricuspid valve, and ventricular septal defect (VSD)—tricuspid atresia with VSD.

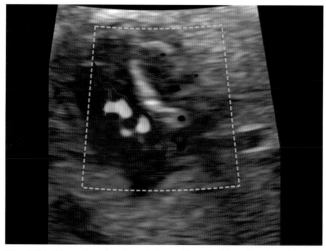

Fig. 9.21: Four-chamber heart view with color Doppler showing very small right side of the heart with no flow across the tricuspid valve and intact ventricular septum—right hypoplastic heart.

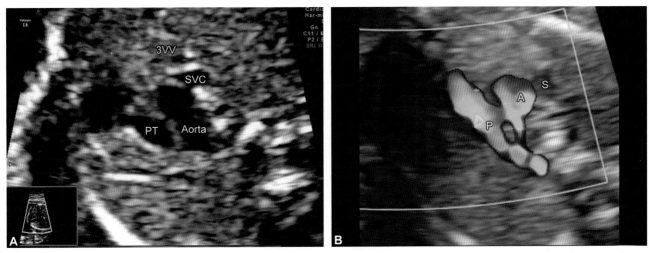

Figs. 9.22A and B: (A) Three-vessel view on B mode shows smaller diameter of pulmonary trunk (PT) as compared to that of aorta; (B) Confirms the findings.

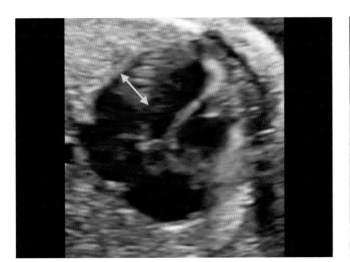

Fig. 9.23: Four-chamber heart view on B-mode ultrasound showing a thick muscular wall of the left ventricle—hypertrophic left ventricle, may be seen in aortic stenosis or coarctation.

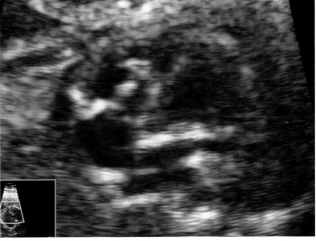

Fig. 9.24: Four-chamber heart view showing hyperechogenicities of the wall and the valve leaflets—endocardial fibroelastosis.

LVOT and cause subvalvular stenosis where valve may appear normal. This is very difficult to diagnose in utero. The hypertrophic ventricle goes into decreased contractility due to fatigue of the myometrium and, therefore, results into dilated left ventricle. At times, aortic stenosis is associated with endocardial fibroelastosis (Fig. 9.24). Aortic stenosis may be progressive in utero and, therefore, often may not be diagnosed on early scan and may progress into hypoplastic left heart syndrome.

Valvular: On systole, also valve does not open fully-thickened valves usually

Postvalvular: Normal valve, but turbulent flow beyond.

Subaortic stenosis: Muscular or membranous, but is usually very rare in fetus.

Color Doppler shows increased flow velocity through aortic valve with turbulence (Fig. 9.25). Following the path of the aorta further with Doppler, reversed flow is seen in aortic arch. This may be noticed on three vessel view. Three vessel view also shows a narrow aorta as compared to the pulmonary trunk. In cases with dilated left ventricle, decreased velocity is seen in aorta and this is suggestive of left ventricular failure.[7]

In cases with left ventricular dilatation and left ventricular failure, mitral regurgitation may be present.

Critical aortic stenosis is ductus-dependent and may be a cause of evolving hypoplastic left heart syndrome. Because of severe stenosis, the aorta is filled through ductus arteriosus by reverse flow (Fig. 9.26). This is seen on color Doppler on three vessel view. The aortic valve may be thickened with poststenotic dilatation and systole jet of PSV more than 200 cm/s. It leads to dilated left ventricle and reduced contractility. Mitral regurgitation may be present. This may result into left ventricular failure and decrease the velocities across the stenotic lumen of aorta.[8] In severe aortic stenosis, reverse flow through the foramen ovale to RA and reversed flow in the DV may be seen (*see* Fig. 9.18).

Coarctation of Aorta

Localized narrowing of the juxtaductal arch is known as coarctation of aorta (Fig. 9.27). This narrowing is between left subclavian artery and ductus arteriosus. Though this lesion is in the arch of the aorta, it is best and most easily suspected on the three vessel view as narrowing of the transverse arch and aortic isthmus (Fig. 9.28). Aorta appears

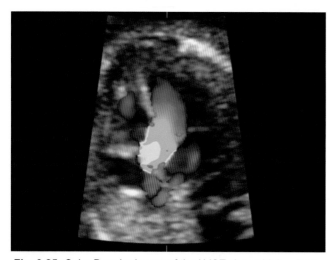

Fig. 9.25: Color Doppler image of the LVOT shows high velocity flow and turbulence due to subaortic stenosis.

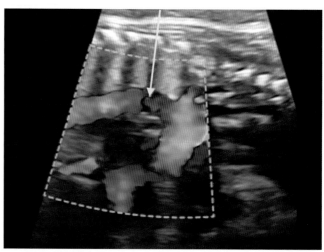

Fig. 9.27: Arch of aorta with color Doppler showing narrowing of the lumen at the isthmic level as shown by arrow—coarctation of aorta.

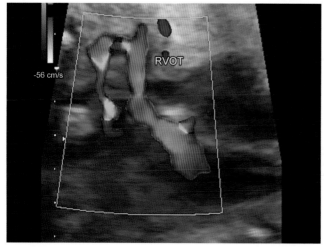

Fig. 9.26: Three vessel view with Doppler showing smaller diameter of the aorta and the reverse color as compared to pulmonary trunk, suggestive of retrograde filling of aorta.

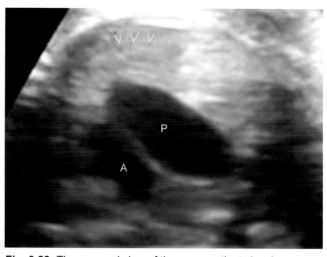

Fig. 9.28: Three vessel view of the same patient showing narrow aorta-arch as compared to the pulmonary trunk.

smaller than pulmonary trunk on three vessel view. There is relative right ventricular and pulmonary trunk enlargement without right heart disease.[9]

Actually there is thickening and hypertrophy of the left ventricular myometrium (Fig. 9.29). On color Doppler, there is high velocity flow in proximal descending aorta as seen in the aortic arch (sagittal) view (Figs. 9.30A and B). Coarctation leads to increased overload in left ventricle and, therefore, it leads to decreased right to left atrial shunt. The flow velocity in the narrow aortic arch in fetal life is not increased in contrast to what is seen in adult life—high velocity flow.

Interrupted Aortic Arch

Aorta is not at all formed beyond the arch. The descending aorta is a continuation of ductal arch. Most common site

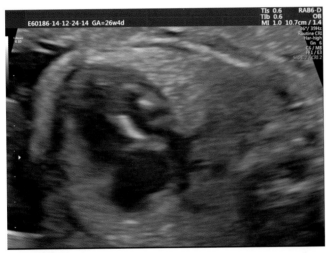

Fig. 9.29: Four-chamber heart showing thickened left ventricular wall.

is between the second vessel and third vessel of the arch. Type B-ascending aorta may show a two-pronged fork appearance. But it may also be at isthmus (type A). Both types are associated with small ascending aorta. This is a difficult diagnosis but the clue is straight ascending aorta on aortic arch view. Branches may or may not be present depending on the type of interruption. This abnormality is almost always associated with VSD.

Hypoplastic Left Heart Syndrome

Left ventricle is small on four-chamber view with poor contractility (Fig. 9.31A). Left atrium may be small or normal in size. There is no forward flow through mitral or aortic valve. Aortic size and origin site are important for postnatal prognosis.

On ultrasound, heart may appear normal at 16–18 weeks as disease may be progressive in utero. On B-mode, the opening and closing of the mitral valve is not seen. On color Doppler, therefore, no flow is seen across the mitral valve from left atrium to the ventricle during diastole (Fig. 9.31B). The LVOT may be very difficult to identify as it may be very narrow especially in the cases where there is no VSD. Because in this, there is no flow across the aortic valve also and may be at times noncanalization of the LVOT. These are then ductus-dependent cases, because since there is no forward flow through the aortic valve, the aortic filling is by reverse flow from the ductus arteriosus. On three vessel view, therefore, the aorta is thin and on this view, color shows reverse flow in it (*see* Fig. 9.26). When there is a VSD, there is a variable degree of canalization of the left ventricle depending on the side of the VSD, because then the inflow into the left ventricle is only through the defect.

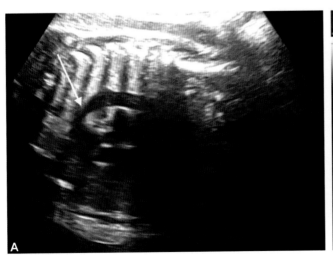
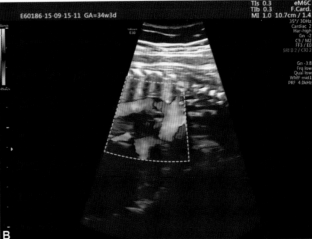

Figs. 9.30A and B: (A) B mode; and (B) Color Doppler image of the aortic arch showing narrowing of the aorta (arrow in Fig. A) with turbulence of the flow on Doppler-coarctation of the aorta.

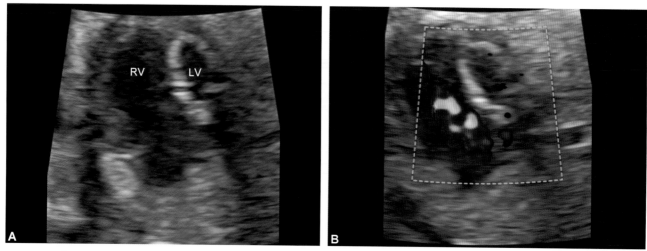

Figs. 9.31A and B: (A) Four-chamber heart view with left heart hypoplasia on B-mode; and (B) Same patient on color no flow is seen across the mitral valve on diastole.

Mitral Valve Defects

Mitral valve defects are rare as isolated abnormalities in the antenatal life, though a dysplastic mitral valve may be seen as a valve with thickened cusps on B-mode. It may often be a part of generalized fibroelastosis. Regurgitation through this valve is seen as blood flow from ventricle to atrium during ventricular systole.

Less common causes of small left ventricle are:

- *Ductal constriction (ductus arteriosus)*: Use of antiprostaglandin drugs like indomethacin may lead to ductal obstruction between 28 weeks and 34 weeks. Evaluation for the same is to be done within 48–72 hours of starting the drug. Total ductal closure may be associated with fetal demise. Ductal obstruction will lead to restriction to the right ventricular outflow. As it has to push the blood against resistance, the myometrium undergoes hypertrophy initially and later on due to afterload leads to dilatation. These changes are reflected back into the atrium leading to RA enlargement and tricuspid regurgitation and ultimately may lead to right heart failure (Fig. 9.32). On color Doppler aliasing is seen in the RVOT, most noticeable at ductus arteriosus. Pulse Doppler normal velocity in ductus arteriosus is 150 cm/s (systole), 40 cm/s (diastole). Its constriction causes higher systolic and diastolic velocities. Only high systolic velocity may be seen in last 4–6 weeks and in conditions with increased fetal cardiac output, but high diastolic velocity is diagnostic of ductal constriction.[10] Ductal arch patency must always be checked when doing a fetal

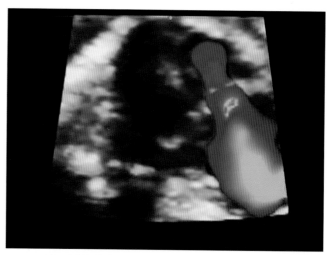

Fig. 9.32: Color Doppler image showing tricuspid regurgitation on systole in blue color.

echocardiography especially when the mother is given indomethacin at any time during pregnancy.

- *Vein of Galen aneurysm*: Though the primary lesion is not in the heart, this hypercirculatory lesion like leads to increased circulatory load through the SVC to the RA, ultimately leading to enlargement of the right ventricle. This evidently may only appear as a small left atrium (chamber asymmetry) (Fig. 9.33A). The enlarged right ventricle and increased venous return in the RA may lead to increased flow across the tricuspid valve in the right ventricle and enlargement of the right ventricle also. There may be tricuspid regurgitation documented on color Doppler across the tricuspid valve. Reverse flow

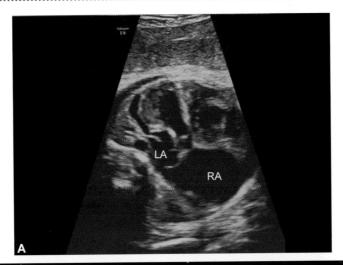

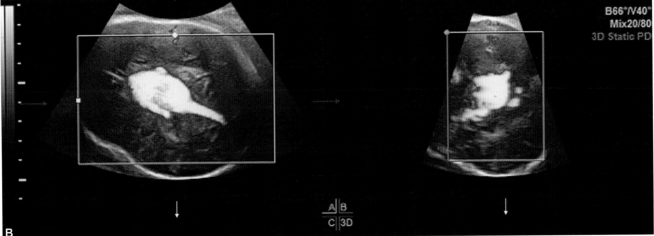

Figs. 9.33A and B: (A) B-mode ultrasound image of four chamber heart showing chamber asymmetry with right atrial enlargement; and (B) Power Doppler image of the fetal head shows a large vascular shadow in the midline—aneurysm of vein of Galen.

in the ductus venosus may also be seen in the later stages (*see* Fig. 9.18), due to increased return in the RA through SVC. The actual lesion also can be diagnosed by Doppler. Vein of Galen aneurysm appears as a cystic lesion in the midline on the transthalamic or transcerebellar planes of the fetal head (Fig. 9.33B).

- *Total anomalous pulmonary venous drainage (TAPVD)*: There are in all four pulmonary veins entering into the left atrium. But in the antenatal life on fetal echocardiography, it is possible to identify only the two lower ones. Anomalous pulmonary venous drainage may affect one or more of these veins. If all the four veins drain out of left atrium, it is TAPVD, otherwise it is partial. Since only two are seen on the fetal echocardiography, only total anomalous drainage can be excluded antenatally.

  Pulmonary veins instead of emptying into left atrium, may empty in RA or any other systemic veins. These may be portal-hepatic veins, innominate vein, SVC, or coronary sinus. TAPVD has obligatory right to left atrial shunt.

  On ultrasound, no pulmonary veins seen on four-chamber view entering the left atrium (Fig. 9.34). Pulmonary venous confluence is seen behind the RA. Increased distance is seen between descending aorta and left atrium (Fig. 9.34). When these veins drain above the heart (supracardiac type), this vein/veins may drain into left innominate vein and is seen as a fourth vessel on the three vessel trachea view, with the fourth vessel to the left of the pulmonary artery. This has cardiofugal flow whereas SVC has cardiopetal flow, this can be appreciated on color Doppler. Right ventricle is large, if TAPVD is present, but enlargement is not seen if there is ASD or infradiaphragmatic drainage. When drainage is infracardiac, the draining vein is seen parallel to esophagus and runs through the diaphragm

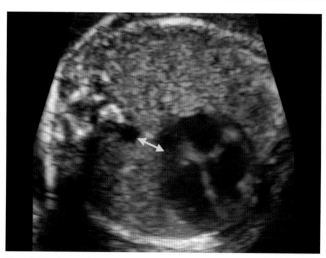

Fig. 9.34: B-mode ultrasound image of the four chamber heart showing no pulmonary veins entering the left atrium and asymmetry between the two atria (larger right atrium) and increased distance between the left atrium and the descending aorta as marked by the arrowed line.

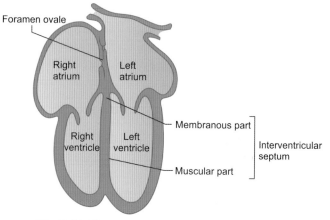

Fig. 9.35: Diagrammatic demonstration of different types of ventricular septal defects.

to drain into the portal venous system. Color Doppler may show the PV drainage precisely. If it is below the diaphragm, it appears as a very high velocity flow spot, as the venous confluence opens into IVC or hepatic vein. But this needs to be differentiated from turbulence in DV. Cardiac drainage of the abnormal pulmonary vein is through the coronary sinus resulting in dilated coronary sinus. Another cause of dilated coronary sinus is persistent left SVC. This may be differentiated from the supracardiac TAPVD on three vessel view by the flow direction, that is same as that in SVC in case of persistent left SVC and the opposite in TAPVD.

Chamber asymmetry, thus, tells us about the abnormalities of the AV valves and the ventricular outflow tracts. Apart from the chambers, the septae are to be evaluated on four-chamber view. The septal defects can be discussed as:

• Ventricular septal defect
• Atrial septal defect
• Atrioventricular septal defect (AVSD).

• *Interventricular septal defects* are most common and consist of 30% of cardiac defects. They cause no hemodynamic disturbances in utero if not too large. This is because there otherwise also is a communication between the right heart and left heart circulation.

Ventricular septal defects can be further classified according to their location in the ventricular septum. Let us, therefore, revise the anatomy of the IV septum once (Fig. 9.35). The IV septum can be divided into muscular part (the ventricular septum that is seen on the

four-chamber heart view), the membranous part of the septum (that is seen on the LVOT view), the outflow tract part (that is between the two outflow tract, appreciated on the short-axis view), and the inlet part (that is just apical to the crux between the two AV valves). 46% of nonmalaligned VSDs close in antenatal life and 23% during the 1st year of life. Only 31% remain patent.[11] Malaligned defects are less likely to be corrected without surgery. Large muscular and large perimembranous defects and inlet and subpulmonary defects usually require surgery.

– *Muscular ventricular septal defect:* Lateral or oblique four-chamber view is the best to diagnose these defects. It is seen as dropout in septal shadow (Fig. 9.36A). But, small defects are difficult to diagnose without color Doppler. This is because these defects especially when small may close during systole.

Color Doppler may be used to demonstrate these defects better. Though even on color Doppler, no through flow may be seen as there is no pressure gradient between the two ventricles during intrauterine life. When present, flow may be from left to right, or from right to left (Fig. 9.36B).

As pressures in both ventricles are similar and there may or may not be significant shunting of blood. Defects that are well-aligned (both ends of the defect maintain the axis of the main septum) (Fig. 9.36C) and are less than 3 mm are known to heal during intrauterine life.

– *Membranous ventricular septal defect:* Left ventricular outflow tract view may demonstrate this defect. It is seen as a breach in the continuity of

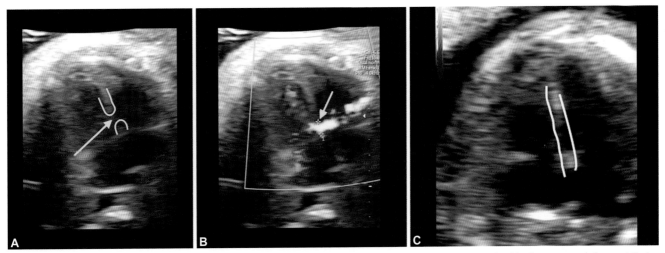

Figs. 9.36A to C: (A) Oblique four-chamber view of the heart showing dropout in septal shadow as marked by lines—muscular ventricular septal defect; (B) On Doppler, this shows the flow across the defect confirming the diagnosis; and (C) The same image as Figure 9.36A, the two parallel lines demonstrate that the two ends of the gap in the septum are well-aligned.

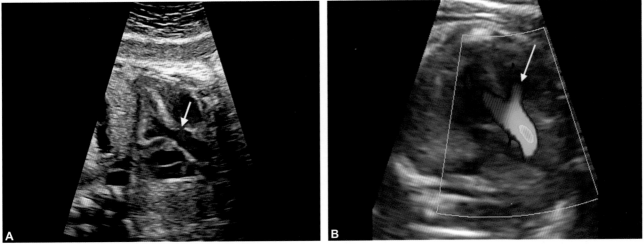

Figs. 9.37A and B: (A) B-mode ultrasound image of left ventricular outflow tract (LVOT) showing the membranous septal defect as marked by the arrow; and (B) Color Doppler image of the same showing the aorta draining the blood from both the ventricles.

the medial wall of the LVOT, apical to the aortic valve (Fig. 9.37A). Color Doppler typically shows a color strand extending from the right ventricle to the aorta (Fig. 9.37B). If it is well-aligned and isolated, and less than 3 mm in size, it has a tendency to heal on its own in intrauterine or early neonatal life. If these defects are malaligned, the chance of spontaneous closure is significantly low. The malaligned ones are often associated with conotruncal defects but may even be isolated. It is typically seen as deviation of the distal wall of the defect toward right ventricular lumen instead being in line with the IV septum and

leads to overriding of aorta. On color Doppler, the aorta is seen to drain blood from both the ventricles. If overriding results in more than 50% of the aortic lumen width arising from the right ventricle, instead of overriding of aorta, it is called double outlet right ventricle (DORV) with VSD.

– *Inlet defects:* This defect is in the inlet part of the septum, close to AV valves' septal cusp insertion. On apical and basal four-chamber view, the part of the septum close to the crux is often not seen. This must not be misinterpreted as septal defect always. It is a defect only if the end of the septal line shows

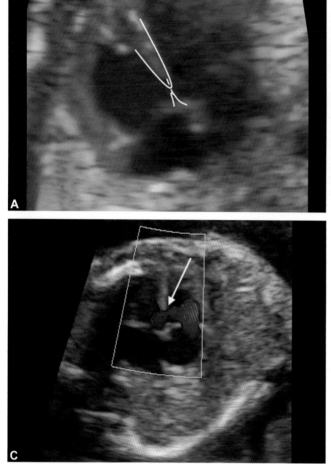

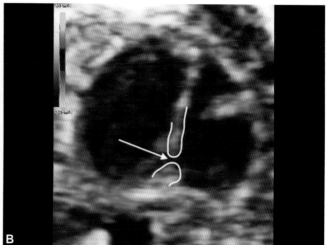

Figs. 9.38A to C: (A) Four chamber heart showing tapering of the ventricular septum just apical to the atrioventricular (AV) valves with an apparent gap in continuity of the septum. This is an artifact and not a true ventricular septal defect; (B) Similar appearance as Figure 9.37A, but the margins that show gap in the ventricular septum are broadened and bold suggesting a true inlet ventricular septal defect; and (C) The same case when color Doppler is used shows the flow across the defect, confirming the diagnosis.

a thickened end or is also appreciated on the lateral four-chamber view, otherwise it is an artifact (Figs. 9.38A and B). Color Doppler may help to confirm the diagnosis (Fig. 9.38C). Bidirectional flow may be seen in systole and diastole on color Doppler in lateral four-chamber view. It may be associated with Down syndrome.

– *Subpulmonary (outflow defect):* It is seen under the pulmonary valve and above the supraventricular crest. It can be demonstrated only on short-axis view below the pulmonary valve (Fig. 9.39).

- *Atrial septum defects:* Consists of 8% of congenital cardiac defects. ASDs can be present at three locations: (1) secundum, (2) sinus venosus, and (3) primum (Fig. 9.40).

– Secundum defects are most common but cannot be diagnosed antenatally. These may be isolated or with VSD/pulmonary valve stenosis. This defect appears as larger than expected area of dropout in the central portion of the septum secundum, close to foramen ovale or it appears as a short foraminal flap that cannot cover the foramen ovale completely. It is to be differentiated from foramen ovale thickening. Small defects may close spontaneously (Fig. 9.41A).

– Redundancy of the foramen ovale flap is known as aneurysm of foramen ovale commonly associated with atrial arrhythmias (Fig. 9.41B).

– Sinus venosus defects are difficult to diagnose. 5–10% of ASDs are sinus venosus defects, situated posterior to foramen ovale and inferior to SVC.

– Primum defects are mostly a part of AV defect (Fig. 9.41C)

Atrial septal defects do not require alteration in obstetric care.

- *Atrioventricular septal defects:* These are the defects of endocardial cushion causing primum ASD with VSD.

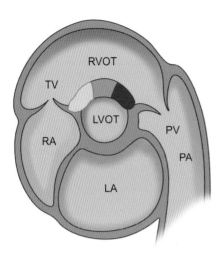

Fig. 9.39: Diagrammatic presentation of the outflow part ventricular septal defect.

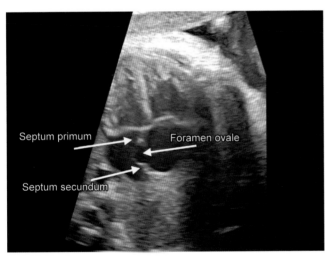

Fig. 9.40: Four-chamber heart view showing anatomy of the interatrial septum.

These defects are common with chromosomal abnormalities. The risk of recurrence is 7–17% in families with normal karyotype.[12] Isolated defects have 85–90% survival rates after surgical repair.

On ultrasound, complete AVSD will show single AV valve on four-chamber view which is better demonstrated in diastole (Fig. 9.42A). In partial AVSD, both valves are attached at the same level on the septum instead of slight apical attachment of tricuspid valve normally. This leads to a typical "T"-shaped configuration formed by two valve cusps and (Fig. 9.42B). Color Doppler shows mixture of flow to ventricles (Fig. 9.42C). This anomaly can be diagnosed in

late 1st trimester. It is often associated with increased nuchal translucency and trisomy 21. It may be associated with Fallot's tetralogy, DORV, coarctation of aorta, ventricular hypoplasia subaortic, or pulmonary valve stenosis.

Atrioventricular septal defect can be balanced or unbalanced. Balanced when both ventricles are equal in size and this has a good prognosis. Unbalanced AVSD shows asymmetrical ventricles due to selective drainage to one of the ventricles from the atria through AV valve. AV regurgitation is demonstrated arising from the center of the AV valve. It has a poor prognosis. This condition must be differentiated from single ventricle.

– *Obstructed foramen ovale:* Commonly associated with left heart obstructive defects. It may also be associated with mitral regurgitation, supra-ventricular tachycardia, or fetal hydrops.

This can lead to prenatal right heart failure, hydrops, and fetal death. Postnatally, it leads to persistent fetal circulation, right heart failure, and death.

OUTFLOW TRACT DEFECTS

These are also known as conotruncal defects.

These are commonly associated with deletion of chromo-some 22q11.2 which can be diagnosed by fluorescence in situ hybridization (FISH). This group of abnormalities includes:

- Fallot's tetralogy
- Double outlet right ventricle
- Truncus arteriosus
- Transposition of the great arteries (TGA)
- Corrected TGA.

Fallot's Tetralogy

It is the most common cyanotic heart defect and almost always missed if only four-chamber heart view is obtained as cardiac screening. The only positive sign on four-chamber view may be increased by cardiac axis. It has four components—(1) membranous VSD, (2) overriding of aorta, (3) pulmonary stenosis, and (4) hypertrophic right ventricle. But it is a progressive condition and the last component becomes evident in late pregnancy or after birth.

On ultrasound, increased angle of cardiac axis is seen on four-chamber view (Fig. 9.43A). Long-axis view shows VSD in the membranous part, with large aortic root and overriding of the aorta. RVOT view shows small pulmonary artery but it depends on the amount of overriding of

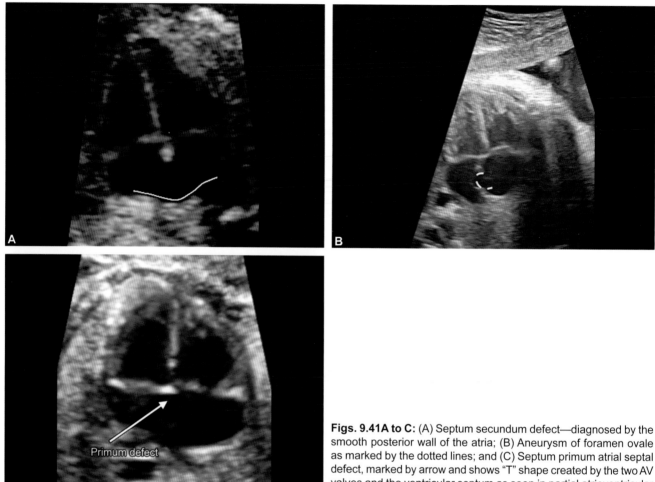

Figs. 9.41A to C: (A) Septum secundum defect—diagnosed by the smooth posterior wall of the atria; (B) Aneurysm of foramen ovale as marked by the dotted lines; and (C) Septum primum atrial septal defect, marked by arrow and shows "T" shape created by the two AV valves and the ventricular septum as seen in partial atrioventricular septal defect (AVSD).

the aorta. More the overriding, smaller is the pulmonary artery. Three vessel view shows inverse PA/aorta ratio when the caliber of pulmonary trunk is significantly small. Color Doppler shows increased velocity in PA due to RVOT obstruction and aorta is fed by two ventricles (Fig. 9.43B). Many a times only membranous VSD may be evident in early gestation.[13] It is the extent of pulmonary stenosis that decides the prognosis of the patients.

At times, there may be total atresia of the pulmonary valve with only the annulus. If this is stenotic, there may be poststenotic dilatation of the pulmonary trunk. Prognosis is extremely bad with this. In such extreme cases, the important differential diagnosis is truncus arteriosus and this is based only on the presence or absence of the pulmonary trunk. In cases of severe pulmonary stenosis, the pulmonary trunk still fills up with aortopulmonary collaterals, which can only be mapped on color Doppler. This especially occurs in cases with absent ductus arteriosus.

Double Outlet Right Ventricle

Both the great arteries arise from right ventricle and depending on the site of origin, one of the two may show variable degree of stenosis when both arteries are arising side by side. Its differentiation from other outflow tract anomalies with large VSD may be difficult.

On ultrasound, deviation of cardiac axis may be present but four-chamber view is otherwise normal. VSD may or may not be present but color Doppler is confirmatory, though presence of VSD in this condition may have a better prognosis. The outflow tracts may be shifted to the right ventricle as such or as a mirror image (Figs. 9.44A to C). Aorta can be on right side or left side of pulmonary trunk.

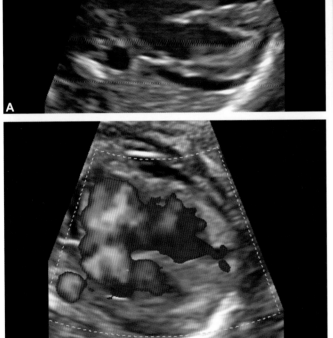

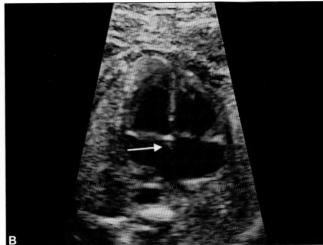

Figs. 9.42A to C: (A) B-mode ultrasound image of complete atrioventricular septal defect (AVSD); (B) Partial AVSD; and (C) Complete AVSD on power Doppler.

When aorta is to the right of the pulmonary trunk, it is Taussig-Bing type of DORV (or a transposition like). When the aorta is posterior and to left, it is a Tetralogy of Fallot like DORV.

In such cases with pulmonary trunk toward the septum, and with VSD may also sometimes show overriding of the pulmonary trunk on the septum. Color Doppler is the modality of choice for confirmation of the diagnosis, to diagnose associated VSD and overriding, and also to confirm the orientation of the vessels. It is commonly seen with right atrial isomerism also.

Truncus Arteriosus

Both the arteries arise as a single trunk from the ventricles. It is a result of incomplete or complete absence of the sprial septum, it is usually associated with outflow type of VSD.

It is usually associated with a large VSD with the trunk overriding the septum. Types of truncus have been shown in the Figure 9.45.

On ultrasound, increased cardiac axis is seen on otherwise normal four-chamber view. Malaligned large VSD is seen in outlet part, and may also at times extend into muscular part of ventricular septum. Truncal root is seen arising from RV or overriding the septum (Fig. 9.46). Abnormal truncal valve may or may not be present. The origin of PA must be confirmed to exclude pulmonary stenosis.

On color Doppler, VSD is seen with origin of truncus overriding the septum. Origin of pulmonary artery from the main trunk must be diagnosed. If dysplastic valve is present, it shows holodiastolic regurgitation on pulse Doppler.

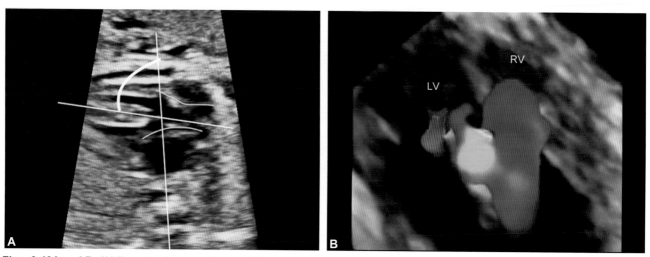

Figs. 9.43A and B: (A) B-mode ultrasound image of the heart showing its transverse orientation and also overriding of the aorta; and (B) Color Doppler showing blood being drained into the aorta through both the ventricles.

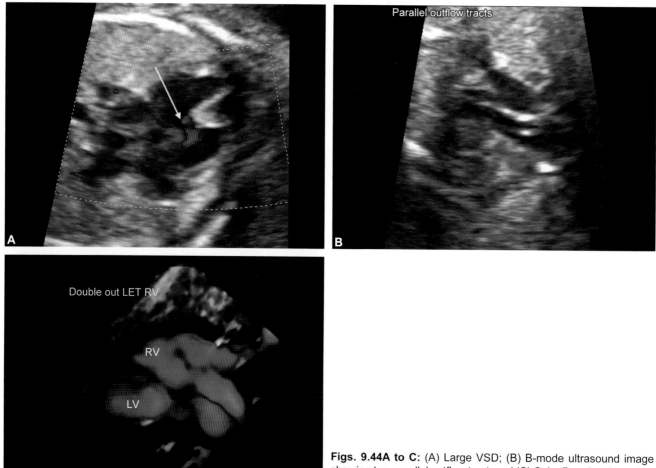

Figs. 9.44A to C: (A) Large VSD; (B) B-mode ultrasound image showing two parallel outflow tract; and (C) Color Doppler shows two parallel outflow tracts, both arising from the right ventricle—DORV. (DORV: double outlet right ventricle; VSD: ventricular septal defect)

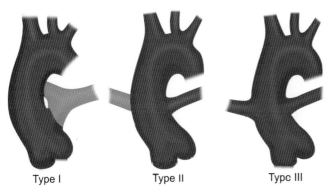

Fig. 9.45: Diagrammatic presentation of different types of truncus arteriosus.

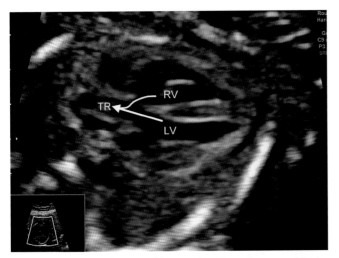

Fig. 9.46: B-mode ultrasound image showing a large ventricular septal defect (VSD) and truncus arising overriding the septal defect.

Complete Transposition of Great Vessels

Normally aorta arises from left ventricle and courses cranially and to right and then curves to left to form the arch and the RVOT arises from right ventricle and takes a route posteriorly. Complete transposition of great vessels is when aorta arises from right ventricle and lies anteriorly and to left of pulmonary trunk and pulmonary trunk arises from left ventricle. This means two great arteries arise side by side at the base of the heart instead of crossing over of great vessels.

On ultrasound, normal four-chamber view is seen. Outflow tracts show parallel great vessels at the roots. There is no crossing over of vessels. Vessel arising out of left ventricle takes posterior course and bifurcates so is pulmonary artery. Vessel arising out of right ventricle takes long upward course and curves. This is aorta (Figs. 9.47A and B). If associated with VSD and overriding, the diagnosis is difficult. This can be demonstrated on ultrasound by tracing the outflow tracts

up and color Doppler is more useful for establishing the vascularity of individual vessel and also for confirmation of overriding and VSD.[13] Three vessel view may show only aorta and the SVC as the pulmonary trunk is hidden by aorta. In cases, therefore, in which only two vessels are seen instead of three, the color Doppler PRF is decreased to see the remote possibility of a narrow pulmonary trunk as in case of hypoplastic right heart.

Corrected Transposition of Great Vessels

This is a very rare abnormality. RA opens into morphological left ventricle which gives out pulmonary trunk and left atrium opens into morphological right ventricle and gives out aorta. These patients may have dextrocardia.

On ultrasound, four-chamber view shows increased cardiac axis. Evidently normal looking heart shows ventricular inversion. AV discordance is confirmed by looking at the morphology of the chambers. Flap of foramen ovale opens in left atrium which opens in a ventricle which is morphologically right containing chordae tendineae and moderator band. Great vessels do not show crossing over, but are parallel. Ventriculoarterial discordance can be confirmed by tracing the outflow tracts. AV complete heart block may be seen on M-mode.[14]

Aorto-left Ventricular Tunnel

No aortic valve is formed leading to marked aortic regurgitation. It may sometimes be associated with a single arterial trunk.

Narrow Pulmonary Artery

It refers to pulmonary atresia or pulmonary valvular stenosis. Pulmonary atresia and stenosis both lead to a smaller diameter of the duct also. There is also a possibility of a reverse flow if there is atresia or severe stenosis. Pulmonary artery may also be narrow if the blood flow is less because of tricuspid valve obstruction.

Large Pulmonary Artery

Absent pulmonary valve syndrome or dysplastic pulmonary valve syndrome, dilated right ventricle.

ABNORMALITIES SEEN ON THREE-VESSEL VIEW: ROLE OF DOPPLER

- Reversal of P to A ratio:
  - Pulmonary stenosis
  - Fallot's tetralogy.

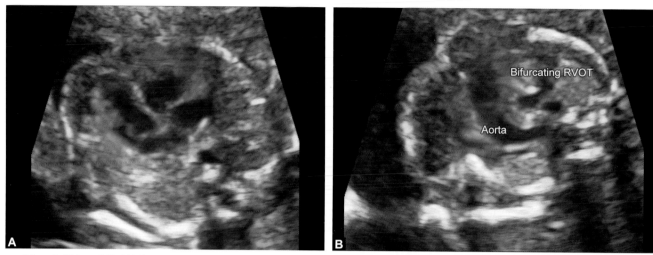

Figs. 9.47A and B: (A) On ultrasound, normal four-chamber view is seen; and (B) Vessel arising out of left ventricle (LV) takes posterior course and bifurcates so is pulmonary artery as seen on B-mode ultrasound.

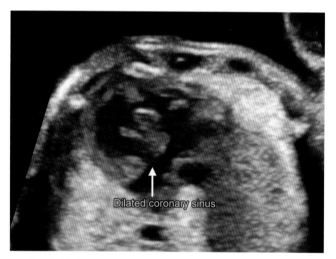

Fig. 9.48: B-mode image of fetal heart, four-chamber view showing dilated coronary sinus.

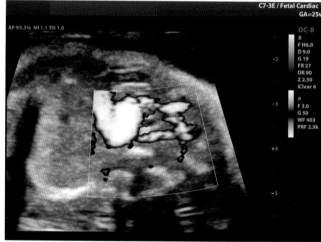

Fig. 9.49: Color Doppler showing incomplete vascular ring formed by persistent right aortic arch.

- Narrow aorta:
  - Coarctation of the aorta
  - Critical aortic stenosis.
- Only two vessels instead of three:
  - Truncus arteriosus
  - Critical aortic stenosis
  - Pulmonary atresia.
- Four vessels instead of three:
  - Persistent left SVC
  - Persistent azygos
  - Persistent right aorta.
- Vessels forming "U" instead of "V":
  - Right-sided aorta.

Persistent Left Superior Vena Cava

Proximal part of the left SVC is seen on three vessel view as the fourth vessel. Right SVC is smaller than normal. This may lead to dilated coronary sinus as left SVC opens in coronary sinus and drains into RA. On four-chamber view, distal part of left SVC is seen and also the dilated coronary sinus (Figs. 9.48 and 9.49).

Right-sided Aorta

It may be isolated or associated with other cardiac abnormalities like Fallot's tetralogy or truncus arteriosus or situs inversus. On three-vessel view, the aorta remains

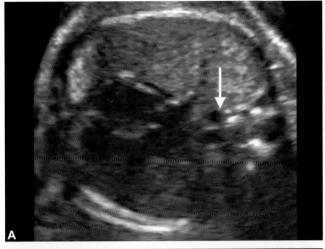

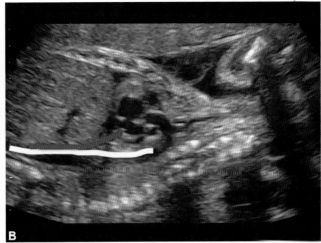

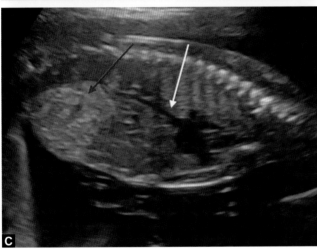

Figs. 9.50A to C: (A) Four-chamber heart view showing azygos placed just by the side of the aorta, anterior to the spine; (B) Sagittal section of the fetus showing the aorta as white line and IVC as blue line; (C) Sagittal section of the thorax and abdomen show anterior deviation of the inferior vena cava (IVC) to enter the heart and this is normal.

on the right of the aorta. But the duct is still on the left side and connects with the descending aorta behind the trachea. Duct may be on the right side with mirror image branching pattern in the right-sided aortic arch. In this case, left brachiocephalic artery crosses in front of the trachea.

Double Aortic Arch (Persistent Right-sided Aortic Arch)

Right-sided aortic arch may also be a part of double aortic arch and shows a complete vascular ring surrounding the trachea (*see* Fig. 9.49).

The ring may not be complete between the left carotid and the left subclavian artery.

Aberrant Right Subclavian Artery

Though can be demonstrated at 11–13 + 6 weeks scan, might not be used as a marker for T21 when isolated.[15] It is seen in 10–20% of T21 fetuses but is also seen in

1.4% of normal fetuses also.[16] Normally, right subclavian artery arises from the right brachiocephalic trunk (first branch of aortic arch), but when aberrant, it arises from the descending aorta. It courses behind trachea and esophagus.

Absence of Ductus Venosus

Umbilical vein is connected to either IVC, iliac vein or renal vein, RA, or coronary sinus. When draining into IVS or iliac vein, it may lead to significant dilatation of IVC since midgestation. Umbilical vein takes an inferior course. A long aberrant vessel is seen from liver to right abdominal wall crossing the diaphragm. Whichever of these sites it drains, it leads to cardiac volume overload. This can be recognized in upper abdominal plane. In another subgroup of patients with absent DV, which is actual absence of DV the connection of the umbilical vein to the portal sinus is normal, but DV is absent and is often associated with aneuploidies and other cardiac and extracardiac anomalies and syndromes like (Noonan's syndrome, VACTERL, Smith–Lemli–Opitz syndrome, etc.).

Dilated Inferior Vena Cava with Absent Ductus Venosus

A dilated vessel is seen as a direct connection between umbilical vein and IVC on color Doppler used on the sagittal section for the right atrial inflow tracts. This leads to mild right atrial and ventricular dilatation. This may sometimes lead to cardiac failure and fetal hydrops.

Dilated Azygos

It is suspected by seeing two vessels instead of one behind the heart. A vessel that is just by the side of and posterior to aorta on four-chamber view (Fig. 9.50A). On abdomen sagittal section, it is seen as a vein running parallel to and posterior to aorta (Fig. 9.50B). This is unlike IVC which is anterior to the aorta, slightly to right and deviating more anteriorly as it approached RA (Fig. 9.50C). Azygos may traverse the diaphragm to join SVC. On three vessel view, azygos is seen and dilated SVC is also seen. It is better demonstrated by color Doppler. Persistent azygos may also be seen in interrupted IVC at the level of kidneys usually. Persistent azygos vein is also likely in left isomerism (90%). As the upper part of the IVC is not present, the hepatic vein directly opens into the RA in this case.

CONCLUSION

Since heart is a blood pumping organ, its detailed study must include the study of the blood flows across its valves and into its outflow tracts. Abnormal flows through the septal defects or abnormal valves need to be documented by the doppler. This abnormalities may include abnormalities of flow direction as well as abnormalities of the velocities. Thus, Doppler is indispensible for fetal echocardiography.

REFERENCES

1. Yagel S, Cohen SM, Achiron R. Examination of the fetal heart by five short axis views: a proposed screening method for comprehensive cardiac evaluation. Ultrasound Obstet Gynecol. 2001;17(5):367-9.
2. Navadia C. Fundamentals of Cardiology: Concise Review for USMLE and General Medical Boards, 2nd edition. India: MedRx Education; 2016.
3. Hornberger LK, Sahn DJ, Kleinman CS, et al. Tricuspid valve disease with significant tricuspid insufficiency in the fetus: diagnosis and outcome. J Am Coll Cardiol. 1991;17(1):167-73.
4. Yagel S, Arbel R, Anteby EY, et al. The three vessels and trachea view (3VT) in fetal cardiac scanning. Ultrasound Obstet Gynecol. 2002;20(4):340-5.
5. Berning RA, Silverman NH, Villegas M, et al. Reversed shunting across the ductus arteriosus or atrial septum in utero heralds severe congenital heart disease. J Am Coll Cardiol. 1996;27(2):481-6.
6. Todros T, Paladini D, Chiappa E, et al. Pulmonary stenosis and atresia with intact ventricular septum during prenatal life. Ultrasound Obstet Gynecol. 2003;21(3):228-33.
7. Jouk PS, Rambaud P. Prediction of outcome by prenatal Doppler analysis in a patient with aortic stenosis. Br Heart J. 1991;65(1):53-4.
8. Hornberger LK, Sanders SP, Rein AJ, et al. Left heart obstructive lesions and left ventricular growth in the midtrimester fetus. A longitudinal study. Circulation. 1995;92(6):1531-8.
9. Sharland GK, Chan KY, Allan LD. Coarctation of the aorta: difficulties in prenatal diagnosis. Br Heart J. 1994;71(1):70-5.
10. Huhta JC, Moise KJ, Fisher DJ, et al. Detection and quantitation of constriction of the fetal ductus arteriosus by Doppler echocardiography. Circulation. 1987;75(2):406-12.
11. Alpert BS, Mellitis ED, Rowe RD. Spontaneous closure of small ventricular septal defects: probability rates in the first year of life. Am J Dis Child. 1973;125(1):194-6.
12. Digilio MC, Marino B, Cicini MP, et al. Risk of congenital heart defects in relatives of patients with atrioventricular canal. Am J Dis Child. 1993;147(12):1295-7.
13. Kirklin JW, Barratt-Boyes BG. Complete transposition of great arteries. In: Kirklin JW, Barratt-Boyes BG (Eds). Cardiac Surgery. New York: Churchill Livingstone; 1993. pp. 1383-467.
14. Lee W, Smith RS, Comstock CH, et al. Tetralogy of Fallot: prenatal diagnosis and postnatal survival. Obstet Gynecol. 1995;86(4 Pt 1):583-8.
15. Borenstein M, Minekawa R, Zidere V, et al. Aberrant right subclavian artery at 16 to 23 + 6 weeks of gestation: a marker for chromosomal abnormality. Ultrasound Obstet Gynecol. 2010;36(5):548-52.
16. Zalel Y, Achiron R, Yagel S, et al. Fetal aberrant right subclavian artery in normal and Down syndrome fetuses. Ultrasound Obstet Gynecol. 2008;31(1):25-9.

Role of Doppler in Intrauterine Growth Restriction and Pregnancy-induced Hypertension

INTRODUCTION

Intrauterine growth restriction (IUGR) or fetal growth restriction (FGR) is one of the major concerns in the fetomaternal health. Fetal growth is influenced by genetic predisposition, parental influence, ethnic differences,[1] environment (altitude), and fetal gender also. IUGR is a very loosely used term. It is very important to clear the concepts of the similar terms used interchangeably. These are low birth weight (LBW), small for gestational age (SGA) fetuses, and IUGR fetuses. Another school classifies these fetuses into normal SGA, abnormal SGA, and IUGR.[2] Though all these terms have been used interchangeably at times, but clearly identify different groups of patients. LBWs are the neonates that are born with a weight of less than 2,500 grams. These LBW patients may be due to prematurity or may be constitutional or may be due to circulatory derangements, infections, or genetic diseases in their intrauterine life.

Most common causes for LBW babies are:
- *Maternal*:
  - Pregnancy-induced hypertension (PIH)
  - Antiphospholipid antibody syndrome/prothrombotic states
  - Chronic hypertension
  - Severe diabetes mellitus
  - Collagen vascular disease
  - Cardiac or renal disease
  - Smoking and poor nutrition
  - Previous history of IUGR baby.
- *Uterine—Placental*:
  - Uteroplacental dysfunction

  - Placental infarct
  - Chronic abruption
  - Multiple gestation—twin-to-twin transfusion
  - Confined placental mosaicism
  - Placental bleeding
  - Placental infections
  - Immunological causes.
- *Fetal*:
  - Chromosomal abnormalities
  - Confined placental mosaicism
  - Major structural anomalies
  - Skeletal dysplasias
  - Multiple anomaly syndromes
  - Infections
  - Teratogens.

Of all these, if the aneuploidies are excluded, the most common causes of LBW are PIH and uteroplacental vascular dysfunction.

Let us understand a more precise usage of the terms, SGA and IUGR. SGA fetuses are those who have a fetal weight of less than 10th centile. Those fetuses that are constitutionally small but have normal fetal and umbilical circulatory parameters and no other cause for restricted growth are normal SGA fetuses. But those that have infections or genetic causes or other causes that may lead to restriction of growth in these fetuses are abnormal SGA fetuses. Whereas those fetuses that have restricted growth due to circulatory abnormalities are IUGR or FGR fetuses. This means that the fetuses that do not grow to their inherited growth potential due to derangement in their cerebral and/or placental circulation are IUGR fetuses. Another simpler method of differentiating SGA from IUGR fetuses is to plot the growth of these fetuses on the nomogram chart. If the growth curve of the fetus follows the curve of the nomogram, may be even lower than the nomogram curve, it is indicative of SGA fetus, but if the fetal growth curve crosses across the nomogram curve, it is indicative of IUGR. It is, therefore, necessary to have serial measurements of biometric parameters at least 2 weeks intervals to diagnose growth abnormalities of the fetus.[3]

The incidence of IUGR varies from 1% to 12%, and the risk is higher in the females who had a history of IUGR or PIH or stillbirth in previous pregnancy or have hypertension, are exposed to toxic substances like alcohol or tobacco, or to infections like cytomegalovirus (CMV) or rubella, etc. or have autoimmune, renal, or vascular diseases. Approximately 20–30% of all SGA fetuses are true growth restricted fetuses,[4] whereas only 10–20% are abnormal SGA fetuses.[5] It is essential to diagnose IUGR because these fetuses have lots of immediate and late consequences like higher perinatal morbidity and mortality, perinatal asphyxia, hypothermia, persistent fetal circulation, hypoglycemia, polycythemia and some neurological deficits, and learning and behavioral problems.[6] To decide whether the fetus is IUGR or not, it is essential to first establish the correct gestational age and to assess the fetal growth by biometric measurements. The gestational age can be established by either last menstrual period (LMP), which has a higher error rate or by 1st trimester or possibly earliest USG–crown-rump length (CRL) measurement, which has lowest deviations from standard measurements. CRL is measured in the midsagittal plane from top of the head to the end of the rump of the embryo on transvaginal scan.[7]

The fetal age is best decided between 9 weeks and 11 weeks based on CRL. CRL is considered to be more reliable after it reaches 18–22 mm,[8] provided CRL should be correctly measured. The CRL must be measured in the true midsagittal plane of the fetus (confirmed by nonvisualization of the proximal parts of the limbs in that image planes), with the fetus in neutral position (neither extended, nor flexed, and no rotation of the neck) (Figs. 10.1A and B). Later in the pregnancy, other biometric parameters like biparietal diameter, head circumference, femur length, etc. are used for dating (Figs. 10.2A to C). Standardized planes/sections are achieved and standard methods are used to achieve correct measurements to assess the fetal age. The first scan done to assess the fetal age is known as pregnancy dating scan. Even if the dating is done in the 2nd trimester, it is reliable because acceleration of normal fetal growth does not begin till the 3rd trimester. If the fetus is assessed for the first time in the 3rd trimester, the transcerebellar diameter[9] (Fig. 10.3) and the clavicular length[10] (Fig. 10.4) can be taken to exactly assess the gestational age, because these are the ones which show the gestational age most accurately and are not affected by IUGR. When there is a discrepancy of 7 days or more in the 1st trimester between the gestational age calculated by LMP and gestational age calculated by ultrasound, the dates are reassigned. From 14 weeks to 20 weeks of gestational age when the difference between the dates calculated according to LMP and ultrasound

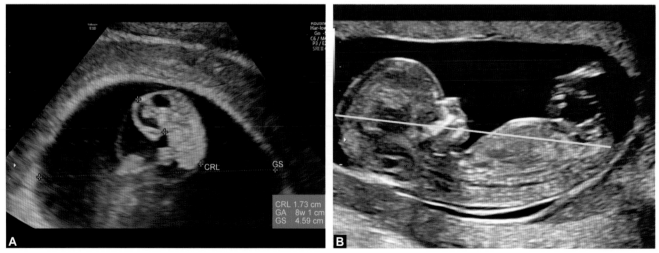

Figs. 10.1A and B: Crown-rump length measurement on B mode in 8 weeks embryo (A) and 12 weeks fetus (B).

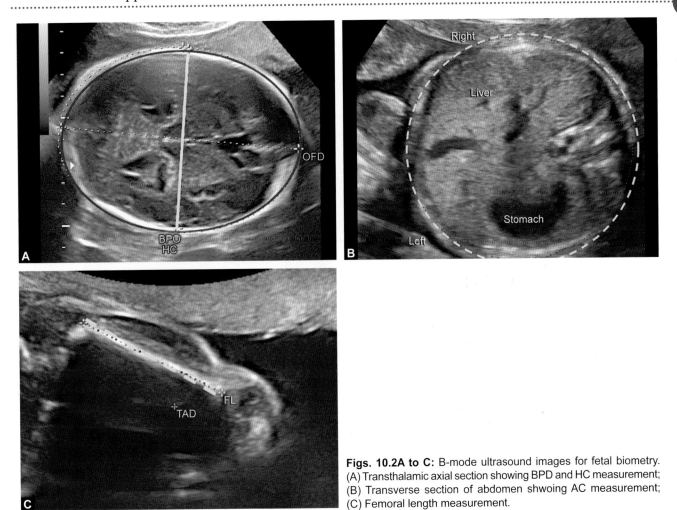

Figs. 10.2A to C: B-mode ultrasound images for fetal biometry.
(A) Transthalamic axial section showing BPD and HC measurement;
(B) Transverse section of abdomen shwoing AC measurement;
(C) Femoral length measurement.

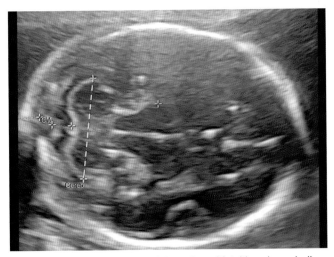

Fig. 10.3: Transcerebellar axial section of fetal head-cerebellar diameter.

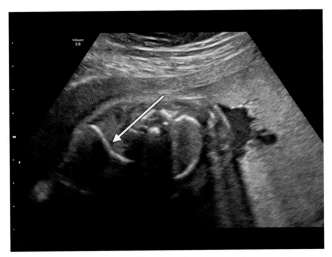

Fig. 10.4: B-mode ultrasound image showing clavicle measurement.

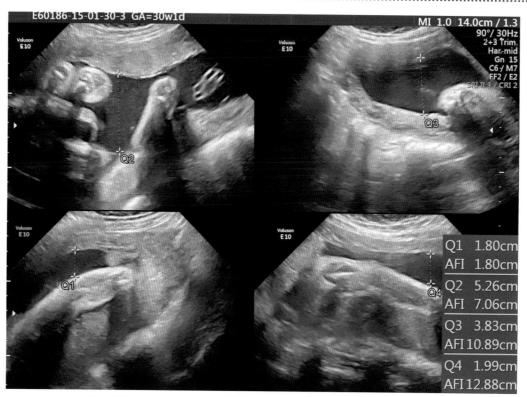

Q1	1.80cm
AFI	1.80cm
Q2	5.26cm
AFI	7.06cm
Q3	3.83cm
AFI	10.89cm
Q4	1.99cm
AFI	12.88cm

Fig. 10.5: B-mode ultrasound image showing amniotic fluid assessment.

assigned gestational age is more than 10 days, the dates are reassigned according to the gestational age assigned by ultrasound. From 20 weeks to 26 weeks, the difference allowed is 14 days. Another method used to decide whether the dates need to be reassigned or not is by following the rule of 8%. Maximum 8% of discrepancy is acceptable during pregnancy between the gestational age calculated by LMP and that calculated by biometric parameters on ultrasound. If the difference between the gestational age calculated by LMP and by ultrasound is more than 8% of the ultrasound calculated age, the dates are reassigned. For example, according to LMP, the gestational age is 149 days and that according to ultrasound is 133 days. The difference between the two is 16 days. The expected margin of error 8% of 133 days is 10.64 days. Since 16 is more than 10.64, the dates will be reassigned according to the gestational age calculated by ultrasound, i.e. 133 days. Dates once assigned have to be followed throughout the pregnancy and have to be taken as a standard to further judge growth derangements. In spite of the fact that for the pregnancy, dating head and long bone biometric parameters are considered more reliable for the birth weight assessment and prediction of IUGR, AC is considered to be more reliable. Estimated fetal weight (EFW) has a more stronger association with birth weight

below 10th centile.[11] EFW could be assessed against birth weight and has a random error of 8%.[12]

Apart from the growth discrepancy, uteroplacental circulatory derangement also leads to oligohydramnios. It is, therefore, essential to assess the amniotic fluid in all the pregnancies that show growth discrepancy or are at a risk for IUGR. It may be measured as a single largest vertical measurement of fluid pouch, free of cord or fetal parts or as a sum of vertical depth of the deepest fluid pocket, free of cord loop or limbs, in all the four quadrants of the uterus, named as amniotic fluid index (AFI) (Fig. 10.5). When a single pocket is considered less than 5 cm is considered abnormal and then AFI should be checked. When AFI is assessed, it normally should be between 15 cm and 25 cm near term, but less than 10 cm is considered oligohydramnios.

It is in IUGR fetuses that Doppler plays an important role for monitoring and management planning. This is so because IUGR is due to uteroplacental vascular dysfunction.

UTEROPLACENTAL VASCULAR ANATOMY

On implantation of the embryo in the endometrium and development of the chorionic villi, the high resistance spiral vessels are converted into low resistance chorionic villous vessels. It is because of this conversion that the placental vessels have a low resistance flow. The key area in the placenta is intervillous space, filled with maternal blood, in which the tertiary villi are immersed and across these vessel walls, there is exchange of blood, nutrients for the fetal nutrition. Any decrease in the blood supply to the placenta leads to decrease in oxygenated blood in intervillous space and, therefore, decrease oxygen supply to fetus.

Normal umbilical artery flow velocity waveform (FVW) is the indicator of normal mother to fetus blood supply. Increase in umbilical artery flow velocities and decreased resistance are seen as the pregnancy advances seen with normally advancing pregnancy are due to:

- Continuous maturation of placental villi
- Widening of placental vessels
- Continuous rise in fetal cardiac output
- Continuous changes in vessel compliance
- Continuous rise in fetal blood pressure.

This conversion chiefly occurs in two phases, at 8–9 weeks of gestation and at 18–20 weeks of gestation. When the conversion of high resistance system into low resistance system is inadequate or incomplete (Fig. 10.6), more pressure is required for the large quantities of blood to be pushed through the high resistance spiral vessels for fetal support, leading to increased uterine artery resistance and ultimately reduction in the umbilical artery flow. This is inadequate placentation and it leads to PIH and/or IUGR (Flowchart 10.1).

So, primarily the flows in uterine and the umbilical arteries are to be assessed in IUGR fetuses. Uterine artery Doppler is the main screening method for prediction of IUGR. Normally the uterine artery and umbilical artery flow velocity increases in the normal pregnancy and resistance decreases as pregnancy advances (Figs. 10.7 and 10.8).[13] Abnormal umbilical artery Doppler correlates with histological evidence of placental vascular pathology. Therefore, umbilical artery Doppler indices correlate with the fetal levels of glucose, amino acids, and blood gases.[14]

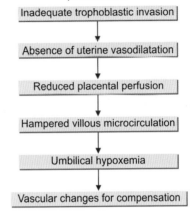

Flowchart 10.1: Schematic representation of abnormal placentation.

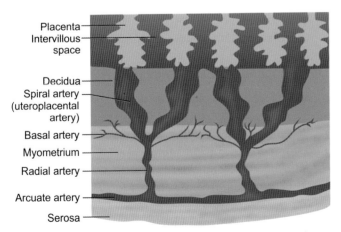

Fig. 10.6: Diagrammmatic representation showing vascular changes in placentation.

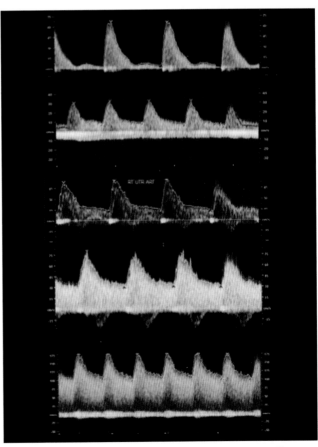

Fig. 10.7: Progressive changes in the uterine artery flow spectrum from early pregnancy to term.

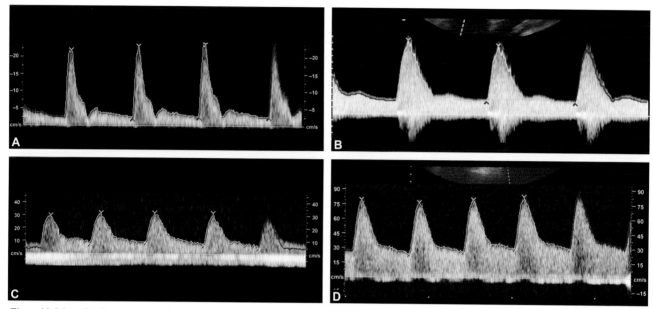

Figs. 10.8A to D: Spectral Doppler images of umbilical artery flow with the progressing pregnancy from (A) very early pregnancy to (D) full term.

There is also a strong evidence to show that SGA fetuses with abnormal umbilical artery flow are at a higher risk of abnormal perinatal outcome.[15] And perinatal death with normal umbilical artery flow is very uncommon.[16] Decreased umbilical vein flow is also documented in otherwise asymptomatic fetuses with decreased placental volume.[17] But to study the oxygenation status of the fetus, it is essential to evaluate the fetal vessels, and middle cerebral artery (MCA) is the one that is considered to be representing the fetal oxygenation status because the cerebral cortex reflects to hypoxia and MCA is the vessel that supplies more than 50% of the cerebral cortex.

Hypoxia leads to cellular dysfunction as the cells loose their ability for oxidative phosphorylation. This changes aerobic metabolism to anaerobic metabolism, accumulation of lactic acid and hydrogen ions, and decreased adenosine triphosphate (ATP) generation. This leads to failure of sodium-potassium pump and cellular edema. Activation of phospholipases also leads to accumulation of free fatty acids. All these lead to cell death and are the basis for neurological deficit in hypoxic fetuses.

TECHNIQUE OF DOPPLER ASSESSMENT

Uterine Artery Doppler

Uterine artery can be best located as it crosses the internal iliac vessels perpendicular to their path.

- Place the probe on the symphysis pubis and slide it laterally, holding vertically.
- Iliac artery and vein are seen as two easily recognizable vessels in their long axis.
- Switch on the color with pulse repetition frequency (PRF) of 0.6–0.9 and a low wall motion filter.
- Rotate the probe laterally and angulate medially and Doppler will show a pulsatile vessel crossing the iliac vessels perpendicularly. This is uterine artery (Fig. 10.9).
- Sample volume should be 2 mm.
- Switch on the pulse Doppler and align the angle almost parallel to iliac vessels.
- Adjust the PRF to get a complete spectrum on one side of the baseline.
- Calculate pulsatility index (PI) of uterine artery.

Umbilical Artery Doppler (Fig. 10.10)

- In a free loop of umbilical cord
- On a zoomed image
- Pulsed Doppler sample volume of 1–2 mm
- Sample volume on one umbilical artery
- Adjust power Doppler scale for velocity
- Obtain at least five waveforms for measurement of indices
- To be assessed when fetus is not breathing and not moving

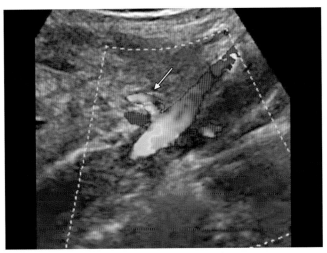

Fig. 10.9: Transabdominal scan with Doppler showing iliac artery and uterine artery crossing over it (arrow).

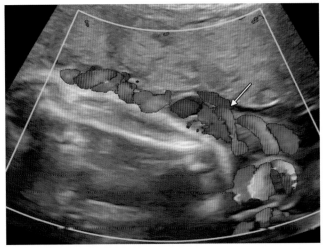

Fig. 10.10: Doppler showing color filled umbilical cord vessels. Arrow shows an unpaired vessel, umbilical vein, blue paired vessels are umbilical arteries.

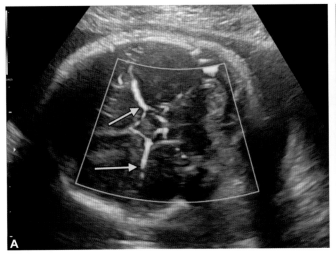

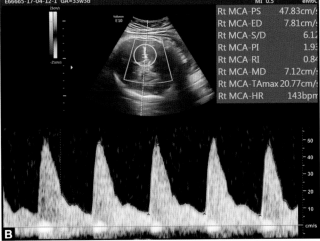

Figs. 10.11A and B: (A) Doppler image of circle of Willis, with arrows showing middle cerebral artery (MCA) on both the sides; and (B) Shows its spectrum.

- As low as reasonably achievable (ALARA) principle is followed.

   Umbilical artery flow assessment is to monitor IUGR fetus but is not reliable screening tool for prediction of IUGR.[18]

Middle Cerebral Artery Doppler

- Locate the MCA closest to the transducer on the circle of Willis section
- Magnify the image for MCA to occupy more than 50% of the image
- Pulse Doppler sample volume of 1–2 mm
- Sample volume is placed close to its origin (Figs. 10.11A and B)
- Adjust pulse Doppler scale to fit the velocity
- Angle between ultrasound beam and blood flow should be smallest possible
- Obtain at least five waveforms
- Ensure no fetal movements or breathing
- Follow ALARA principle
- Take at least three traces and use the highest peak systolic velocity (PSV) for clinical care.

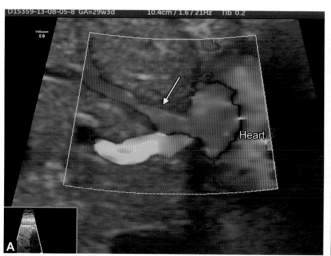

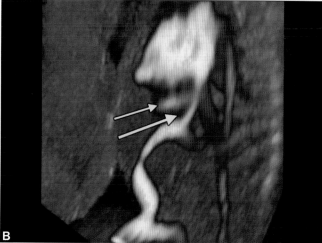

Figs. 10.12A and B: (A) Color Doppler on the fetal midsagittal section showing ductus venosus (arrow); (B) Power Doppler on the fetal mid sagittal section. Larger arrow—ductus venosus, smaller arrow—hepatic vein.

SILENT PERIOD OF INCREASED RESISTANCE

Pathophysiology

Till decreased villous microcirculation up to 50%, no change is seen in the umbilical artery flow, if there is no defect in maternal supply.

During this stage, no change is seen in the Doppler parameters of umbilical artery or MCA that are the most commonly interrogated vessels in mothers with PIH or fetuses with IUGR. If growth parameters of the fetus are normal and umbilical artery waveform is normal, then no other Doppler studies are required.

Stage of Hypoxemia

When the placental circulatory compromise progresses beyond that, fetal hypoxemia starts developing, and fetal partial pressure of oxygen (pO_2) may fall up to 18–19 mm of Hg and pH reaches 7.20–7.25. As primary compensatory mechanism to hypoxemia, there is reopening of the ductus venosus to divert blood from liver toward the heart (Figs. 10.12A and B) and increase in the MCA flow in the distal segment for better peripheral cerebral circulation (Fig. 10.13). This leads to decreased MCA PI in sector 2, the distal segment of MCA as compared to the proximal segment of MCA, M1/M2 more than 1, and increased velocity and low resistance in DV.

Reduction in circulatory oxygen level is sensed by peripheral chemoreceptors and leads to vagal stimulation of heart with preferential shift of cardiac circulation toward

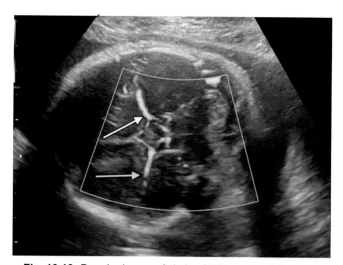

Fig. 10.13: Doppler image of circle of Willis, with white arrow showing the MCA 1 and yellow arrow showing MCA 2.

left ventricle (LV) leading to increased umbilical artery resistance and lower resistance MCA flow. But aortic and carotid chemoreceptors are mostly not affected. Fetal hypoxemia is reflected by reduced heart rate variation and heart rate decclerations.[19]

Mild increase in umbilical artery PI is the cause of hypoxemia, whereas lower resistance in MCA flow is the indication of the adaptation to hypoxemia.

The third phase is the phase of hypoxia that can be divided into:
- Initial phase
- Advanced phase
- Terminal phase.

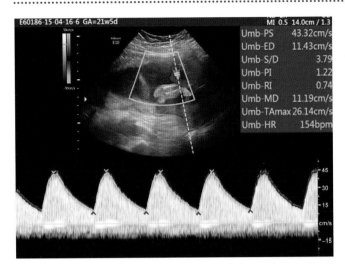

Fig. 10.14: Umbilical artery flow spectrum with low but positive diastolic flow.

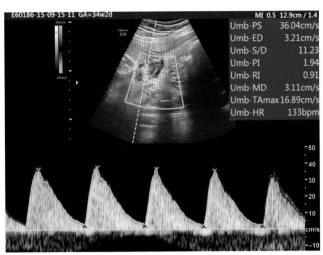

Fig. 10.16: Umbilical artery flow spectrum with very minimal diastolic flow.

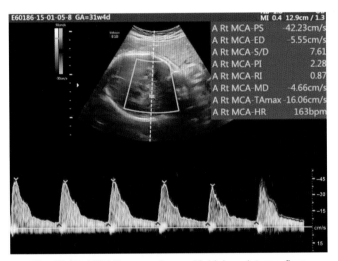

Fig. 10.15: MCA flow spectrum with high resistance flow.

Initial Phase

Vascular changes during this period are: There is rise in umbilical artery PI but still positive flow is seen throughout the cardiac cycle in the umbilical artery (Fig. 10.14). Due to fall in resistance in the cerebral circulation, presence of end-diastolic flow is seen at 32–34 weeks along with low MCA PI (Fig. 10.15). Umbilical artery PI/MCA PI ratio [cerebroplacental ratio (CPR)] is the best indicator for fetal hypoxia. Prediction of the adverse outcome is improved using umbilical and cerebral parameters in combined ratio is 70%. CPR is the single most sensitive parameter

for assessment of the IUGR and has a single cutoff value of one.[20] Biophysical profile (BPP) may be unaltered at this stage and the biophysical score is usually less than 7. This phase lasts for 9–60 days, but its length is usually about 2–3 weeks.

Other progressive changes that occur during this period are: Reduced fetal respiratory and somatic movements, reduced AFI (5–8 cm), and raised aortic PI. It gives the summation of blood supply information to kidneys, abdominal organs, lower limbs, and placenta. It must be remembered that fetal aortic flow is a direct reflection of the cardiac output and the peripheral resistance of systemic circulation. It is to divert the blood flow to the heart and brain, the circulation to the periphery is decreased. This is a compensatory mechanism. Renal artery PI is also raised as a consequence to rise in aortic resistance.

Advanced Phase

When the placental villous circulation is compromised to about 80%, this is an advanced stage of fetal hypoxia. The vascular changes observed on Doppler at this stage are:

- Absent end-diastolic flow in umbilical artery (Fig. 10.16). But it is to be remembered that, although umbilical artery waveform is a good reflector of placental resistance, it does not give any information as to fetus is coping up with the compromised blood supply or not.
- Absent end-diastolic flow in aorta is seen and this leads to significantly decreased circulation to the abdominal organs thus, leading to high risk of necrotizing

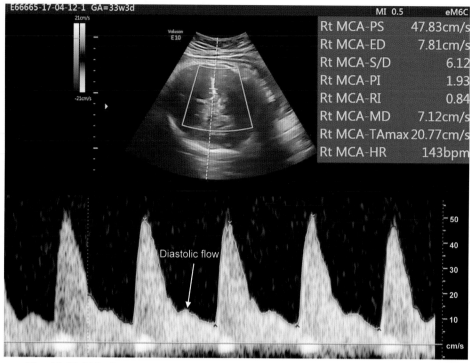

Fig. 10.17: MCA flow spectrum with high diastolic flow—abnormal low resistance flow.

enterocolitis. Thus, increasing the risk of morbidity and mortality.

- Low MCA PI values (Fig. 10.17) are seen as a compensation to cerebral hypoxia by cerebral vasodilatation. But it must be kept in mind that prolonged cerebral vasodilatation and low MCA PI cannot be taken as a compensatory mechanism, as in the second phase of vasodilatation deoxygenated blood floods the brain and could lead to cerebral edema. There is also a higher risk of intracranial hemorrhages in the neonatal life in these cases. Fetus will also show loss of reactivity at this stage due to cerebral hypoxia.

Terminal Phase

This is a phase of acidosis. Doppler shows reversed end-diastolic flow in umbilical artery and aorta (Fig. 10.18). MCA resistance may start rising due to cerebral edema. Severe hypoxia in the myocardium leads to failing of cardiac muscle and, therefore, marked reduction in ventricular ejection fraction. This leads to marked reduction in intracardiac flow velocities. To compensate for myocardial hypoxia, there is dilatation of the coronary vessels to the extent that sometimes blood flows in the coronaries may

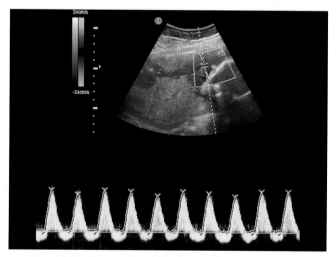

Fig. 10.18: Abnormal umbilical artery flow spectrum with reversed diastolic flow.

be documented. The dysfunction of the myocardium leads to decreased ventricular compliance, therefore incomplete emptying of the atrium and increasing preload reflecting as reversed flow or decreased telediastolic velocity values (Fig. 10.19A) in ductus venosus. But this stage precedes the stage when there is increase in the ductus venous PI (Fig. 10.19B).

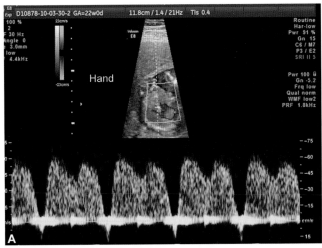 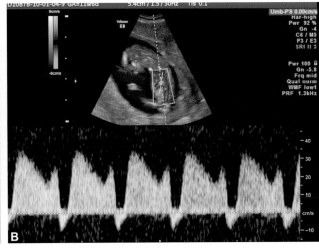

Figs. 10.19A and B: (A) Abnormal ductus venosus flow with absent A wave; (B) With reversed A wave.

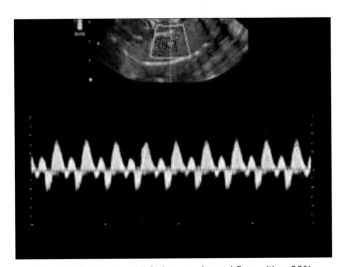

Fig. 10.20: Abnormal inferior venal caval flow with > 30% reversal of A wave.

Fig. 10.21: Umbilical cord vessels spectral Doppler. Spectrum above the baseline showing abnormal umbilical artery flow with absent diastolic flow and spectrum below the baseline is the abnormally pulsatile umbilical venous flow.

Inferior vena cava (IVC) normally also shows negative flow during atrial contraction up to 10% but rises up to 30% in terminal phase of centralization (Fig. 10.20). Umbilical vein flow may also show pulsatility (Fig. 10.21). Venous Doppler reflects the physiological status of right ventricle giving specific information regarding the ventricular preload, myocardial compliance, and right ventricular end-diastolic pressure.

These findings with reversed flow in hepatic vein and deceleration in heart rate are indicators of acidosis.

Fetal acidemia reliably presents as very short term and low value variations in fetal heart rate (FHR), and precedes intrauterine fetal death.

In about 90% of cases, DV flow also becomes abnormal only 48–72 hours before abnormal BPP.[21] Longitudinal studies have demonstrated that AFI and FHR are the only two parameters that may change a little earlier in fetal compromise.

Abnormal ductus venosus flow may be seen as (Figs. 10.22A to D):

- Deep "A" nadir (atrial contraction)
- Reduced second peak (diastole)
- Reduced diastolic flow
- Reversed diastolic flow
- PI 0.5 is normal, more than 0.9 is very bad.

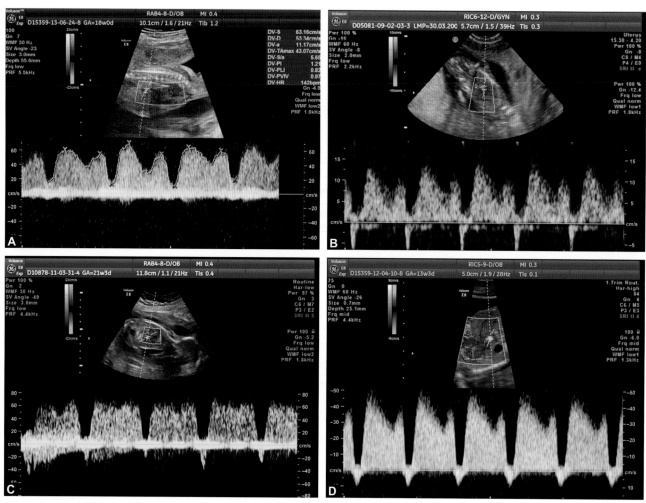

Figs. 10.22A to D: The progressive deteriorating ductus venosus flow patten. (A) Normal; (B) Reduced A wave velocity; (C) Absent A wave; (D) Reversed A wave.

Progressively increasing umbilical artery PI leads to impaired fetal cardiac performance, increased central venous pressure, and reduced diastolic flow in DV. Vasodilatation of DV diverts flow to the heart, further increasing the arterial pressure and leads to further decrease in DV flow during atrial contraction.

This follows the phase of fetal decompensation: Severe tissue hypoxia leads to anaerobic metabolism for energy production. This leads to acidemia and then acidosis. In the brain, it leads to lactic acid accumulation and cerebral edema due to altered cell membrane permeability. Severe hypoxemia and hypoxia leads to irreversible interference in the central mechanism of the arterial tone in severe hypoxemia pO$_2$ [less than 4 standard deviation (SD) of mean], leading to generalized fetal vascular paralysis.

This results in myocardial cell necrosis phenomena and replacement of myocardial tissue with fibrous tissue, affecting myocardial compliance and increase in telediastolic pressure in both the ventricles.

Doppler studies show:

- Reversed end-diastolic flow in umbilical artery (Fig. 10.23), aorta, and renal artery.
- Regaining PI values in MCA with reduced or even absent end-diastolic flow (Figs. 10.24A and B). Porencephaly or ventriculomegaly due to hypoxic necrosis of brain may develop due to severe oxygenation and vascular insult to the cerebral tissue.
- Fixed fetal cardiac frequency and no alteration in heart rate even with oxytocin test.

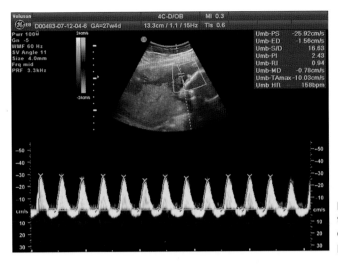

Fig. 10.23: Umbilical cord vessels spectral Doppler. Spectrum above the baseline showing abnormal umbilical artery flow with absent diastolic flow and spectrum below the baseline is the abnormally pulsatile umbilical venous flow.

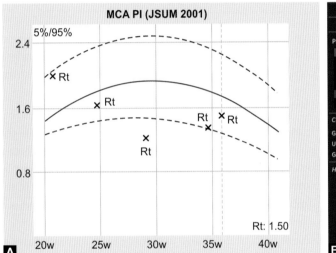

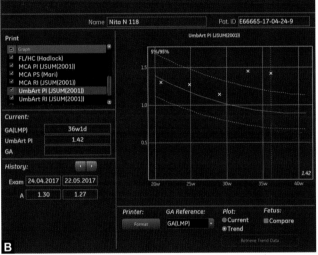

Figs. 10.24A and B: (A) Plotting of progressive changes in MCA flow on nomogram, shows abnormal trend as from 20 to 30 weeks the resistance is decreased, goes below the 5th centile indicating fetal hypoxia and then again rises indicating paradoxical rise of decompensating fetal hypoxia; (B) Plotting of progressive changes in umbilical artery flow on nomogram, shows abnormal trend as from 30 weeks onwards with increasing resistance.

Aortic Isthmus Flow

Aortic isthmus is the part of aorta, just beyond the origin of brachiocephalic trunk (Figs. 10.25A and B). The flow in this part of the aorta is usually a continuous positive flow with high velocity. Aortic isthmus flow represents the balance between right and left ventricular outputs. In systolic phase, forward flow indicates LV output and reverse flow indicates RV output. Whereas in diastole, forward flow indicates upper body resistance and reverse flow indicates lower body resistance. Retrograde flow in the aortic isthmus represents increased right ventricular afterload and decreased left

ventricular afterload, though a small flow reversal in early diastole is normal in 3rd trimester. Normal peak velocities in aortic isthmus are 30–100 cm/s from 11 weeks to term as compared to ductus arteriosus that is 40–120 cm/s. Low velocities and high resistance in aortic isthmic flow are seen in IUGR fetuses. Abnormality of this flow occurs about a week before the changes of hypoxia are seen in ductus venosus.[22]

Abnormal ductus venosus flow indicates high morbidity and mortality of the fetus. And therefore, if delivery of the fetus is done after ductus venosus, flow becomes abnormal,

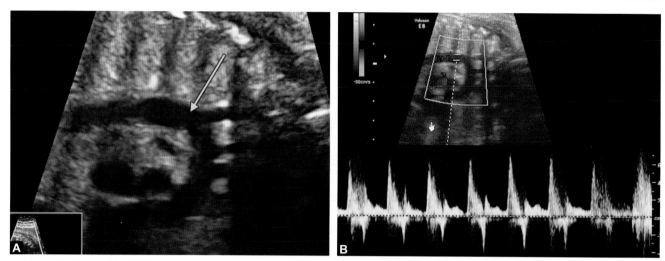

Figs. 10.25A and B: (A) B-mode image of aortic arch showing the aortic isthmus; (B) Spectral Doppler of the aortic isthmic flow.

the chances of fetal survival is very low. But, if the delivery of the fetus can be done before this stage, fetal survival and chances of its well-being can be improved significantly. Abnormal aortic isthmic flow impedance is an intermediate step between placental insufficiency—hypoxemia and cardiac decompensation.[23] Abnormality of aortic isthmus flow can be recorded a week before abnormality in the DV flow.[22] Retrograde flow in the aortic isthmus in growth restricted fetuses correlated strongly with adverse perinatal outcome.[24] Reversed diastolic flow in aortic isthmus clearly indicates poor neurological outcome. Abnormal aortic isthmus flow is a better marker than abnormal ductus venosus flow for predicting bad perinatal outcome, whereas abnormal ductus venosus flow is a better marker for predicting fetal mortality.

The aortic isthmic flow can be quantitatively rated by the isthmic flow index as follows:
- *Type 1*: Isthmic flow index (IFI) less than 1: Antegrade systolic and diastolic flow
- *Type 2*: IFI = 1: Absent diastolic flow
- *Type 3*: IFI = 0–1: Predominant systolic but some reversed diastolic flow
- *Type 4*: IFI = 0: Some antegrade and some retrograde flow
- *Type 5*: IFI more than 1: Chiefly retrograde flow
- IFI types 3–5 have bad to worst prognosis.

Applying this Knowledge for the Assessment of Fetal Well-being

These tests could be classified as chronic or acute. Chronic tests progressively become abnormal due to increasing hypoxemia and/or hypoxia. Whereas acute tests correlate with the acute changes occurring in advanced stages of fetal compromise due to severe hypoxia and metabolic acidosis.

Umbilical Artery

It is known that with the functional damage in the placental villi, the umbilical artery resistance increases. But the placental histological changes cannot always be correlated with the severity of increased resistance in the umbilical artery. Though, when the umbilical artery shows a reverse end-diastolic flow, it is considered that there is a severe placental damage and there is an increased risk of perinatal death. And this has a sensitivity and specificity of about 60%.[25] Studies have shown that 80% of the fetuses have abnormal umbilical artery flow, 2 weeks before acute deterioration of fetal condition, and, therefore, this may be considered a chronic marker for fetal non-well-being. The same study has also shown that up to 1 week before fetal death, the umbilical artery diastolic flow may be present.[26] Absent or reversed end-diastolic flow in the umbilical artery respectively has a relative risk of 4 and 10.6 for prediction of fetal morbidity and mortality and is also associated with long-term abnormal neurodevelopment.[27] A multicentric randomized trial on the Growth Restriction Intervention Trial (GRIT) has concluded that early delivery for fetuses with reversed end-diastolic flow does not improve the outcome and 24–48 hours of interval after corticosteroids injection for lung maturation and then delivery should be planned.[28]

Middle Cerebral Artery

In deteriorating IUGR, MCA PI progressively becomes abnormal.[29] Up to 80% of fetuses have vasodilatation 2 weeks before acute deterioration in one study[26] and less than 50% in other.[28] Moreover, the paradoxical reversal of the MCA flow that is explained to be due to terminal cerebral edema, has also not been documented in few other studies.[29] In near-term SGA fetuses, MCA could be useful to predict adverse outcome, independently of umbilical artery Doppler. But its value in overall SGA population is not proved in another study.[30] Some studies have also shown that MCA vasodilatation may be a protective mechanism against hypoxia, but is associated with suboptimal neurological development[31] and in one study, its association is also shown with impaired visual function and visual motor capabilities at 11 years.[32] Brain sparing effect can also be considered a chronic marker of IUGR.

Ductus Venosus

Acidemia, acidosis, and abnormal venous Doppler are acute markers. Increasing PI in the ductus venosus may occur early but reversal of A wave represents the terminal changes. In preterm fetuses, a 3 SD cutoff optimizes the sensitivity and specificity.[33] With absent or reversed A wave, perinatal mortality ranges from 60% to 100%.[33] However, its sensitivity for perinatal death is 40–70%. Abnormal venous flow may be ductus venosus or IVC or hepatic vein identifies about 90% of newborns with acidosis.[34] But in about 90% of cases, a ductus venosus flow shows reverse A wave only 48–72 hours before the BPP shows changes.[21]

Heart rate deceleration or loss of variability in heart rate is not a reliable guide to predict perinatal morbidity or mortality according to one study,[35] but other longitudinal studies have proved its potential role as acute marker.[29]

Intrauterine growth restriction can be divided into two types depending on the time of initiation of the manifestations. In some patients, IUGR sets in as early as 26–28 weeks of pregnancy and this is known as early-onset IUGR, whereas when IUGR sets in at about 32–33 weeks, it is late-onset IUGR. It is important to differentiate between the two because the behavior of the fetus and deterioration pattern in the two situations is different. In the early-onset IUGR, the fetal adaptation is better and in spite of redistribution of circulation, or marked circulatory changes, the fetus does survive the situation. But in late-onset IUGR, the fetus does not get sufficient time to get adapted to the circulatory derangements and, therefore, the fetal deterioration is fast. In the early-onset IUGR cases,

TABLE 10.1: Characteristic features of early-onset and late-onset intrauterine growth restriction (IUGR).

Early-onset IUGR	Late-onset IUGR
Problem: Management	Problem: Diagnosis
Severe placental disease (abnormal, umbilical, arterial, assessed with preeclampsia)	Mild placental disease (normal, umbilical, arterial Doppler, less assessed with preeclampsia)
Hypoxia-systemic cardiovascular adaptation	Hypoxia may or may not be there, cardiovascular adaptation is central
Better fetal tolerance and adaptation to hypoxia	Lower fetal tolerance to hypoxia and poor adaptation
High morbidity and mortality, lower prevalence	Low mortality (but common cause of late stillbirth)

Source: Adapted from Mureşan D, Rotar IC, Stamatian F. The usefulness of fetal Doppler evaluation in early versus late onset intrauterine growth restriction. Review of literature. Med Ultrason. 2016;18(1):103-9.

therefore, one can wait even with absent umbilical artery diastolic flow and also at times till ductus venosus flow becomes abnormal. Because of fast deterioration in the late-onset cases, the entire cascade of vascular changes may not be followed and may result into unexplained fetal death. Unfortunately, 70–80% of IUGR fetuses are late-onset IUGR (Table 10.1).[36]

The management strategies, therefore, in both the situations have to be different.

When and how often should these patients be monitored by Doppler?

It is very important to understand that a single Doppler assessment cannot be relied upon for decision making on the fetal oxygenation as well as obstetric management. One has to observe the trend of the vascular resistance in MCA and umbilical artery. Therefore, a baseline Doppler at about 30–32 weeks will be helpful to serve as a guide for further Doppler changes in IUGR fetuses. The follow-up would depend on gestational age at the onset of disease, severity of vascular changes at the primary examination, and presence of deterioration on subsequent assessment. The deterioration may be in the form of discrepancy in growth, reducing amount of liquor, abnormal nonstress test (NST), or worsening of Doppler parameters. The monitoring intervals may also vary depending on whether it is an early-onset IUGR or a late-onset IUGR.

For example, in an early-onset IUGR even with umbilical showing absent end-diastolic flow, once a weekly Doppler follow-up may be maintained till the MCA flow and in turn, the DV flow becomes abnormal, or fetus reaches 34 weeks or more of gestation or even with reversed end-diastolic flow in umbilical artery and DV PI more than 95th centile, time can be bought to give steroids and plan a delivery. Whereas in late-onset IUGR, even with umbilical artery PI more than 95th centile or MCA PI less than 5th centile, monitoring may be required much more often and any new development in Doppler finding is considered an emergency and especially when the fetus has already reached 34 weeks, no unnecessary delay in delivery is advisable. In short, in early-onset IUGR, the sequential changes that take about 7–10 days, and in late-onset IUGR, the same changes may occur in 7–24 hours.

OBSTETRIC MANAGEMENT DEPENDING ON DOPPLER FINDINGS

- *Intrauterine growth restriction with normal hemo-dynamic profile*: No immediate action and repeat Doppler and BPP every 2 weeks.
- *Intrauterine growth restriction with hemodynamic redistribution 32–34 weeks*: Early stage of centralization, Doppler and BPP monitoring. With late stage of centralization, termination of pregnancy.
- If IUGR with hemodynamic redistribution is seen between 28 weeks and 32 weeks, termination of pregnancy with advanced and terminal stages of centra-lization but expectant management with early stage of centralization with Doppler and BPP monitoring every 5 days.
- Same is true for the gestational age of less than 28 weeks. All chances are taken to allow the pregnancy to reach 30 weeks.

It was believed that as long as the fetal growth and the umbilical artery indices are normal, no further hemodynamic study is required. Though, there are situations in which in spite of normal umbilical artery flow, the fetal circulation is affected and reflects as abnormal MCA flow. This is especially common, when the causes for fetal hypoxia are nonplacental. Therefore, as a rule in all high-risk cases for fetal hypoxia, MCA flow must be assessed with umbilical artery flow. Doppler findings must be evaluated in conjunction with gestational age, fetal weight, liquor, BPP, fetal activity, and cardiotocography (CTG). Delivery must be considered if one of these parameters are persistently abnormal.[29]

Role of Biophysical Profile

When used alone, it has 50% false positive rate and so has a limited value clinically.[37] A meta-analysis has also not shown its significant benefit in high-risk pregnancies. But both Doppler and BPP effectively stratifies IUGR into risk categories.[38]

Advances

The myocardial performance index (MPI) is a novel method in fetal medicine that assesses both systolic and diastolic functions by including the measurement of isovolumetric and ejection times and would be useful in assessing the progressive hemodynamic deterioration. It has been reported to be associated with perinatal mortality in very preterm IUGR fetuses.[38]

Prediction of Intrauterine Growth Restriction

If predicted, pregnancies with IUGR fetuses can be better managed. Uterine artery Doppler has an effective application for the same. Several workers have published on the importance and efficacy of biochemical markers along with uterine artery Doppler for prediction of IUGR. 1st trimester high uterine artery resistance index (RI) (0.74) and bilateral uterine artery diastolic notch can be significant predictors for IUGR. High uterine artery resistance at 11–14 weeks with low pregnancy-associated plasma protein-A (PAPP-A) can provide early assessment of risk for uteroplacental insufficiency.[39] Uterine artery PI and PAPP-A have negative linear correlation. Low PAPP-A in 1st trimester in euploid fetus with growth restriction at 18–24 weeks predicts high chance of PIH, IUGR, and preterm birth.[40] It has been shown that low placental growth factor (PIGF) and high uterine artery PI have a sensitivity of 89.5% and specificity of 95% for prediction of early-onset preeclampsia and IUGR.[41] According to another study, combination of 1st trimester low placental protein 13 (PP13), high uterine artery PI, and uterine artery notch can be promising signs for prediction of preeclampsia in women with high priori risk of PE.[42] One more study shows that persistent early diastolic notch increases predictive value from 4.3% to 23% for IUGR and 68-fold increased risk of developing pre-eclampsia.[43]

Low PAPP-A (<0.3 MoM), small placental size (<10 cm), and elevated alpha-fetoprotein (AFP) (>2.0 MoM) even in the absence of abnormal uterine artery indices (PI > 1.45), identify women with high risk of IUGR, extreme preterm delivery, and stillbirth.[44]

At 22–24 weeks if Doppler shows high resistance in uterine artery, a 24-fold increased chances of preeclampsia and IUGR are estimated. It has an overall sensitivity of growth restriction of 16%. But its sensitivity for preeclampsia related or no preeclampsia growth restriction with risk of requiring delivery before 32 weeks is 93% and 56%, respectively with specificities of 95%.[45] A systematic review with meta-analysis showed that uterine artery Doppler had limited accuracy in predicting IUGR and perinatal death.[46]

Combining all together, effective screening for early preeclampsia can be provided by a combination of maternal factors:

- Low PAPP-A
- Low PP13
- High-soluble endoglin
- Low PIGF
- Uterine artery resistance
- Uterine artery notch.

SUMMARY

Doppler is an important modality for predicting IUGR. It has an important role in deciding the progress and prognosis of the fetuses having IUGR and thus, has an important role in taking management decisions. For long-term monitoring, it is better than CTG. It warns for the potential of intrauterine oxygen deprivation. Though it is important to understand that definite cutoffs that may accurately predict the outcome of the patient is still not available. Association of abnormal intrafetal Doppler study and poor fetal outcome does not equate to cause. Our Doppler fetal tests do not measure the potential for damage. Damage to fetus may occur without gross alterations in hemodynamics.[47]

REFERENCES

1. Alexander GR, Kogan MD, Hims JH, et al. Racial differences in birth weight for gestational age and infant mortality in extremely low risk US populations. Pediatr Perinat Epidemiol. 1999;13(2):129-43.
2. Todros T, Plazztta C, Patorin L. Body proportionality of small-for-date fetus: is it related to etiological factors? Early Hum Dev. 1996;45(1-2):1-9.
3. Mongelli M, Ek S, Tambyrajia R. Screening for fetal growth restriction: a mathematical model of the effect of time interval and ultrasound error. Obstet Gynecol. 1998;92(6) 908-12.
4. Wilcox AJ. Intrauterine growth retardation: beyond birth weight criteria. Early Hum Dev. 1983;8(3-4):189-93.
5. Snijders RJ, Sherrod C, Gosden CM, et al. Fetal growth retardation: Associated malformations and chromosomal abnormalities. Am J Obstet Gynecol. 1993;168(2):547-55.
6. Spinillo A, Capuzzo E, Piazzi G, et al. Significance of low birthweight for gestational age among very preterm infant. Br J Obstet Gynecol. 1997;104(6):668-73.
7. Illescas T. 11-14 weeks' scan. In: Illescas T (Ed). Advanced Ultrasound in Obstetrics and Gynecology, 1st edition. New Delhi: Jaypee Brothers Medical Publishers (P) Ltd; 2015.
8. Honemeyer U, Kurjak A, Monni G. Normal and abnormal early pregnancy In: Kurjak A, Monni G (Eds). Donald School Textbook of Ultrasound in Obstetrics and Gynecology, 2nd edition. New Delhi: Jaypee Brothers Medical Publishers (P) Ltd; 2011. pp. 106-29.
9. Altman DG, Chitty LS. New charts for ultrasound dating of pregnancy. Ultrasound Obstet Gynecol. 1997;10(3):174-91.
10. Stebbins B, Jaffe R. Fetal biometry and gestational age estimation. In: Jaffe R, Bui TH (Eds). Textbook of Fetal Ultrasound. Texas: Parthenon Publishing; 1999. pp. 47 57.
11. Chang TC, Robson SC, Boys RJ, et al. Prediction of the small for gestational age infant: which ultrasonic measurement is best? Obstet Gynecol. 1992;80(6):1030-8.
12. Hadlock FP, Harrist RB, Sharman RS, et al. Estimation of fetal weight with the use of head, body and femur measurements: a prospective study. Am J Obstet Gynecol. 1985;151(3):333-7.
13. Wherry KL, Dubinsky TJ, Waitches GM, et al. Low resistance endometrial arterial flow in the exclusion of ectopic pregnancy revisited. J Ultrasound Med. 2001;20(4):335-42.
14. Nicolaides KH, Bilardo CM, Soothill PW, et al. Absence of end-diastolic frequencies in umbilical artery: a sign of fetal hypoxia and acidosis. Br Med J. 1988;297(6655):1026-7.
15. McCowan LM, Harding JE, Stewart AW. Customized birthweight centiles predict SGA pregnancies with perinatal morbidity. Br J Obstet Gynecol. 2005;112(8):1026-33.
16. McCowan LM, Harding JE, Stewart AW. Umbilical artery Doppler studies in small for gestational age babies reflect disease severity. Br J Obstet Gynecol. 2000;107(7):916-25.
17. Trudinger BJ, Cook CM, Giles WB, et al. Fetal umbilical artery velocity waveforms and subsequent neonatal outcome. Br J Obstet Gynecol. 1991;98(4):378-84.
18. Society for Maternal-Fetal Medicine Publications Committee, Berkley E, Chauhan SP, et al. Doppler assessment of the fetus with intrauterine growth restriction. Am J Obstet Gynecol. 2012;206(4):300-8.
19. Bekedam DJ, Visser GH, Mulder EJ, et al. Heart rate variation and movement incidence in growth retarded fetuses: the significance of antenatal late heart rate decelerations. Am J Obstet Gynecol. 1987;156(6):126-33.
20. Odibo AO, Riddick C, Pare E, et al. Cerebroplacental Doppler ratio and adverse perinatal outcomes in intrauterine growth restriction: evaluating the impact of using gestational age-specific reference values. J Ultrasound Med. 2005;24(9):1223-8.
21. Baschat AA, Gembruch U, Harman CR. The sequence of changes in Doppler and biophysical parameters as severe fetal growth restriction worsens. Ultrasound Obstet Gynecol. 2001;18(6):571-7.
22. Figueras F, Benavides A, Del Rio M, et al. Monitoring of fetuses with intrauterine growth restriction: longitudinal changes in

ductus venosus and aortic isthmus flow. Ultrasound Obstet Gynecol. 2009;33(1):39-43.

23. Bachat AA, Guclu S, Kush ML, et al. Venous Doppler in prediction of acid-base status of growth-restricted fetuses with elevated placental blood flow resistance. Am J Obstet Gynecol. 2004;191(1):277-84.

24. Del Rio M, Martinez JM, Figueras F, et al. Doppler assessment of the aortic isthmus and perinatal outcome in prenatal fetuses with severe intrauterine growth restriction. Ultrasound Obstet Gynecol. 2008;31(1):41-7.

25. Sebire NJ. Umbilical artery Doppler revisited: Pathophysiology of changes in intrauterine growth restriction revealed. Ultrasound Obstet Gynecol. 2003;21(5):419-22.

26. Ferrazzi E, Bozzo M, Rigano S, et al. Temporal sequence of abnormal Doppler changes in the peripheral and central circulatory systems of severely growth-restricted fetus. Ultrasound Obstet Gynecol. 2002;19(2):140-6.

27. Cosmi E, Ambrosini G, D'Antona D, et al. Doppler cardiotocography and biophysical profile changes in growth-restricted fetuses. Obstet Gynecol. 2005;106(6):1240-5.

28. Thornton JG, Hornbuckle J, Vail A, et al. Infant well-being at 2 years of age in the Growth Restriction Intervention Trial (GRIT): Multicentred randomised controlled trial. Lancet. 2004;18(6):571-7.

29. Hecher K, Bilardo CM, Stigter RH, et al. Monitoring of fetuses with intrauterine growth restriction: a longitudinal study. Ultrasound Obstet Gynecol. 2001;18(6):564-70.

30. To WW, Chan Am, Mok KM. Use of umbilical-cerebral Doppler ratios in predicting fetal growth restriction in near-term fetuses. Aust N Z J Obstet Gynecol. 2005;45(2):130-6.

31. Scherjon S, Briet J, Oosting H, et al. The discrepancy between maturation of visual-evoked potentials and cognitive outcome at five years in very pre-term infants with and without hemodynamic signs of fetal brain-sparing. Pediatrics. 2000;105(2):385-91.

32. Kok JH, Prick L, Merckel E et al. Visual function at 11 years of age in preterm-born children with and without fetal brain sparin. Pediatrics. 2007;119(6):e1342-50.

33. Bilardo CM, Wolf H, Stigter RH, et al. Relationship between monitoring parameters and perinatal outcome in severe, early intrauterine growth restriction. Ultrasound Obstet Gynecol. 2004;23(2):119-25.

34. Baschat AA, Cosmi E, Bilardo C, et al. Predictors of neonatal outcome in early-onset placental dysfunction. Obstet Gynecol. 2007;109(2 Pt 1):253-61.

35. Pattison N, McCowan L. Cardiotocography for antepartum fetal assessment. Cochrane Database Syst Rev. 2000(2);1: CD001068.

36. Muresan D, Rotar IC, Stamatian F. The usefulness of fetal Doppler evaluation in early versus late onset intrauterine growth restriction. Review of literature. Med Ultrason. 2016;18(1):103-9.

37. Baschat AA, Galan HL, Bhide A, et al. Doppler and biophysical assessment in growth restricted fetuses: distribution of test results. Ultrasound Obstet Gynecol. 2006;27(1):41-7.

38. Hernandez-Andrade E, Crispi F, Benavides-Serralde A, et al. Contribution of the modified myocardial performance index and aortic isthmus blood flow index to refine prediction of mortality in preterm intrauterine growth restricted fetuses. Ultrasound Obstet Gynecol. 2009;34(4):430-6.

39. Pilalis A, Souka AP, Antsaklis P, et al. Screening for pre-eclampsia and fetal growth restriction by uterine artery Doppler and PAPP-A at 11-14 weeks' gestation. Ultrasound Obstet Gynecol. 2007;29(2):135-40.

40. Fox NS, Shalom D, Chasen ST. Second trimester fetal growth as a predictor of poor obstetric and neonatal outcome in patients with low first trimester serum pregnancy associated plasma protein-A and a euploid fetus. Ultrasound Obstet Gynecol. 2009;33(1):34-8.

41. Crispi F, Llurba E, Dominguez C, et al. Predictive value of angiogenic factors and uterine artery Doppler for early-versus late onset preeclampsia and uterine artery growth restriction. Ultrasound Obstet Gynecol. 2008;3(3)1:303-9.

42. Khalil A, Cowans NJ, Spencer K, et al. First trimester markers for the prediction of pre-eclampsia in women with a-priori high risk. Ultrasound Obstet Gynecol. 2010;35(6):671-9.

43. Giguere Y, Bujoid E, Charland N, et al. Literature Review. Ann de Biologieclinique. 2011;69(3):257-71.

44. Proctor, LK, Toal, M, Keating, S, et al. Placental size and the prediction of severe early-onset intrauterine growth restriction in women with low pregnancy-associated plasma protein-A. Ultrasound Obstet Gynecol. 2009;34(3):274-82.

45. Papageorghiou AT, Yu CK, Bindra R, et al. Multicenter screening for pre-eclampsia and fetal growth restriction by transvaginal uterine artery Doppler at 23 weeks of gestation. Ultrasound Obstet Gynecol. 2001;18(5):441-9.

46. Chien PF, Amott N, Gordon A, et al. How useful is uterine artery Doppler flow velocimetry in the prediction of pre-eclampsia, intrauterine growth retardation and perinatal death? An overview. Br J Obstet Gynecol. 2000;107(2): 196-208.

47. Tridinger B ISUOG. Editorial. 2007;29(3):243-6.

Fetal Anemia: Role of Doppler

INTRODUCTION

Fetal anemia is *defined as* hematocrit or hemoglobin concentration greater than 2 standard deviations (SDs) below the mean gestational age. Anemia in fetus is calculated by calculating multiples of median (MoM), of hematocrit or hemoglobin values because no single cutoff can be used for a fetus of any age. Hemoglobin value is different in fetus of different gestational age that can be seen in Table 11.1.[1,2]

According to Table 11.1, when fetal hemoglobin is less than 0.84 MoM, it is mild anemia, between 0.84 and 0.65 it is moderate anemia and less than 0.55 is severe anemia.

It is true that the fetuses with anemia have a significantly increased morbidity and mortality. If the diagnosis is done early, before hydrops occurs, fetal survival is up to 80–90%, but if the hydrops has already occurred, the survival reduces to almost one-third.

The *incidence* of fetal anemia is high and the exact numbers are difficult to calculate in India because of several home deliveries, in which hardly any antenatal care also is sought/seeked.

The *common causes* of fetal anemia may be immune, nonimmune (parvovirus infection, alpha-thalassemia twin-to-twin transfusion syndrome, fetomaternal hemorrhage or Kell-related fetal anemia) or idiopathic.

Rhesus (Rh) isoimmunization is the common cause for the same, leads hemolysis and therefore anemia. Rh isoimmunization is likely in fetuses of Rh[-ve] women with Rh[+ve] husband/partner. The incidence of fetuses affected by Rh isoimmunization can be controlled by anti-D prophylaxis, both antenatally and postnatally.

TABLE 11.1: Hemoglobin values at differnet gestational ages.

Weeks of gestation	Multiples of median				
	1.16	1.00 (median)	0.84 (g/dL)	0.65 (g/dL)	0.55 (g/dL)
18	12.3	10.6	9.9	6.9	5.8
20	12.9	11.1	9.3	7.2	6.1
22	13.4	11.6	9.7	7.5	6.4
24	13.9	12.0	10.1	7.8	6.6
26	14.3	12.3	10.3	8.0	6.8
28	14.6	12.6	10.6	8.2	6.9
30	14.8	12.8	10.8	8.3	7.1
32	15.2	13.1	10.9	8.5	7.2
34	15.4	13.3	11.2	8.6	7.3
36	15.6	13.5	11.3	8.7	7.4
38	15.8	13.6	11.4	8.9	7.5
40	16.0	13.8	11.6	9.0	7.6

The risk is more in patients who had previous pregnancy affected by isoimmunization. This may be a successful pregnancy or may be an abortion. The risk is also more in Kell-sensitized patients, in fetuses of mothers with high serum titers of antibodies, mismatched transfusions or in fetuses with other pathologies that may lead to anemia.

PATHOPHYSIOLOGY OF SIGNS AND SYMPTOMS OF FETAL ANEMIA

Anemia leads to decreased oxygen-carrying capacity of blood, thus requiring increased cardiac output. Moreover because of hemolysis, the viscosity of the blood is also reduced. Both these factors together lead to hyperdynamic circulation. This leads to initially increase in the myocardial thickness and then as it progresses toward failure, there is cardiac enlargement. This is followed by accumulation of fluid in the body cavities and hydrops fetalis. The contributory factors for the development of this may be increasing hepatic erythropoiesis, interfering with the protein production—hypoproteinemia and also portal hypertension due to compression of blood vessels by proliferating erythropoietic tissue.

In Rh isoimmunization, maternal antibodies cross the placental barrier and attach to fetal red blood corpuscles (RBCs) leading to their destruction in fetal reticuloendothelial system and increased bilirubin in fetal blood. Hemolysis also leads to extramedullary erythropoiesis in liver and spleen.[3]

DIAGNOSIS

Confirmation of the diagnosis of the fetal anemia can be done by *cordocentesis* and assessment of fetal hemoglobin. But this invasive procedure cannot be used to screen the patients at risk. *Amniotic fluid* can be aspirated by amniocentesis and by assessing the spectral absorption curve of amniotic fluid at 450 nm (ΔOD 450). Rh sensitization can be quantified and has proved to be a reliable predictor for hemolytic causes of fetal anemia.[4] But amniocentesis has a potential for fetomaternal hemorrhage and therefore may worsen sensitization in 2–11% of amniocentesis, apart from 1% to 2% of procedural risk of amniocentesis.[5]

Indirect Coombs test[6] has been used as a screening test for the pregnancies with risk factors. Titers above 1:16 are considered as positive for hemolytic fetal anemia. Rising titers do suggest progressive hemolysis, but unfortunately it cannot predict hemoglobin level or severity of anemia.

As fetuses with anemia have hyperdynamic circulation and extramedullary erythropoiesis, leading to hepatosplenomegaly, *ultrasound* (US) can be used for the diagnosis of fetal anemia.

B-MODE SIGNS OF FETAL ANEMIA

- Increase in umbilical vein and intrahepatic portal vein diameter (>5 mm) is a result of hyperdynamic circulation. This is measured in the true transverse section of the fetal abdomen at the stomach level, measured from inner wall to inner wall, perpendicular to its long axis (Fig. 11.1). Umbilical vein diameter increases to satisfy the oxygenation need, which occurs due to hemolysis.

- Hepatosplenomegaly is a result of extramedullary hemopoiesis. Liver length is measured in sagittal plane on the right side of the fetus from the dome of diaphragm till the tip of the right lobe of liver (Fig. 11.2). Spleen is visualized in the transverse section of the abdomen at stomach level and spleen perimeter is calculated as (longitudinal diameter + transverse diameter) × 1.57 (Fig. 11.3).

- Hyperdynamic circulation leads to cardiomegaly. Enlargement of the right atrium occurs first due to long-term high flow state and then enlargement of the whole heart follows due to overload failure. Cardiac size is always measured in the true four-chamber heart section (Fig. 11.4).

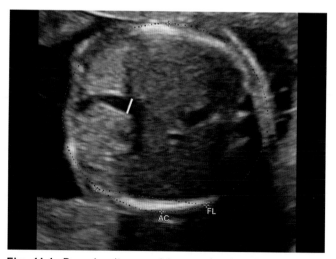

Fig. 11.1: B-mode ultrasound image showing the abdominal transverse section with the white line showing the diameter assessment of the umbilical vein.

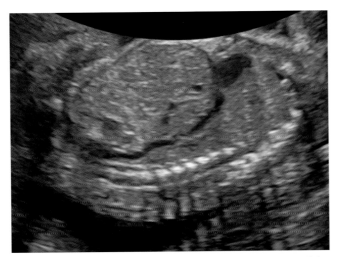

Fig. 11.2: B-mode ultrasound image of longitudinal section of the fetus showing hepatomegaly.

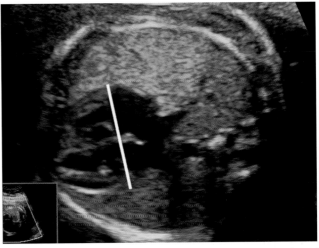

Fig. 11.4: B-mode ultrasound image of the transverse section of the thorax—four chamber view. White line shows measurement of transverse cardiac diameter.

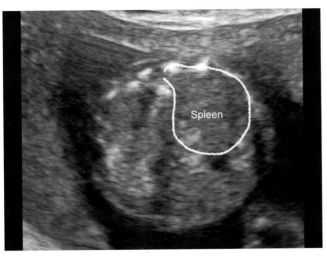

Fig. 11.3: B-mode ultrasound image of the transverse section of the fetus with the white line outlining the spleen.

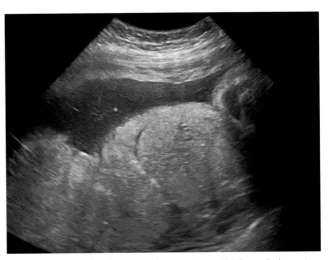

Fig. 11.5: B-mode ultrasound image shows thickened placenta.

- When hematocrit fall less than 6 g/dL fluid starts accumulating in the serous cavities and also in the extracellular space leading to ascites, pleural effusion and pericardial infusion and fetal edema can also be documented on US as thick skin layer (Fig. 11.5). Therefore using hydrops as a sign of fetal anemia, it would be a very late diagnosis.
- Normal placental thickness in millimeters is not more than number of weeks of gestation. Large placenta (>5 cm in thickness) with ground glass echogenicity is seen in fetal anemia (Fig. 11.6). In severe anemia, thickness may be two to three times the normal.
- *Polyhydramnios/oligohydramnios*: Polyhydramnios is seen in earlier stage due to hyperdynamic circulation but in the later stage with development of congestive cardiac failure (CCF), the renal circulation is hampered and leads to decreased urine output.

  But both the placental thickness and the amniotic fluid volume have been shown to have a poor predictive power for diagnosis of fetal anemia.[7]

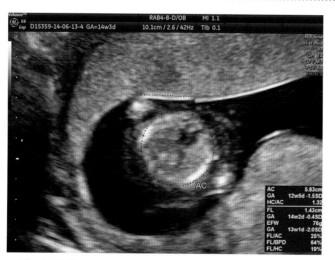

Fig. 11.6: Transverse section of fetal trunk with fetal edema, seen on B-mode ultrasound.

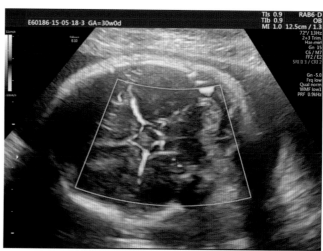

Fig. 11.8: Cerebral circulation—circle of Willis seen on the HD flow.

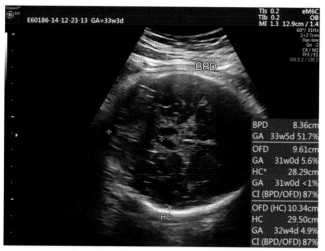

Fig. 11.7: B-mode ultrasound image of the axial section of the head showing hyperechoic star shaped shadow, which indicates circle of Willis.

ROLE OF DOPPLER IN FETAL ANEMIA

Rightmire et al. developed a method of assessing the fetal hematocrit by combining Doppler measurements of aorta, inferior vena cava (IVC) and umbilical vein with an error of 3.8 hematocrit units.[8]

They also showed that in fetuses with anemia, portal vein showed high-velocity flow with sawtooth waveform.

Mari et al. reported that middle cerebral artery (MCA) peak systolic velocity (PSV) measurements could accurately predict fetal anemia in pregnancy.[1] More than

seven prospective studies have proved the importance of MCA PSV for detection of fetal anemia in pregnancies complicated by red cell alloimmunization and parvovirus B19 infection. Mari G et al. also published reference tables for fetal hemoglobin and MCA PSV.[9] This means actual hemoglobin levels also can be predicted by MCA PSV values.

Why Middle Cerebral Artery?

Fetal brain is the organ of preference for oxygen supply in the fetal body. MCA supplies 80% of cerebral tissue, and so it is the vessel of choice to study the fetal cerebral circulation. Moreover, it is a large vessel, easy to identify with color Doppler. It can be insonated with an optimum Doppler angle of between 0° and 20°, which gives most accurate PSV values. These can be easily and reliably reproduced.

How to Correctly Measure the Middle Cerebral Artery Flow?

Middle cerebral artery can be located on the axial section of the head, just caudal to the transthalamic plane. On this plane, the circle of Willis is seen (Fig. 11.7) as an echogenic star-shaped structure on which pulsations may be seen also on B-mode. Once this section is achieved, High definition (HD) zoom is used for magnification. The axial section of the head should cover two-thirds of the image. Color Doppler is then switched on. It shows the entire circle of Willis (Fig. 11.8). The color Doppler settings required are pulse repetition frequency (PRF) 0.9 and wall motion

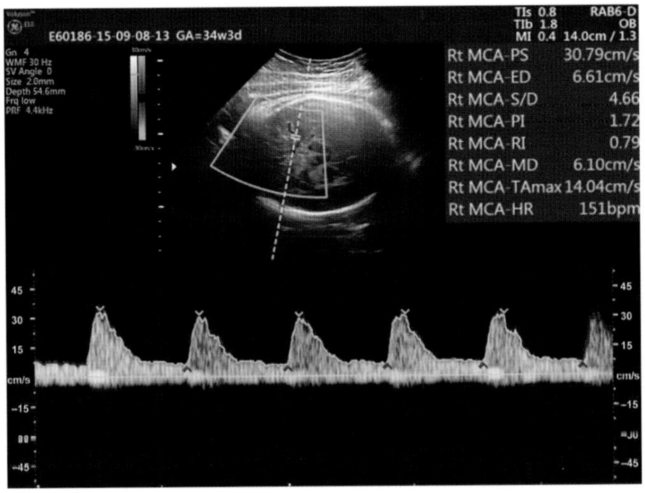

Fig. 11.9: Spectral Doppler of middle cerebral artery flow.

filter (WMF) low. Pulsed wave Doppler is then switched on. The pulsed wave gate is placed 2 mm from the origin from internal carotid artery: proximal segment. Sample volume is small enough not to include the internal carotid artery, usually 2 mm in 2nd or 3rd trimester. The spectrum should be tall enough to cover two-thirds of the height of the space dedicated to spectrum and speed should be adjusted to show 4–5 complete waveforms (Fig. 11.9). The auto or manual calculations can be used on the spectrum to calculate the velocities and ratios to assess the flow resistance.

There is a correlation between fetal hemoglobin and MCA PSV when fetus is nonanemic, but the correlation becomes stronger as the hemoglobin level decreases. Though in mild anemia, evident difference might not be seen. MCA PSV of 1.5 times the median or higher indicates high risk of anemia. This predicts moderate or severe anemia with sensitivity—100%, positive predictive value (PPV)—65%, false positive rate 12%, and negative predictive value (NPV)—100%.[9] For detection of moderate to severe fetal anemia, MCA PSV greater than 1.5 MoM had a sensitivity of 88% and specificity of 87%.[10] But its sensitivity decreases after 35 weeks of gestational age. Mari et al. have also developed an equation to calculate fetal hemoglobin from the fetal MCA PSV values.[11] Though the equation is a little too complicated to be discussed. The MoM values can be calculated from Table 11.2 given by Mari et al.[9]

Based on the MoM values, the severity of the anemia can be judged and based on that the surveillance and the treatment plan can be made. The treatment of moderate to severe fetal anemia consists of intrauterine fetal blood transfusion. A comprehensive plan has been suggested by Moise et al.[6]

- Less than 1.29 MoM repeat US every 10–14 days till 34–35 weeks
- If MCA PSV between 1.29 and 1.5 MoM and worsening, repeat US every 2–7 days till 34–35 weeks
- In case of MCA PSV greater than 1.5 MoM, or hydrops repeat scan in 24 hours and cordocentesis as soon as possible.

This strategy has been charted out to simply the decision making on management strategy of fetal anemia (Fig. 11.10).

TABLE 11.2: Middle cerebral artery peak systolic velocity (MCA PSV) according to gestational age and multiples of the median (MoM) values.

Gestational age in weeks	*Multiples of median*			
	1.00 (median)	*1.29 (cm/sec)*	*1.50 (cm/sec)*	*1.55 (cm/sec)*
18	23.2	29.9	34.8	36.0
20	25.5	32.8	38.2	39.5
22	27.9	36.0	41.9	43.3
24	30.7	39.5	46.0	47.5
26	33.6	43.3	50.4	52.1
28	36.9	47.6	55.4	57.2
30	40.5	52.2	60.7	62.8
32	44.4	57.3	66.6	68.9
34	48.7	62.9	73.1	75.6
36	53.5	69.0	80.2	82.9
38	58.7	75.7	88.0	91.0
40	64.4	83.0	96.6	99.8

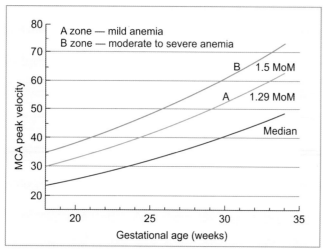

Fig. 11.10: Graph nomogram of the MCA peak systolic velocity at different gestational age and 1.29 and 1.5 MoM values.

On the Figure 11.10, if the values are plotted in zone A, it indicates mild anemia and Doppler is repeated every 5–7 days. If the values fall in zone B, it indicates moderate to severe anemia and the management call should be to transfuse the fetus.[6]

If the transfusion is required, how much to transfuse and how to transfuse?

How much blood to transfuse in fetal anemia is a crucial decision, because the total fetal blood volume changes with the growing fetal age and also because the transfusion given is of adult blood that contains adult hemoglobin and the fetal blood contains fetal hemoglobin. The exact calculation therefore requires assessment of total fetal blood volume and exact fetal hematocrit. The exact hematocrit can only be calculated by cordocentesis and fetal blood aspiration.

Cordocentesis is preferably done in the 2nd trimester, under transabdominal US guidance. A 20 gauge, long spinal needle (8–12 cm) is inserted through maternal abdominal wall and anterior uterine wall into the gestational sac to pierce the umbilical vessel at placental insertion or in free loop. Free loop is safe. Fetal insertion may be enervated and is not a preferred puncture site. The procedure is done when the mother is sedated and/or local anesthetic agent is given. Umbilical vein is preferred to umbilical artery. Using several 1 cc syringes for aspiration is a preferred approach to prevent collapse of the umbilical vein. If fetus is too active, fetal paralysis may be achieved by pancuronium 0.03 mg/kg injected in fetal deltoid/fetal portal vein and this leads to temporary fetal paralysis in 5–10 minutes.

After the hematocrit is calculated the fetal blood volume and the conversion of how much adult blood is required to correct the fetal anemia can be calculated by: fetoplacental blood volume × number calculated by a graph of donor hematocrit to fetal hematocrit.[12]

The transfusion is done with O[-ve] packed cells with high hematocrit value. Red cells are cross matched with mother's serum before transfusion and preferably it should be washed and irradiated before transfusion. It is better to use fresh samples compared to the stored ones. Transfusions can be done intraperitoneal or intravascular.

The details of the method of transfusion are out of the scope of this book. But the follow-up of these patients is done by MCA Doppler. After transfusion repeat scan is done every 2–7 days till 3 transfusions or till 35 weeks. After three transfusions or after 35 weeks the Doppler sensitivity for prediction of fetal hematocrit reduces significantly and therefore then onward we need to revert to conventional management by US and amniocentesis ΔOD 450 for further surveillance. Multiple intrauterine transfusions (IUTs) increase fetal blood viscosity, which may alter the predictive accuracy of MCA PSV.[13] This is so because with transfusions the adult hemoglobin enters the fetal circulation and the oxygen-carrying capacity of the adult hemoglobin is lower than the oxygen-carrying capacity of the fetal hemoglobin. Moreover, the size of adult RBCs is also lower than the RBCs of the fetus. This also leads to decreased viscosity of the adult blood as compared to fetal blood. It is for these reasons that after a transfusion is given, the threshold for decision on further transfusions changes. Cutoff for IUT:

- 1st IUT = 1.5 MoM[11]
- 2nd IUT = 1.69 MoM[14]

Each transfusion decreases hemolysis and improves MCA PSV. Interval between transfusions increases with number of transfusions, and the success rate for the effective treatment of fetal anemia is 85–90%.

Limitations of MCA PSV as a Predictor of Fetal Anemia

- Accuracy diminishes after 35 weeks of gestation, leading to higher false positive rates for prediction of anemia.[10] MCA PSV is not a good predictor of fetal anemia in cases with structural heart disease where left ventricular (LV) output is compromised or in fetuses with hydrops who have low cardiac output.
- MCA PSV may be altered with:
  - Fetal tachycardia/bradycardia
  - Fetal movements
  - Active labor
  - Severe intrauterine growth restriction (IUGR)

CONCLUSION

Peak systolic velocity in the MCA is a very good predictor of moderate and severe anemia. It does not predict hemoglobin levels in normal and mildly anemic fetus well. It can be used for treatment and management of fetal anemia—calculation of the volume of transfusion required and also for post-transfusion surveillance—to decide the interval between transfusions.

It is useful in the noninvasive diagnosis of fetal anemia and has reduced number of invasive tests required.

REFERENCES

1. Mari G, Adrignolo A, Abuhamad AZ, et al. Diagnosis of fetal anemia with Doppler ultrasound in the pregnancy complicated by maternal blood group immunization. Ultrasound Obstet Gynecol. 1995;5(6):400-5.
2. Mari G. Middle cerebral artery peak systolic velocity for the diagnosis of fetal anemia: the untold story. Ultrasound Obstet Gynecol. 2005;25(4):323-30.
3. Patel BS. Diagnosis of fetal anemia. In: Malhotra N, Shah PK, Kumar P, Acharya P, Panchal S, Malhotra J (Eds). Ultrasound in Obstetrics and Gynecology, Federation of Obstetrics and Gynecological Societies of India, 4th edition. New Delhi: Jaypee Brothers Medical Publishers (P) Ltd.; 2014. pp. 416-9.
4. Nishie EN, Brizot ML, Liao AW, et al. A comparison between middle cerebral artery peak systolic velocity and amniotic fluid optical density at 450 nm in the prediction of fetal anemia. Am J Obstet Gynecol. 2003;188(1):214-9.
5. Bowman JM, Pollock JM. Transplacental fetal hemorrhage after amniocentesis, Obstet Gynecol. 1985;66:749-54.
6. Moise KJ Jr. Management of rhesus alloimmunization in pregnancy. Obstet Gynecol. 2008;112:164-76.
7. Nicolaides KH, Rodeck CH. Maternal serum anti-D antibody concentration and assessment of rhesus isoimmunization. BMJ. 1992;304:1155-6.
8. Rightmire DA, Nicolaides KH, Rodeck CH, et al. Fetal blood velocities in Rh isoimmunization: relationship to gestational age and to fetal hematocrit. Obstet Gynecol. 1986;68:223-6.
9. Mari G, Deter RL, Carpenter RL, et al. Noninvasive diagnosis by Doppler ultrasonography of fetal anemia due to maternal red-cell alloimmunization. Collaborative Group for Doppler Assessment of the Blood Velocity in Anemic Fetuses. N Engl J Med. 2000;342:9-14.
10. Zimmerman R, Durig P, Carpenter RJ, et al. Longitudinal measurement of peak systolic velocity in the fetal middle cerebral artery for monitoring pregnancies complicated by red cell alloimmunization: a prospective multicentre trial with intention-to-treat. Br J Obstet Gynecol. 2002;109:746-52.
11. Mari G, Detti L, Oz U, et al. Accurate prediction of fetal hemoglobin by Doppler ultrasonography. Obstet Gynecol. 2002;99:589-93.
12. Leduc L, Moise KJ Jr, Carpenter RJ Jr, et al. Fetoplacental blood volume estimation in pregnancies with RH alloimmunization. Fetal Diagn Ther. 1990;5(3-4):138-45.
13. Stefos T, Cosmi E, Detti L, et al. Correction of fetal anemia on the middle cerebral artery peak systolic velocity. Obstet Gynecol. 2002;99:211-5.
14. Detti L, Oz U, Guney I, et al. Doppler ultrasound velocimetry for timing the second intrauterine transfusion in fetuses with anemia from red cell alloimmunization. Am J Obstet Gynecol. 2001;185:1048-51.

Doppler for Diagnosis of Congenital Fetal Abnormalities

INTRODUCTION

Ultrasound is the modality of choice for assessment of growing fetus and for diagnosis of the fetal abnormalities. Majority of these abnormalities are not only suspected but also confidently diagnosed on B mode or 3D studies. Doppler has an essential role for the diagnosis of certain structural abnormalities, especially those in which there is vascular involvement. In this chapter, we shall divide the discussion of role of Doppler for diagnosis of structural abnormalities depending on the fetal organ system involved in the abnormality. This chapter aims only at the role of Doppler in the diagnosis or differential diagnosis of fetal abnormalities and therefore the discussion will be limited to only those abnormalities for diagnosis of which Doppler is used. But even in fetuses with chromosomal abnormalities, ductus venosus flow and tricuspid valve flow needs to be assessed for which Doppler studies are essential.

DOPPLER FOR DIAGNOSIS OF STRUCTURAL ABNORMALITIES

- Head and spine
- Thorax (excluding cardiovascular system)
- Abdomen
- Cardiac abnormalities
- In twin pregnancies.

Head and Spine

Doppler has a role in differential diagnosis of some lesions in head and spine and not in actually suspecting those abnormalities. Doppler can help differentiate vascular lesions like aneurysms from nonvascular lesions. The common lesions, for the diagnosis of which Doppler can aid the diagnosis are aneurysm of the vein of Galen, arachnoid cysts, agenesis of corpus callosum, holoprosencephaly and sacrococcygeal teratomas.

- *Aneurysm of the vein of Galen:* On ultrasound, it is seen as cystic structure in the midline (Fig. 12.1), anterior to the occipital bone up to the quadrigeminal plate cistern. The lesion shows turbulent color signals on Doppler (Fig. 12.2). It may compress aqueduct, leading to secondary hydrocephalus/ventriculomegaly (Fig. 12.3). It may lead to high output cardiac failure in the fetus. High output failure leads to cardiac enlargement and altered cardio-thoracic ratio. Due to high output failure, the fetus may present with hydrops. This may also lead to a high risk of neonatal mortality.

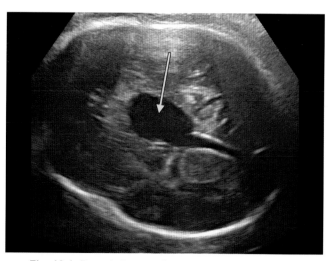

Fig. 12.1: B-mode image of aneurysm of vein of Galen.

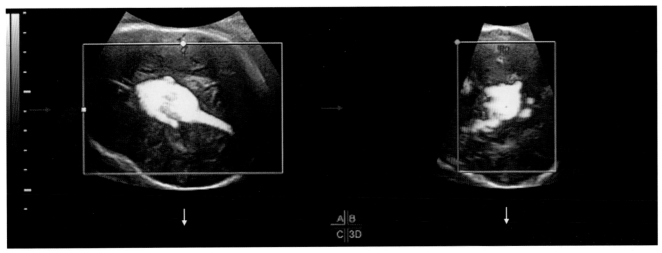

Fig. 12.2: Power Doppler image of aneurysm of vein of Galen.

• *Arachnoid cysts:* These are extra-axial cysts, sonolucent on ultrasound. (Fig. 12.4). The commonest location is supratentorial but also be subtentorial. These cysts typically do not communicate with the ventricles. These may be of various sizes, have regular walls and may or may not have septae. If the cysts are large and compress the aqueduct or foramina of Monro, it may lead to hydrocephalus. On Doppler, arachnoid cysts typically displace the blood vessels and these vessels are seen by the side of these cysts (Fig. 12.5).

• *Agenesis of corpus callosum:* Agenesis of corpus callosum may be complete or partial. When complete, it is easier to diagnose. On B-mode ultrasound, it typically shows absent cavum septum pellucidum on the axial sections (transthalamic, transventricular and transcerebellar sections) (Fig. 12.6) and the lateral ventricles show selective dilatation of the posterior horn (tear-shaped ventricle or colpocephaly) (Fig. 12.7) on transventricular section. On the coronal section, the distance between the frontal horns of the lateral ventricles is increased (Fig. 12.8) and these horns on this section also show convexity laterally. In the third trimester, on midsagittal section, the sulci and gyri are seen converging in the midline around the ventricle and not on the corpus callosum, giving a sunray pattern (Fig. 12.9). On Doppler absence of pericallosal artery is seen (Fig. 12.10). If the agenesis is partial, the ultrasound findings may vary depending on the extent of the lesion. On Doppler, typically the pericallosal artery, instead of extending toward the occipital horn of the lateral ventricle, takes an upturn toward the cortex (Fig. 12.11).

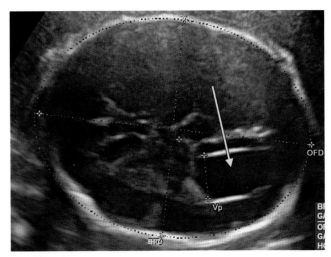

Fig. 12.3: B-mode ultrasound image of ventriculomegaly.

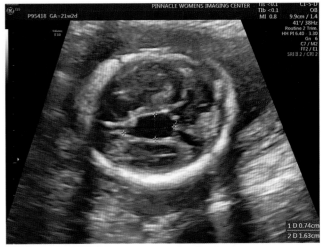

Fig. 12.4: B-mode ultrasound image of the axial section of the head with midline cystic lesion.

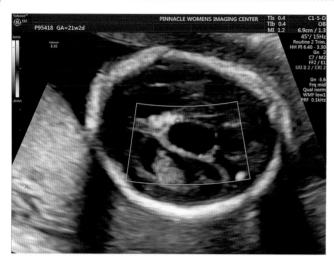

Fig. 12.5: The same lesion as seen in Figure 12.4, with HD flow showing displaced vessels—Arachnoid cyst.

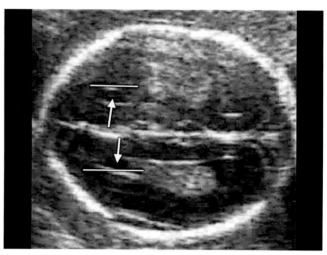

Fig. 12.8: B-mode ultrasound image of transventricular axial section of the head with asent cavum septum pellucidum and parallel orientation of the anterior horns of lateral ventricles.

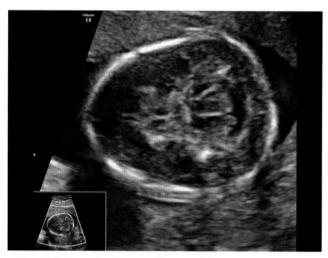

Fig. 12.6: B-mode ultrasound image of the axial section of the head with absent CSP.

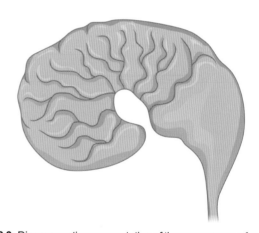

Fig. 12.9: Diagrammatic representation of the appearance of sulci and gyri on the midsagittal plane in patients with absent corpus callosum.

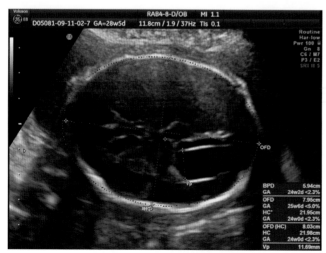

Fig. 12.7: B-mode ultrasound image of transventricular axial section of the head with selective dilatation of posterior horn of the lateral ventricle.

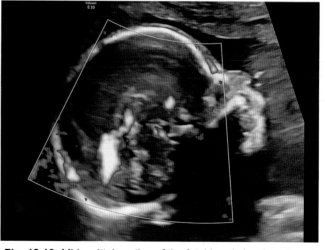

Fig. 12.10: Midsagittal section of the fetal head showing absent pericallosal artery in a fetus with ACC.

- *Holoprosencephaly:* Holoprosencephaly may be alobar, semilobar or lobar, depending on severity of the lesion. Alobar holoprosencephaly is the most severe form and this shows complete absence of the cleavage of the forebrain, leading to incomplete division of the cerebral hemispheres and of telencephalon from diencephalon. Depending on the severity, on ultrasound in axial and coronal sections, there is complete or incomplete fusion of the lateral ventricles, with absence of falx and cavum septum pellucidum (Fig. 12.12). Corpus callosum also shows dysgenesis and there may be associated facial midline abnormalities like cleft lip, palate (Fig. 12.13), cebocephaly, cyclopia, with or without proboscis. Ethmocephaly or hypotelorism may also be seen on axial or coronal section. Though in lobar form, the facial abnormalities and thalamic fusion are not seen and the fusion of the ventricles may be variable.

On Doppler the anterior cerebral artery takes an abnormal route and crawls under the skull on midsagittal section (Fig. 12.14). This is also called the "snake under the skull sign". This is because the anterior cerebral artery is pushed anteriorly along the frontal bone by abnormal bridge of cortical tissue between the two frontal gyri.[1] This is the sign that helps differentiate lobar holoprosencephaly from septo-optic dysplasia, a difficult differential diagnosis. Both these abnormalities show absent cavum septum pellucidum and also convex lateral margin of frontal horn of lateral ventricle.

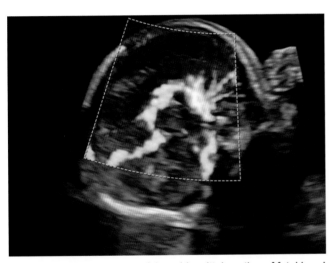

Fig. 12.11: Doppler image of the midsagittal section of fetal head in a patient with partial agenesis of corpus callosum.

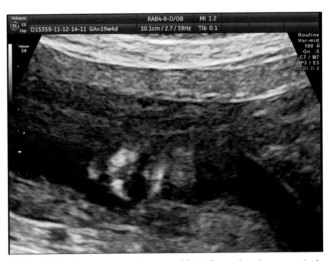

Fig. 12.13: 3D ultrasound image of fetal face showing a central cleft lip.

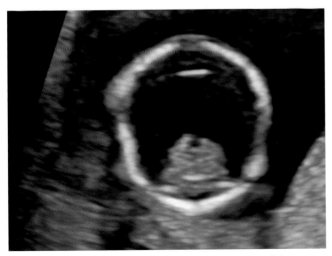

Fig. 12.12: Axial section of the fetal head with alobar holoprosencephaly.

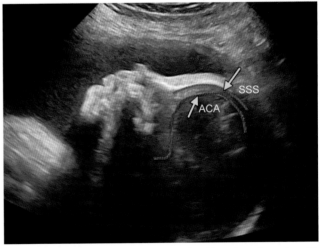

Fig. 12.14: Midsagittal section of the fetal head on B-mode with diagrammatic representation of anterior cerebral artery and the superior sagital sinus in a patient with holoprosencephaly.

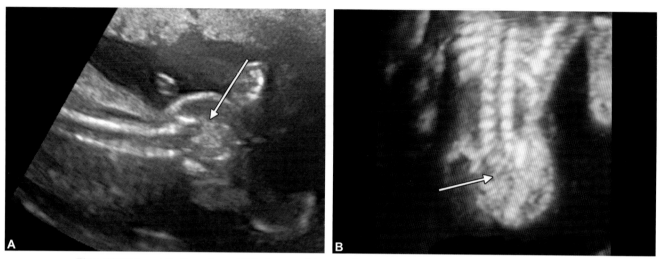

Figs. 12.15A and B: B-mode and 3D ultrasound image of extrapelvic (Type 1) sacrococcygeal teratoma.

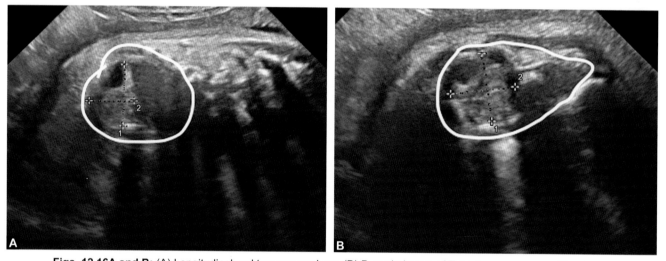

Figs. 12.16A and B: (A) Longitudinal and transverse plane; (B) B-mode image of Type 4 sacrococcygeal teratoma.

- *Sacrococcygeal teratoma*: This tumor arises from the pluripotent cells at the sacrococcygeal area. Since these tumors have variety of tissues, these tumors show heterogeneous echogenicity. These may have cystic and solid components. These tumors may have intrapelvic as well as extrapelvic components. The extrapelvic components are easy to diagnose on ultrasound as these protrude posteriorly beyond the skin (Figs. 12.15A and B) overlying the spine, but the intrapelvic components are easily missed and need a careful assessment to be diagnosed. Intrapelvic tumors project anteriorly from the sacral spine and are situated between the rectum and the sacrum. Increased distance between the rectum and spine may be indicative of diagnosis (Figs. 12.16A and B). Intrapelvic tumor may also erode the vertebral bodies of the affected segments of the spine (Fig. 12.17). Depending on the extent of intrapelvic component, sacrococcygeal teratomas can be divided into four types:[2]

  - *Type 1*: Predominantly external (extrapelvic), minimal presacral component.
  - *Type 2*: Predominantly external with significant presacral component.
  - *Type 3*: Predominantly internal with abdominal component.
  - *Type 4*: Entirely internal (intrapelvic) 80% of sacrococcygeal teratomas are type 1 and 2.[2]

  These tumors are often highly vascular (Fig. 12.18) and especially when large may lead to high output cardiac failure and may also lead to hydrops with large lesions.

Doppler shows vascularity in these tumors and is of special help especially for the diagnosis of the intrapelvic components, between the sacrum and the anal canal.

Thoracic Lesions (Extracardiac)

Among the various thoracic lesions, Doppler has a role in diagnosis pulmonary lesions like, cystic adenomatoid malformation of the lung, Schimitar syndrome, sequestration of the lung, lung aplasia, etc. Moreover, Doppler also plays a role in fetuses with diaphragmatic hernia.

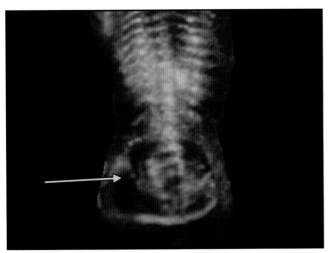

Fig. 12.17: 3D ultrasound image of the spine—vertebral body ossification centers eroded by the sacrococcygeal teratoma (seen in Figure 12.16).

• *Cystadenomatoid malformation of the lung:* This is a result of disordered pulmonary parenchymal lesion, leading to proliferation of terminal bronchioles. Cystadenomatoid malformation of the lung can be classified into type 1, with large cysts, type 2, with small cysts, and type 3 solid or microcystic type.

Depending on the type, the lung may show large cystic lesions in type 1 (Fig. 12.19), small cysts in type 2 or a hyperechoic mass as in type 3 (Fig. 12.20). The later may appear similar to the sequestration of the lung, whereas type 1 may need differentiation from congenital diaphragmatic hernia (CDH). For differentiation of type 3 lesion from the sequestration, Doppler helps. As the only differentiating point between the two is the feeding artery that is ubiquitous in pulmonary sequestration and is seen by power Doppler. This can be seen when the PRF is set at low.

• *Pulmonary sequestration:* Pulmonary sequestration is an island of lung parenchyma that does not communicate with the bronchial tree and is also fed by systemic circulation. The drainage of this artery may be supradiaphragmatic or subdiaphragmatic. The lesion often involves the left lower lobe of the lung, that is seen in the same plane as the four chamber heart view, especially when it is supradiaphragmatic. On B-mode it appears as a homogenous hyperechoic triangular area (Fig. 12.21). It may be seen below the diaphragm in the subdiaphragmatic type. On sagittal section with Doppler, the feeding artery to this part of the lung is seen

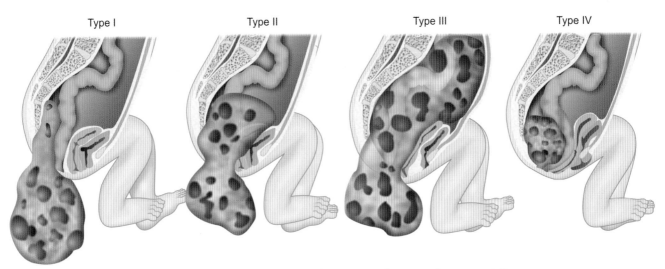

Type I   Type II   Type III   Type IV

Fig. 12.18: Types of sacrococcygeal teratoma—diagrammatic representation.

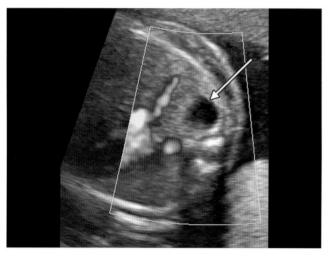

Fig. 12.19: Cystic lesion in the transverse section of the thorax showing no flow on power Doppler is possibly a cystadenomatoid malformation of lung (macrocystic type).

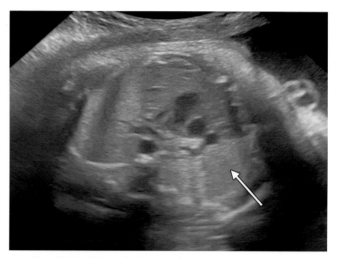

Fig. 12.21: Triangular hyperechoic area of the lung seen posterior to the heart—sequestration of the lung.

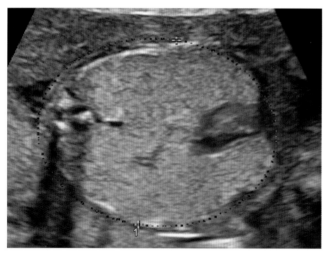

Fig. 12.20: Hyperechoic lungs seen on transverse section of the thorax—microcystic cystadenomatoid malformation of the lung.

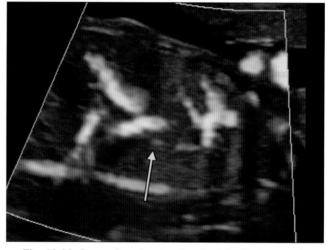

Fig. 12.22: Power Doppler showing the infradiaphragmatic vascular connection of the sequestrate lung.

(Fig. 12.22) and this is a pathognomonic to the diagnosis of pulmonary sequestration.

- *Scimitar syndrome:* Scimitar syndrome is a rare association of congenital cardiopulmonary anomalies consisting of a partial anomalous pulmonary venous connection of the right lung to the inferior vena cava, right lung hypoplasia, dextroposition of the heart, and anomalous systemic arterial supply to the right lung.[3]
- *Congenital diaphragmatic hernia (CDH):* Herniation of the abdominal organs into the thorax through a defect in the diaphragm in the intrauterine life. On B-mode ultrasound in the four chamber heart view, the heart is displaced. In left diaphragmatic hernia, the stomach herniates chiefly and the heart is displaced to right side

(Fig. 12.23A). The herniated stomach appears as an anechoic cystic looking shadow in the thorax. In a few cases, the small bowel may also herniate (Fig. 12.23B). If distended, this may appear like multiple cystic spaces in the thorax displacing the heart and when collapsed, appears as hyperechoic lesion displacing the heart to right side. In right-sided diaphragmatic hernia, heart is further displaced to left (Fig. 12.24). Since the liver is a solid organ, it is often difficult to differentiate from the lung. In the conditions where the heart is displaced to extreme left, color or power Doppler may be used to identify and outline the hepatic vessels in the thoracic cavity to confirm liver herniation (Fig. 12.25). At times colon may also herniate with the liver. Though it is

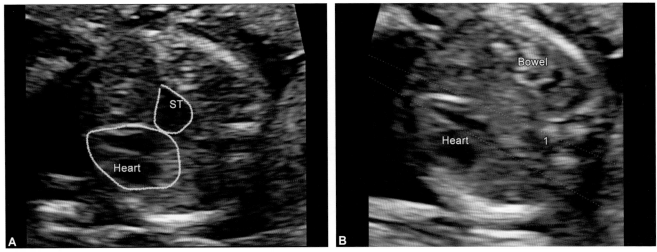

Figs. 12.23A and B: (A) B-mode ultrasound image of the diaphragmatic hernia of the stomach, and of the (B) Bowel, both displacing the heart to left.

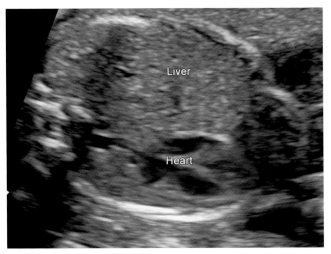

Fig. 12.24: Transverse section of the thorax on B-mode showing diaphragmatic hernia involving the liver and displacing the heart.

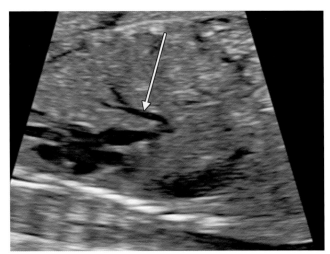

Fig. 12.25: On B-mode also the hepatic vasculature is seen in the thorax which confirms the contents in the hernia.

important to understand and remember that though the diaphragmatic defect appears at 12 weeks, the herniation may present on the second trimester scan and sometimes even in the first few hours of birth. Left CDH with stomach may need to be differentiated from macrocystic cyst adenomatoid malformation of the lung and the right CDH may need to be differentiated from the microcystic type of cystic adenomatoid malformation of the lung. Doppler can be a modality of help to differentiate between the lung and the liver vasculature.

Abnormalities of the Fetal Abdomen

- *Omphalocele:* It is a defect in the closure of the anterior abdominal wall, also involving the cord insertion. This

leads to herniation of the abdominal organs contained in two layers, a peritoneum and amniotic membrane. The umbilical cord typically is inserted on the top of the sac (Figs. 12.26A and B). Presence of umbilical vein within the omphalocele, that can be demonstrated by Doppler, is an indirect sign of the primary closure defect of the anterior abdominal wall. The defect may contain bowel or liver. When it contains bowel, the contents in the herniated sac appear hyperechoic than the intra-abdominal organs. There is also a risk of bowel obstruction leading to polyhydramnios. With bowel herniation, the risk of chromosomal abnormalities is also higher. Omphalocele that contains liver will show the intra-abdominal contents more echogenic than the contents in the herniated sac. Moreover, Doppler

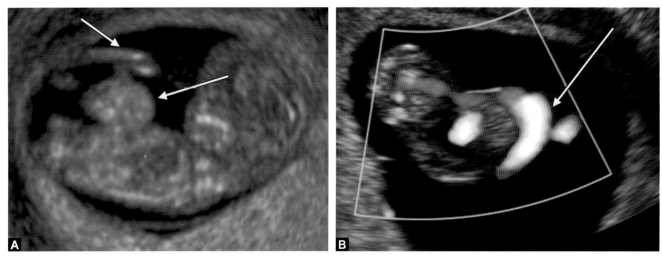

Figs. 12.26A and B: B-mode and Doppler image of omphalocele.

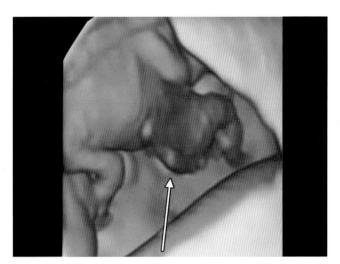

Fig. 12.27: 3D image of gastroschisis with irregular margins of the herniated contents suggestive of the lesion.

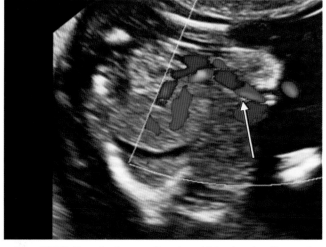

Fig. 12.28: Doppler image of gastroschisis showing the cord insertion by the side of the lesion.

will show the hepatic vasculature in the herniated contents and that may be used as a diagnostic sign of liver containing omphalocele. Omphalocele needs to be differentiated from gastroschisis.

• *Gastroschisis:* This is a paraumbilical defect of anterior abdominal wall. Intestinal loops herniate through the defect and float in the amniotic fluid (Fig. 12.27). Doppler showing umbilical cord inserted in the anterior abdominal wall by the side of the defect differentiates omphalocele from gastroschisis (Fig. 12.28).

• *Umbilical cord abnormalities:* Umbilical cord normally has two arteries and a vein. On B mode on the transverse cut section of the cord, two arteries with smaller diameter and one vein with a larger diameter give a

Mickey mouse appearance (Fig. 12.29). This can be better appreciated on Doppler. Single umbilical artery (Fig. 12.30) was thought to be a marker for chromosomal abnormalities earlier and then a risk factor for PIH and IUGR. There is no evidence that this may affect the development of the fetus. No evidence was found that it was associated with higher risk of aneuploidy.[4]

Now, it has been documented in literature that an isolated single umbilical artery does not increase the risk of chromosomal abnormalities. Though with single umbilical artery, the risk of intrauterine and intrapartum death of the fetus is found to be higher. Single umbilical artery can be most confidently diagnosed by Doppler. In the studies available so far, though fetuses with isolated single umbilical artery were found more likely to be SGA or may suffer perinatal mortality. None of these outcomes has reached statistical significance.[5] Difference in diameter of umbilical arteries of at least 1 mm in three different parts of cord. These arteries also show difference in impedance to blood flow.[6]

Abnormal coiling pattern of the umbilical cord has also been found to be of interest in predicting the prognosis of pregnancy. The total number of coils may be counted in the entire length or the number of coils in a unit length, and that is called coiling index of the umbilical cord. It is easiest to count the coils when the umbilical cord is assessed by Doppler. Uncoiled or hypocoiled cords (Fig. 12.31) are more seen in fetuses with IUGR, maternal hypertensive disorders and aneuploidies. Supercoiled cords (Fig. 12.32) can be associated with pathologic intra-abdominal process leading

to increase in resistance at umbilical ring and venous congestion in extra-abdominal umbilical vein. Even cord round the neck, especially more than two loops may be of significance and that too can be confidently diagnosed by Doppler only (Figs. 12.33A to C). The same is true for the true knot in the cord also (Fig. 12.33D). Knot in the cord may lead to severe fetal hypoxia and intrapartum death. This is usually difficult to identify on B-mode image. Though 3D power Doppler can be diagnostic. Doppler is also a modality of choice for evaluation of normal or abnormal cord insertion in the placenta. Abnormal cord insertions like eccentric or velamentous have a higher risk of IUGR and intrapartum accidents (Figs. 12.34A to C).

- *Adherent placenta*: Abnormally adherent placentas are named as placenta accreta, increta and percreta

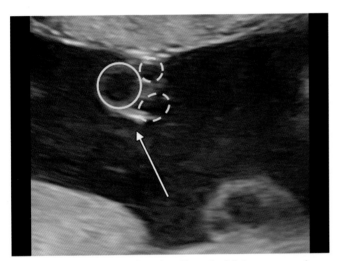

Fig. 12.29: Three vessel cord on B mode: Mickey mouse sign.

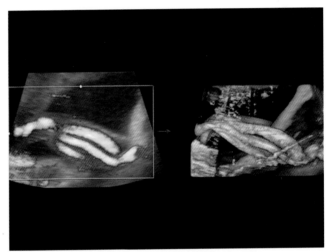

Fig. 12.31: Doppler image of the cord with no coils.

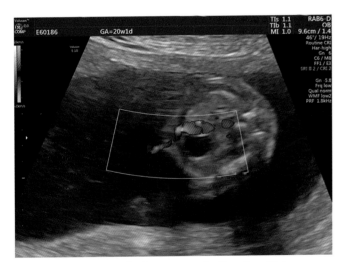

Fig. 12.30: Single umbilical artery on color Doppler with transverse section of fetal abdomen. The cystic structure is fetal urinary bladder.

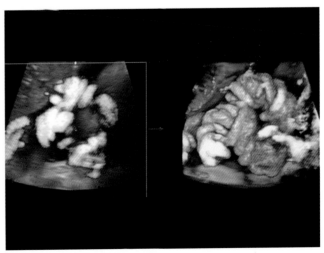

Fig. 12.32: Hypercoiled cord seen on Doppler.

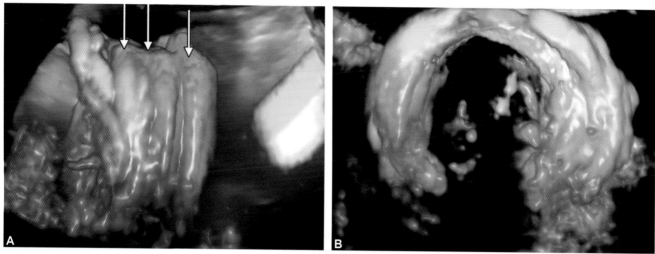

Figs. 12.33A and B: Doppler showing three loops of cord on longitudinal and transverse planes.

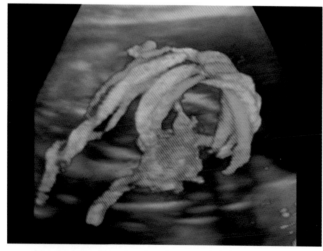

Fig. 12.33C: Doppler showing complete loops of cord.

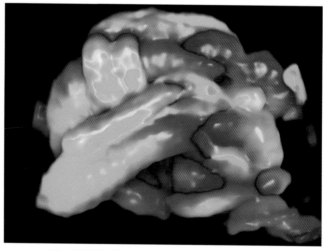

Fig. 12.33D: Doppler showing knot of the cord.

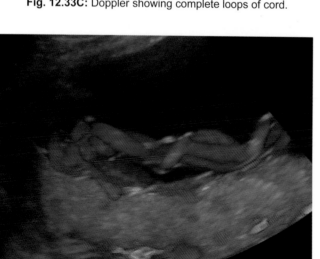

Fig. 12.34A: Eccentric cord insertion seen on Doppler.

depending on the extent of chorionic tissue into the uterine wall.

- *Placenta accreta vera:* Adherent to but not invading the myometrium
- *Placenta increta:* When there is myometrial invasion, and
- *Placenta percreta:* Invasion of placenta beyond uterine serosa and into urinary bladder.

Placenta accreta is the placenta that is adherent to the uterus. It is consequential to a defect in the fibrinoid (Nitabuch's) layer of decidua underlying the placenta.[7] It is common in the uteruses with scar or pathologies underlying the placenta. Doppler is a useful modality for diagnosis and differential diagnosis of the same. The extent of penetration of the placental vessels in the uterine wall can be used as the

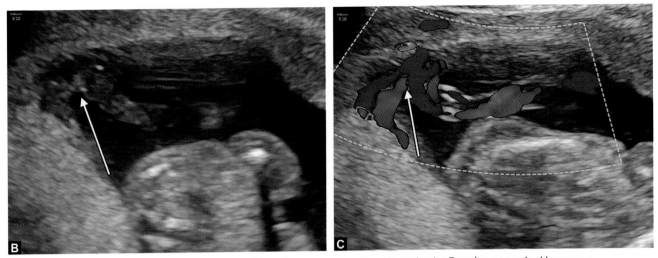

Figs. 12.34B and C: Velamentous cord insertion as seen on B-mode and color Doppler, as marked by arrows.

landmark to assess the penetration of the placental tissue in the uterine wall (Figs. 12.35A to D).

- *Renal agenesis:* Complete absence of one or both kidneys may be defined as unilateral or bilateral renal agenesis. When it is bilateral, it presents with absence of bladder shadow also and severe oligohydramnios. But fetuses with unilateral renal agenesis, usually do show normal bladder shadow as well as amniotic fluid index. In cases with bilateral renal agenesis, because of severe oligohydramnios, the visibility of the intra-abdominal fetal anatomy may be difficult to assess. Color/power Doppler can be used in these cases to confirm the presence or absence of renal arteries (Fig. 12.36), which is an indirect diagnostic sign of renal agenesis. The course of superior vesical arteries may also help to confirm absence of bladder in cases of bilateral renal agenesis. Moreover, Doppler is also used in these cases to assess the umbilical artery flow, that is normal and this rules out fetal growth restriction (FGR) as a cause of oligohydramnios. Diagnosis of unilateral renal agenesis may often be overlooked on the antenatal scans and also at times later in life, till one kidney is functioning normally. It is therefore important to document anechoic spot of both the renal pelvicalyceal systems or so to hyperechoic renal shadows on transverse or coronal section of the abdomen (Fig. 12.37). Inability to do this demands a Doppler to ascertain both the renal arteries are seen in their normal anatomical position. Abnormal anatomical position of one of the renal arteries may be indicative of an ectopic kidney.

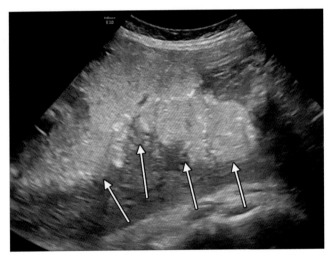

Fig. 12.35A: Ill-defined placental-myometrial interface—adherent placenta.

- *Ectopic kidney:* As just discussed, when one kidney is not seen, there is a strong possibility of an ectopic kidney. Especially when in pelvis, it may be confused with a pelvic mass, both because of its vascularity and also at times due to abnormal origin of renal artery from the mesenteric vessels as seen on color or power Doppler (Fig. 12.38). But carefully studying the vascular pattern will surely be helpful to identify the structure as kidney. In other cases, kidney may be crossed on to the opposite side and may be fused with the other kidney. The evidently seen large size of the kidney may be misinterpreted for a compensatory hypertrophy of the single kidney with unilateral agenesis. But Doppler in compensatory hypertrophy will show only one renal

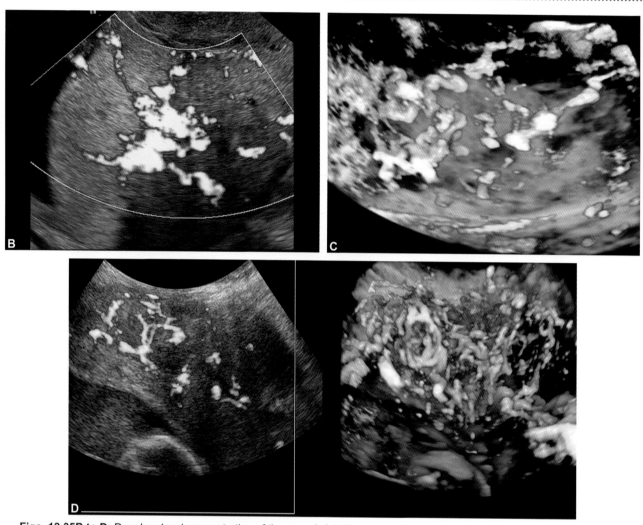

Figs. 12.35B to D: Doppler showing penetration of the vessels into the myometrium in placenta accrete, increta and percreta.

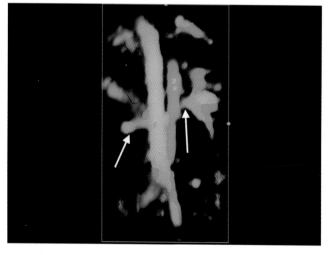

Fig. 12.36: Doppler of fetal vasculature showing renal vessels.

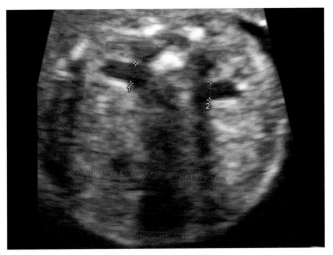

Fig. 12.37: B-mode ultrasound image of the transverse section of the abdomen, showing pelvicalyceal systems.

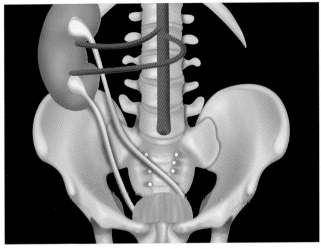

Fig. 12.39: Crossed ectopia with its renal artery also crossed on to the other side.

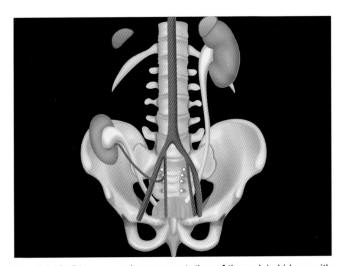

Fig. 12.38: Diagrammatic representation of the pelvic kidney with its vasculature.

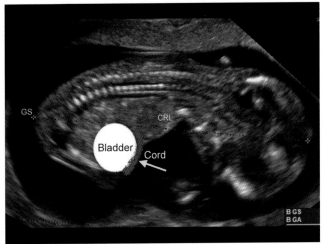

Fig. 12.40: Diagrammatic representation of umbilical cord position and bladder position in bladder exstrophy.

vessel, whereas in crossed fused ectopic (Fig. 12.39), the entire renal complex is supplied by two renal vessels, especially when Doppler also shows the origin of one of the two vessels from the opposite side of the aorta. Pelvic kidney is often associated with other gastrointestinal and/or cardiac abnormalities.

- *Bladder exstrophy:* Incomplete closure of the lower anterior abdominal wall associated with separation of the pubic bones, low set umbilicus and abnormal genitalia is associated with absent anterior wall of the bladder, the posterior wall of which is exposed to the amniotic fluid.[8,9] It may sometimes be a part of exstrophy of the cloaca also. The later will show omphalocele, bowel anomalies, spina bifida and phallus bifidus.

On ultrasound, the bladder is not seen in the pelvis. A small solid mass is seen bulging out of lower abdomen, umbilical cord is inserted low in the anterior abdominal wall (Fig. 12.40). Omphalocele is present and this defect extends to lower abdomen in cloacal atrophy. Among the spinal abnormalities, meningomyelocele may be seen (Fig. 12.41). Lower limbs may also show abnormalities. Doppler shows a typical arrangement of the umbilical arteries. The two umbilical arteries take a parallel course when in the abdomen, instead of converging.

- *Renal tumors:* The most common renal tumor found antenatally is a mesoblastic nephroma. This is a benign tumor, usually unilateral and involves part of the ovary.

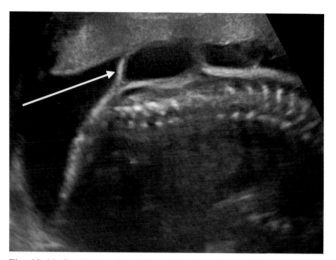

Fig. 12.41: Sagittal section of the spine showing meningomyelocele.

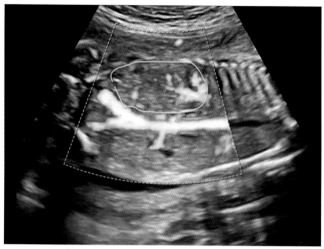

Fig. 12.43: HD flow Doppler of a fetal trunk, coronal section showing large renal shadow with marked vascularity—renal tumor.

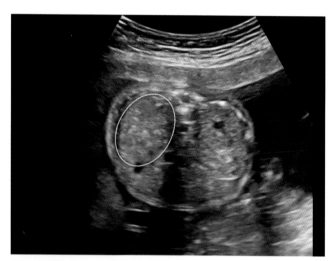

Fig. 12.42: Transverse section of the fetal abdomen at the renal pelvicalyceal system level showing large renal shadow.

It has ill-defined margins and no capsule. The common malignant tumor of the kidney diagnosed antenatally is Wilm's tumor (nephroblastoma). Though on B-mode, this appears as a capsulated neoplasm but with heterogeneous echogenicity (Fig. 12.42). The typical low resistance and heterogeneously distributed increased vascularity suggests its malignant nature (Fig. 12.43).

Cardiac Abnormalities

Heart is an organ that pumps blood and therefore for diagnosis of cardiac anomalies Doppler is an essential modality. Whenever there is a structural defect in the cardiovascular system, there would also be an abnormality in the circulation. There may be blood flow where it should not be, or no blood flow where it should be, or blood flow in reverse direction, or blood flow with a velocity more or less than normal. But for the correct diagnosis and optimum use of color Doppler, relevant Doppler settings are essential. It is essential to remember that heart is a highly mobile, active organ and the blood flow in and out of it is also a high velocity flow. Therefore, to get correct information from the Doppler studies of the heart, it is essential to use high PRF, high wall filter and low persistence settings for fetal echocardiography. Gains and line density should be set so that the color filling of the cardiac chambers is complete and homogeneous. These can all be diagnosed by Doppler. Let us discuss the abnormalities of the heart for the diagnosis of which Doppler plays an important role. But these will be discussed in detail in the chapter dedicated to the same.

Miscellaneous Anomalies

This group especially includes the abnormalities of inflow tracts to the heart and abnormality of major vessels.

- *Anomalous pulmonary venous drainage:* Normally the left atrium drains four pulmonary veins, right and left upper and right and left lower. But normally on four chamber heart view, only the lower pair is seen (Fig. 12.44). The upper pair is difficult to see on antenatal scans. Therefore during antenatal life, only total anomalous pulmonary venous drainage can be confidently diagnosed. In these typical cases, the venous confluence is seen posterior to the left ventricle along with absence of the pulmonary veins that are normally seen on four chamber heart view, are the two diagnostic signs on Doppler (Fig. 12.45). This leads to increased distance between the left atrium and the descending aorta.

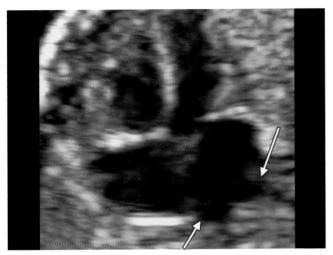

Fig. 12.44: B-mode ultrasound image of the four-chamber heart with the pulmonary veins entering LA shown by arrows.

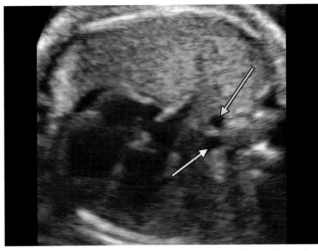

Fig. 12.46: Two vessels placed side-by-side anterior to the spine on the four-chamber heart view. Indicative of persistent azygus.

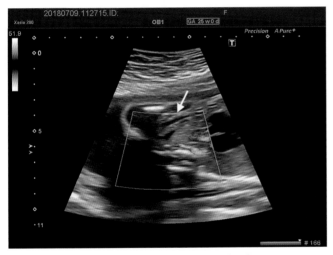

Fig. 12.45: Doppler image showing abnormal pulmonary venous drainage.

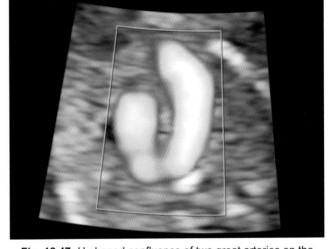

Fig. 12.47: U-shaped confluence of two great arteries on the three vessel view—right sided aortic arch.

- *Persistent azygos:* The azygos is persistent when IVC is absent or interrupted. This is usually most easily diagnosed on the sagittal view for right atrial inflow tracts. On the sagittal section of abdomen, the aorta and IVC are parallel in the lower half of the abdomen but close to the diaphragm; the IVC deviates anteriorly to enter into right atrium. Instead a persistent azygos is documented as a vein parallel to the aorta right up to the diaphragm and even beyond. This on transverse section is seen as two vessels placed side by side anterior to the spine on the four chamber heart view. Doppler helps the clear visualization (Fig. 12.46).
- *Right-sided aortic arch:* It may be isolated or associated with other cardiac abnormalities like Fallot's tetralogy or truncus arteriosus or situs inversus. On 3VV, the aorta remains on the right of the pulmonary trunk.

But if the duct is still on the left side and connects with the descending aorta behind the trachea, it may show as a vascular conduit behind the trachea (Fig. 12.47). If the duct is on the right side, a mirror image branching pattern may be seen.

In this case, left brachiocephalic artery crosses in front of the trachea. This can be documented on Doppler. Right-sided aortic arch may also be a part of double aortic arch. In that case, it shows a complete vascular ring surrounding the trachea on Doppler.

Rare abnormalities like persistent left superior vena cava, absent ductus venosus, etc. will all demand Doppler studies for confirmation.

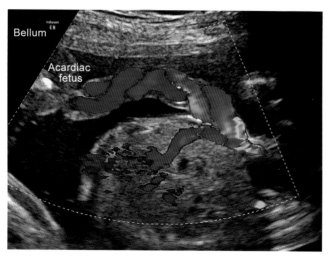

Fig. 12.48: Teversal of blood flow in umbilical artery of acardiac twin seen on the color Doppler.

Doppler for Assessment of Complications of Twin Pregnancies

- *Twin-to-twin transfusion syndrome (TTTS):* It is seen in 5–15% of monochorionic twin pregnancies. It has mortality as high as 60–100% if not treated. Typically there is discrepancy in growth in both the fetuses with small or absent stomach and bladder shadow in the smaller fetus. The sac with the smaller fetus also shows marked oligohydramnios, whereas the larger fetus shows polyhydramnios. The larger fetus shows hyperdynamic circulation and high output failure. This may be presented with abnormal ductus venosus flow and may also show pulsatile umbilical venous flow in the terminal stages.
- *Acardiac twins and TRAP syndrome (Twin reversed arterial perfusion syndrome):* Incidence is 1% of monozygotic twins. The hallmark of the diagnosis is reversal of blood flow in umbilical artery of acardiac twin can be demonstrated by Doppler (Fig. 12.48). In these cases, cord insertions in placenta are close to

each other. As the name suggests, one of the two twins is incompletely formed and does not have the heart and the circulation to this phantom is through the other fetus. This leads to overload on the heart of the other fetus and may lead to cardiac failure.

CONCLUSION

Doppler can be used for diagnosis and confirmation of several vascular and nonvascular abnormalities of the fetus. For the evaluation of cardiac abnormalities Doppler is a must.

REFERENCES

1. Bernard JP, Drummond CL, Zaarour P, et al. A new clue to the prenatal diagnosis of lobar holoprosencephaly: the abnormal pathway of the anterior cerebral artery crawling under the skull. Ultrasound Obstet Gynecol. 2002;19(6):605-7.
2. Altman RP, Randolph JG, Lilley JR. Sacrococcygeal teratoma. American academy of pediatrics surgical section survey. J Pediatr Surg. 1974;9:389-98.
3. Sehgal A, Loughran-Fowlds A. Scimitar Syndrome. Indian J Pediatr. 2005;72:249-51.
4. Voskamp BJ, Fleurke-Rozema H, Oude-rengerink K, et al. Relationship of isolated single umbilical artery to fetal growth, aneuploidy and perinatal mortality: systematic review and meta-analysis. Ultrasound Obstet Gynecol. 2013;42:622-8.
5. Battarbee AN, Palatnik A, Ernst LM, et al. Association of isolated single umbilical artery with small for gestational age and preterm birth. Obstet Gynecol. 2015;26:760.
6. Raio L, Ghezzi F, Di Naro E, et al. The clinical significance of antenatal detection of discordant umbilical arteries. Obstet Gynecol. 1998;91:86-91.
7. Mazouni C, Gorincour G, Iuhan V, et al. Placenta Accreta: a review of current advances in prenatal diagnosis. Placenta. 2006;28(7):599-603.
8. Van Allen MI. Urinary tract. In: Stevenson RE, Hall JG, Goodman RM (Eds). Human Malformations and Related Anomalies. Oxford: Oxford University Press. 1993. pp. 502-62.
9. Lee EH, Shim JY. New Sonographic finding for the prenatal diagnosis of bladder exstrophy: a case report. Ultrasound Obstet Gynecol. 2003;21(5):498-500.

Index

Page numbers followed by *b* refer to box, *f* refer to figure, and *t* refer to table.